Fungal Infections

Diagnosis and Treatment

Fungal Infections

Diagnosis and Treatment

Kabir Sardana MD DNB MNAMS
Professor
Department of Dermatology
PGIMER, Dr Ram Manohar Lohia Hospital
New Delhi

Khushbu Mahajan MD
Associate Professor
North Delhi Municipal Corporation
Medical College and Hindu Rao Hospital

Delhi

Pooja Arora Mrig MD, DNB, MNAMS
Assistant Professor
Department of Dermatology
PGIMER, Dr Ram Manohar Lohia Hospital
New Delhi

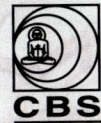

CBS

CBS Publishers & Distributors Pvt Ltd

New Delhi • Bengaluru • Chennai • Kochi • Kolkata • Mumbai
Hyderabad • Nagpur • Patna • Pune • Vijayawada

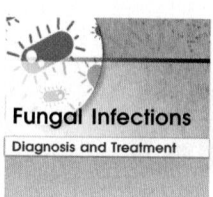

Fungal Infections

Diagnosis and Treatment

ISBN: 978-93-86310-75-0

Copyright © Authors and Publisher

First Edition: 2017

Published by Satish Kumar Jain and produced by Varun Jain for

CBS Publishers & Distributors Pvt Ltd

4819/XI Prahlad Street, 24 Ansari Road, Daryaganj, New Delhi 110 002, India.
Ph: 23289259, 23266861, 23266867 Website: www.cbspd.com
Fax: 011-23243014   e-mail: delhi@cbspd.com; cbspubs@airtelmail.in.
Corporate Office: 204 FIE, Industrial Area, Patparganj, Delhi 110 092
Ph: 4934 4934   Fax: 4934 4935   e-mail: publishing@cbspd.com; publicity@cbspd.com

Branches

- **Bengaluru:** Seema House 2975, 17th Cross, K.R. Road,
  Banasankari 2nd Stage, Bengaluru 560 070, Karnataka
  Ph: +91-80-26771678/79   Fax: +91-80-26771680   e-mail: bangalore@cbspd.com
- **Chennai:** 7, Subbaraya Street, Shenoy Nagar, Chennai 600 030, Tamil Nadu
  Ph: +91-44-26680620, 26681266   Fax: +91-44-42032115   e-mail: chennai@cbspd.com
- **Kochi:** Ashana House, No. 39/1904, AM Thomas Road, Valanjambalam,
  Ernakulam 682 016, Kochi, Kerala
  Ph: +91-484-4059061-65   Fax: +91-484-4059065   e-mail: kochi@cbspd.com
- **Kolkata:** 6/B, Ground Floor, Rameswar Shaw Road, Kolkata-700 014, West Bengal
  Ph: +91-33-22891126, 22891127, 22891128   e-mail: kolkata@cbspd.com
- **Mumbai:** 83-C, Dr E Moses Road, Worli, Mumbai-400018, Maharashtra
  Ph: +91-22-24902340/41   Fax: +91-22-24902342   e-mail: mumbai@cbspd.com

Representatives

- **Hyderabad** 0-9885175004 • **Nagpur**   0-9021734563 • **Patna** 0-9334159340
- **Pune**   0-9623451994 • **Vijayawada** 0-9000660880

Printed at Magic International Pvt. Ltd., Greator Noida, UP, India

to
_____

my parents Amba Sardana and Maj Gen KN Sardana
at Dehradun

my wife Dr Supriya Mahajan and my daughter Zoya

my seniors teachers, colleagues and students at LHMC,
MAMC, CNBC and RML Hospital

Kabir Sardana

my grandfather, whose pure admiration for profession inspired
me to strive harder and dream to be here

my daughter, whose innocence helped me rekindle honesty and
purity in words and actions

my teachers and students, whose questions always inspired
me to constantly seek knowledge to the core of the subject

my friends and family, who by their sheer presence and unending
support have made everything look and feel so simple....

Khushbu Mahajan

my family for their continuous love and support
my parents for being my inspiration since childhood
my husband Dr Sumit Mrig for being the pillar of strength
my guru Dr Kabir Sardana for having faith in me in such projects

Pooja Arora Mrig

Everything is predetermined

Success and failure are due to 'prarabdha karma', and not to willpower or the lack of it. One should try to gain equipoise of mind under all circumstances. That is willpower.

Man is always free not to identify himself with the body, and not to be affected by the pleasures or pains consequent on the body's activities.

Free will and destiny are inconsequential if one understands the transience of the body and mind and the eternity of the spirit

Shri Raman Maharishi

Contributors

Aastha Gupta MD
Senior Resident
Department of Dermatology
PGIMER, Dr Ram Manohar Lohia Hospital
New Delhi

Autar K Miskeen
Director, Dr Miskeen's Central Clinical
Microbiology Laboratory
Thane, India 400601

Bhavna Garg
Professor, Department of Pathology
Dayanand Medical College and Hospital
Ludhiana, Punjab

C Srinivas CMD, DM
Manager Medical Affairs
Global Generics-India
Dr Reddy's Laboratories Ltd.

G Raghu Rama Rao
Prof and HOD, DVL
GSL Medical College
Rajahumandry, AP.

Harpreet Kaur
Professor, Department of Pathology
Dayanand Medical College and Hospital
Ludhiana, Punjab

Khushbu Mahajan MD
Associate Professor
North Delhi Municipal Corporation Medical
College and Hindu Rao Hospital, Delhi

Neena Sood
Prof and Head
Department of Pathology, Dayanand
Medical College and Hospital
Ludhiana, Punjab

Priya Uppuluri
Los Angeles Biomedical Research Institute
Harbor-UCLA, 1124 W. Carson St., Torrance,
CA 90502

Pooja Agarwal MD
Consultant Dermatologist
Shifa Multispeciality Hospital,
Ahmedabad

Pooja Arora Mrig MD, DNB, MNAMS
Assistant Professor
Department of Dermatology
PGIMER, Dr Ram Manohar Lohia Hospital
New Delhi

Shukla Das
Director Professor
Department of Microbiology
UCMS & GTB Hospital
Dilshad Garden, Delhi-110095

SN Bhattacharya
Prof and Head
Department Dermatology & STD
UCMS & GTB Hospital,
Dilshad Garden, Delhi-110095

Suchita Gawde MBBS, MD (Pharmacology.), DBM
Mumbai

Sukriti Sharma
DNB student, Hindu Rao hospital
Delhi

Sumit Mrig MS, DNB, MNAMS
Senior Consultant and Head
Department of ENT and Cochlear Implant
Surgery
Max Smart Superspeciality Hospital
Delhi

Surabhi Sinha MD, DNB
Specialist, Department of Dermatology
PGIMER, Dr Ram Manohar Lohia Hospital
New Delhi

Thurakkal Salim
Clinical Head and Medical Director
Cutis Institute of Advanced Dermatology
Calicut, India

Veena Chandran MD, DNB Dermatology
Medical Officer, Royal Perth Hospital
Perth, WA, Australia

Vineet Narula MS, DNB
Associate Consultant
Department of ENT and Cochlear Implant
Surgery
Max Smart Superspeciality Hospital
Delhi

Vikram Narang
Asstt Professor
Department of Pathology
Dayanand Medical College and Hospital
Ludhiana, Punjab

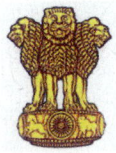

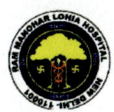

Foreword

It is my privilege to write the Foreword to the book *Fungal Infections: Diagnosis and Treatment* by Dr Kabir Sardana and 18 other contributors who are eminent in the field of microbiology, with special interest in mycology, dermatology, ENT and pharmacology.

Fungal infections are important for dermatologists and nowadays, resistance to treatment for fungal infections is encountered due to various factors, eloquently detailed in this book. This book by Dr Kabir Sardana and others covers all aspects related to superficial and deep fungal infections and also highlights the treatment. This book is yet another compilation on fungal infections and is important for postgraduates as well as the faculty. The photographic documentation of various fungal disorders shall help in identifying these conditions and was much desired from an Indian perspective by an Indian author.

I am sure the book shall not only be read by practitioners, but be recommended for reading to all postgraduates by their teachers. I hope the authors shall also write similar books on bacterial and viral infections.

15/12/16

Dr. (Prof.) RK Gautam MD, MNAMS
Professor and Consultant
Dr RML Hospital, Delhi

Foreword

It gives me immense pleasure and privilege to contribute a foreword for this book, which has been written by an eminent dermatologist, Dr Kabir Sardana.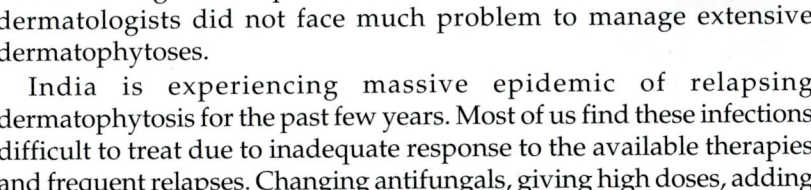

Superficial fungal infections have never been so critical arena for dermatologist for many years. Even during HIV epidemic across India; dermatologists did not face much problem to manage extensive dermatophytoses.

India is experiencing massive epidemic of relapsing dermatophytosis for the past few years. Most of us find these infections difficult to treat due to inadequate response to the available therapies and frequent relapses. Changing antifungals, giving high doses, adding oral retinoids; all have been tried with variable efficacy.

This book is the result of intense hard work and reflects the knowledge and dedication of Dr Sardana in the field of dermatology. The authors have provided a substantial and crystal clear understanding to the "Fungal infections, immunology, pathogenesis, diagnosis, resistance, relapse and management." They have given an in-depth analysis of not just superficial fungal infections but also subcutaneous and deep fungal infections prevalent in India and has offered solutions as well in a very scientific and crisp manner which will be able to clear the prevailing dilemmas.

This book will contribute to the field of mycology greatly and will be useful to the clinicians, academicians and postgraduates in the field. I compliment Dr Sardana and his team for their excellent effort and wish them all the success.

Dr. Bela J. Shah

Dr. Bela J Shah
Professor and Head
Department of Dermatology, STD, AIDS and Leprosy
BJ Medical College and Civil Hospital,
Asarwa, Ahmedabad

Preface

Fungal infections have two basic divisions, the superficial infections and deep infections. The former has always been simple to treat, but in recent times, recalcitrant dermatophytosis has been an issue and a large number of clinicians believe that resistance is a cause but there is very little data to support this with concrete mycological proof in direct proportion to the extent of the problem. The problem lies in the intricate host fungal interaction and a change in the species to anthropophilic from zoophilic which helps it to evade the host immune response.

In this quest we have had the privilege of involving two mycologists in this book to add their views on this issue. Dermatologists both in clinical practice and from institutions have added their wisdom to cover the clinical aspects of superficial infections. A chapter on recalcitrant infections has been added to put this problem in the right perspective.

Of course, some of the readers may have a different perspective which mirrors the eternal truth of life

"Don't believe in everything that you hear.
There are always three sides to a story.
Yours, theirs and the truth".

For the deep infections, we have taken chapters written by authors who have studied and seen these disorders and the list encompasses dermatologists and ENT specialists to make it a multiopinionated input. For the drug section, we have two pharmacologists, working for national companies who have added inputs on itraconazole and terbinafine.

A big thanks to CBS Publishers & Distributors, Mr SK Jain (CMD) and Mr YN Arjuna (Senior Vice President—Publishing, Editorial and Publicity) and their team, Mrs Ritu Chawla (Assistant General Manager—Production), Mr Vikrant Sharma, Neeraj Prasad, Mr Sanjay Chauhan (Sanju), Mr Kshirod Sahoo and Mr Ananda Mohanty, Mr SK Verma and the endless cups of tea and coffee, all of which played a role in this book.

In the end we would like to emphasize that the intricacies of the host immune response and the evasion of the same by the fungus proves that there is a power much more intelligent that all of us that determines the way things run in this world.

Lastly a big thanks to the contributors and the support of the Department of Dermatology at RML Hospital and PGIMER.

Happy reading!

Kabir Sardana
Khushbu Mahajan
Pooja Arora Mrig

Contents

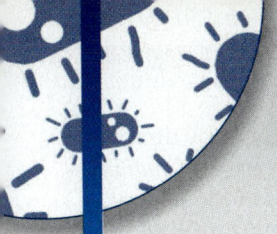

CHAPTER 1

Introduction to Fungal Infections: Focus on Dermatophytoses

Kabir Sardana

Among the 50,000 to 2,50,000 species of fungi that have been described, fewer than 500 have been associated with human disease, and no more than 100 are capable of causing infection in otherwise normal individuals. The remainder are only able to produce disease in hosts that are debilitated or immunocompromised in some way. In general these organisms are free living in nature and are in no way dependent on humans (or animals) for their survival. With a few exceptions, fungal infections of humans originate from an exogenous source in the environment and are acquired through inhalation, ingestion or traumatic implantation.

Some conditions may not be included under fungal disorders but owing to their clinical and biologic similarities with fungal diseases, actinomycetoma and nocardiosis (caused by aerobic actinomycetic bacteria), and rhinosporidiosis (a human pathogen from the DRIPs—dermocystidium, rosette agent, ichthyophonus, and psorospermium) clade, a novel clade of aquatic protistan parasites (Ichthyosporea) have traditionally been included in the classification of subcutaneous fungal diseases; however, they should be studied as separate entities.

Classification

Fungi are conventionally classified as *superficial*, *deep* and *systemic* infections. In recent years, fungal infections have been grouped according to their clinical presentation, subdividing them into *superficial*, *subcutaneous*, *systemic*, and *opportunistic* mycoses. The term "deep" is sometimes used as synonymous for systemic, and at other times, it is used to describe subcutaneous and systemic disease. To clear this it is useful to classify subcutaneous mycoses as mycotic infections that mainly involve subcutaneous tissue, even though they can occasionally spread to other sites because of disseminated or systemic infection.

1

Mycology textbooks state that systemic mycoses are caused by dimorphic fungi and separate them from diseases caused by yeasts (*Candida* spp., *Cryptococcus* spp.), regardless of the immune status of the patient.

The most common classifications separate systemic from opportunistic diseases according to their fungal virulence and the host's immune response. *Histoplasma* spp., *Coccidioides* spp., *Blastomyces dermatitidis*, and *Paracoccidioides brasiliensis* are true pathogenic systemic dimorphic fungi, whereas other less virulent organisms cause opportunistic disease in immunosuppressed individuals.

Superficial Mycosis

The superficial mycoses are infections limited to the outermost layers of the skin, the nails and hair, and the mucous membranes (Table 1.1). The principal infections in this group are the dermatophytoses and superficial forms of candidosis. The dermatophytes are limited to the keratinized tissues of the epidermis, hair and nail. Most are unable to survive as free-living saprobes in competition with other keratinophilic organisms in the environment and thus are dependent on passage from host to host for their survival. These obligate pathogens seem to have evolved from unspecialized saprobic forms. In the process, most are now no longer capable of sexual, and some even asexual, reproduction. In general, these organisms have become well adapted to humans, evoking a little or no inflammatory reaction from the host.

Table 1.1: Superficial cutaneous mycoses*	
Disease	*Causative agent*
Tinea (pityriasis) versicolor, seborrheic dermatitis, including dandruff and *Malassezia* folliculitis	*Malassezia* spp (a lipophilic yeast)
Tinea nigra	*Exophiala werneckii*
White piedra**	*Trichosporon asahii*
Black piedra	*Piedraia hortae*
Dermatophytosis, ringworm of the scalp, glabrous skin, and nails	Dermatophytes (*Microsporum, Trichophyton, Epidermophyton*)
Candidosis of skin, mucous membranes and nails	*Candida albicans* and related species
Dermatomycosis	Nondermatophyte moulds, *Hendersonula toruloidea, Scytalidium hyalinum, Scopulariopsis brevicaulis*

*Arenas R, *et al.*
**White piedra caused by *T. ovoides* earlier called beigelii.

The etiological agents of candidosis, like the dermatophytes, are largely dependent on the living host for their survival, but differ from them in the manner by which this is achieved. These organisms, of which *Candida albicans* is the most important, are normal commensal inhabitants of the human digestive tract or skin. Acquisition of these organisms from another host seldom results in overt disease, but rather in the setting up of a commensal relationship with the new host. These organisms do not produce disease unless some change in the circumstances of the host lowers its natural defences. In this situation, endogenous infection from the host's own reservoir of the organism may result in mucosal, cutaneous or systemic infection.

Subcutaneous Mycoses

Subcutaneous mycoses, previously known as deep mycosis, belong to a group of infections acquired from ubiquitous saprophyte fungi that affect the skin and subcutaneous tissue (Table 1.2). These infections are usually acquired as a result of the traumatic implantation of organisms that grow as saprobes in the soil and on decomposing vegetation. These infections are most frequently encountered among the rural populations of the tropical and subtropical regions of the world, where individuals go barefoot and wear the minimum of clothing. The disease may remain localized at the site of implantation or spread to adjacent tissue. More widespread dissemination of the infection, through the blood or lymphatics, is uncommon, and usually occurs only if the host is in some way debilitated or immunocompromised.

Chromoblastomycosis, sporotrichosis, and eumycetoma are more common. Lobomycosis and conidiobolomycosis (entomophthoromycosis) are rare and have a low association with immunosuppression, even though these fungi are considered to have low virulence.

Systemic Mycoses

These are infections that usually originate in the lungs (Table 1.2), but may spread to many other organs. These infections are most commonly acquired as a result of inhaling spores of organisms that grow as saprobes in the soil or on decomposing organic matter, or as pathogens on plants. The main organisms causing them are depicted in Fig. 1.1.

The organisms that cause systemic fungal infection can be divided into two distinct groups: The *true pathogens* and the *opportunists*. The first of these groups consists of a handful of organisms such as *Histoplasma capsulatum* and *Coccidioides immitis*, that are able to invade and develop in the tissues of a normal host with no recognizable predisposition. Often these organisms possess unique morphological

Table 1.2: Clinical classification of subcutaneous and systemic mycoses*

Disease	Causative agent
Subcutaneous mycoses	
Sporotrichosis	*Sporothris complex*
Chromoblastomycosis	*Fonsecaea, Phialophora, Cladosporium*
Phaeohyphomycosis	*Cladosporium, Exophiala, Wangiella, Bipolaris, Exserohilum, Curvularia*
Eumycetoma	Genera *Madurella, Acremonium, Exophiala, Scedosporium* spp.
Subcutaneous zygomycosis (entomophthoromycosis)	*Basidiobolus ranarum* *Conidiobolus coronatus*
Subcutaneous zygomycosis (mucormycosis)	Genera *Rhizopus, Mucor, Rhizomucor, Mycocladus, Saksenaea*
Lobomycosis	*Lacazia loboi*
Dimorphic systemic mycoses	
Histoplasmosis	*Histoplasma capsulatum, Histoplasma capsulatum* var *duboisii*
Coccidioidomycosis	*Coccidioides immitis, Coccidioides posadasii*
Blastomycosis	*Blastomyces dermatitidis*
Paracoccidioidomycosis	*Paracoccidioides brasiliensis*
Opportunistic systemic mycoses	
Candidiasis	*Candida albicans* and related spp.
Cryptococcosis	*Cryptococcus neoformans* (var neoformans, var *gattii*)
Aspergillosis	*Aspergillus fumigatus,* other spp.
Pseudallescheriasis	Genera Scedosporium (*Pseudollescheria boydii*)
Zygomycosis (mucormycosis)	Genera *Rhizopus, Mucor, Rhizomucor, Mycocladus*
Fusariosis	*Fusarium* spp.
Penicilliosis	*Penicillium marneffei*
Trichosporonosis	*Trichosporon* spp.
Hyalohyphomycosis	Genera *Penicillium, Paecilomyces, Beauveria, Fusarium, Scopulariopsis*
Phaeohyphomycosis	Genera *Cladosporium, Exophiala, Wangiella, Bipolaris, Exserohilum, Curvularia*

*Arenas R, *et al.*

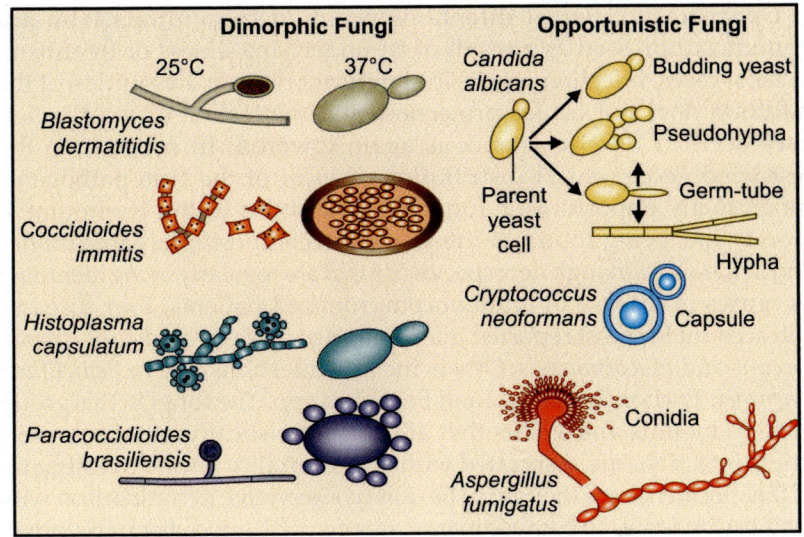

Fig. 1.1: A diagrammatic depiction of common organisms causing systemic fungal infections

features that appear to contribute to their survival within the host. The second group, the opportunists, consists of less virulent and less well-adapted organisms, such as *Aspergillus fumigatus*, that are only able to invade the tissues of an immunocompromised host.

In many instances, infections with *true pathogenic* fungi are asymptomatic or mild and of short duration. Most cases occur in geographical regions where the aetiological agents are found in nature and follow inhalation of spores that have been released into the environment. The host must encounter the fungus while sporulation occurs. After this, the fungi exhibit a morphologic transition from the mycelial (saprophytic) form to the parasitic form found in infected tissues. This transformation is determined by the temperature of incubation (called thermal dimorphism), which is seen in most fungi that cause systemic infections. Individuals who recover from these infections enjoy marked and lasting resistance to reinfection, while the few patients with chronic or residual disease often have a serious underlying illness. In addition to their well-recognized manifestations in otherwise normal persons, infections with true pathogenic fungi have emerged as important diseases in immunocompromised individuals. Histoplasmosis and coccidioidomycosis, for instance, have been recognized as AIDS-defining illnesses. Both have been seen in significant numbers of human immunodeficiency virus (HIV)-infected persons.

Opportunistic fungal infections occur in individuals who are immunosuppressed as a result of an underlying illness or treatment. In most cases, infection results in significant disease. Resolution of the infection does not confer protection, and reinfection or reactivation may occur if host resistance is again lowered. In contrast to the restricted geographical distribution of most of the true pathogenic fungi, many opportunistic fungi are ubiquitous in the environment worldwide, being found in the soil, on decomposing organic matter and in the air. Although new species of fungi are regularly being identified as causes of disease in immunocompromised patients, four diseases still account for most reported infections: *Aspergillosis, candidosis, crypto-coccosis* and *mucormycosis*. Others include infections due to *Penicillium marneffei*, Trichosporon spp., and Fusarium spp. The fungi in this group include moulds and yeasts that are characteristically not dimorphic. These infections are associated with high mortality rates, but estimates of their incidence are thought to be quite conservative in comparison with their true magnitude because many cases go undiagnosed or unreported.

THE CHANGING PATTERN OF FUNGAL INFECTION

Over the past few years, major advances in health care have led to an unwelcome increase in the number of life-threatening infections due to true pathogenic and opportunistic fungi. These infections are being seen in ever increasing numbers, largely because of the increasing size of the population at risk. This population includes persons with HIV infection, transplant recipients, cancer patients and other individuals receiving immunosuppressive treatment. Among patients undergoing transplants or treatment for malignancies, novel and more intensive regimens have resulted in more profound levels of immuno-suppression that are sustained for longer periods.

In addition to the rise in prevalence of opportunistic fungal infections due to such well-recognized organisms as *A. fumigatus* and *C. albicans,* an everincreasing number of fungi, hitherto regarded as harmless saprobes, are being reported as the cause of serious or lethal infection in immunocompromised individuals. For instance, *Fusarium* species, long recognized as a cause of nail and corneal infections, are now well documented as the aetiological agents of lethal disseminated infections in neutropenic cancer patients and hematopoietic stem cell transplantation (HSCT) recipients. The emergence of these organisms as significant pathogens has important implications for diagnosis and management, not only because the clinical presentation can mimic a more common disease, aspergillosis, but also because the organisms are usually resistant to amphotericin B, the drug of choice for empirical treatment of suspected fungal infections in febrile neutropenic patients.

Dermatophytosis: A Recalcitrant "Epidemic"

Although dermatophytes are found throughout the world, the most prevalent strains and the most common sites of infection vary by region. Countries like India with their hot and humid climates and overcrowding predispose populations to skin diseases, including tinea infections. Developing countries have high rates of tinea capitis, while developed countries have high rates of tinea pedis and onychomycosis.

Dermatophyte diseases recur at a high rate following treatment with an antifungal [Gupta AK, Cooper EA (2008)]. It is currently unknown whether this is due to insufficient clearing of the fungus during treatment and reemergence of disease, and thus an example of *relapse*, or if these represent *new infections* (Fig. 1.2). In fact most cases belong to the former and herein the immunity may be more important than resistance (Fig. 1.2). The high false-negative culture rate from clinical samples contributes to this problem. The advent of molecular biology tools may provide a means by which clinicians can more accurately determine the presence (or absence) of dermatophytes. Such tools will help determine whether a new infection is indeed caused by the same strain as a previous infection in the same patient.

Is it drug-resistant dermatophytes? Surprisingly, drug resistance among dermatophytes is *rare*. Two large clinical studies looking at drug susceptibility in dermatophytes did not find significant increases in the minimum inhibitory concentration of several antifungal drugs used to treat dermatophytes [Ghannoum M, et al.]. Occasional cases

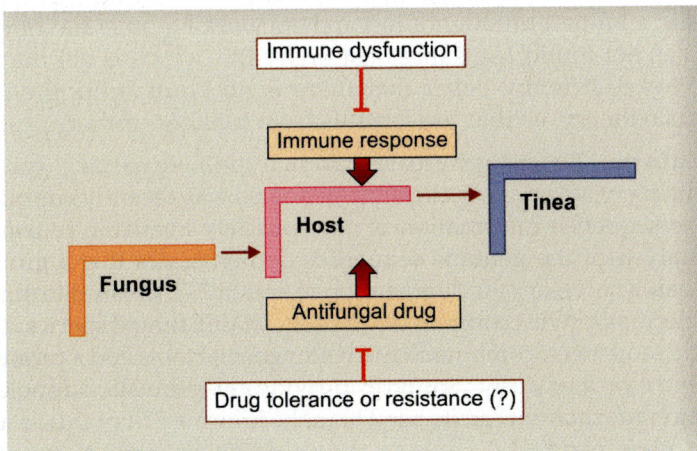

Fig. 1.2: A depiction of the role of host immunity and antifungal drug in the causation of tinea infection

of drug resistance have been documented. For example, a single amino acid substitution in the target enzyme was found to confer resistance to terbinafine in a clinical isolate from a patient with onychomycosis [Mukherjee PK, Osborne CS]. Why is it that such mutations conferring drug resistance are not a more widespread occurrence? One possibility is that dermatophytes are able to tolerate drugs without acquiring point mutations in the target enzyme.

Issues with dermatophytes research: Despite the prevalence of dermatophyte infections worldwide, a sophisticated understanding of how they cause disease is lacking [White TC]. The historic difficulties in working with dermatophytes have been twofold: Technical difficulties due to poor virulence models and a lack of genetic tools, and an under-appreciation of the need to study these organisms.

Currently, the most common animal model for studying dermatophyte virulence is the guinea pig. Although this has been useful for zoophiles, guinea pigs and other dermatophyte animal models do not provide accurate infection models for most anthropophilic species [Achterman RR]. Other virulence models include determining the ability of the organism to grow on keratinized surfaces such as sterilized nail fragments, which is a non-quantitative model. Recently, skin explants have been used to study dermatophyte adherence and invasion. Human epidermal tissues are commercially available and represent a possible virulence model to study the initial stages of dermatophyte infection.

Another reason is that many mycologists do not consider dermatophytes as important as other infectious diseases. Therefore, there are a limited number of researchers working on it and our own work has not found resistance, just high MIC, which is not the same thing, hence it is my belief that there is no point "whipping" the resistance theory, as that prevents us from looking further.

The future: Dermatophyte research is poised to take off. The sequencing of seven dermatophyte genomes was recently completed, and the sequence information is now publicly available [Burmester A]. Analysis of the genome sequences demonstrates that a group of proteinases necessary for degradation of keratin is increased in number in the dermatophytes compared to closely related fungal species. These genome sequences, combined with better genetic tools and a promising model in which to study virulence, provide an optimistic outlook. The sequence information can be used to make informed hypotheses about which gene products, such as the proteinases, are important to virulence, and these genes can be deleted and tested in virulence models. These experiments will contribute to our understanding of how dermatophytes interact with human cells and cause disease. Knowing the fungal factors involved will allow development of better therapeutics and will inform preventative treatments.

A deeper understanding of the pathogenesis (*see* Chapter 2) can make one appreciate that it is the host factors and particularly the fungi-immune interaction that can explain the recalcitrant dermatophyte infection in our country.

Bibliography

1. Achterman RR, White TC. Dermatophyte virulence factors: identifying and analyzing genes that may contribute to chronic or acute skin infections. Int J Microbiol 2012: 305–358.

2. Arenas R, Moreno-Coutiño G, Welsh O. Classification of subcutaneous and systemic mycoses. Clin Dermatol. 2012 Jul-Aug;30(4):369–71. doi: 10.1016/j.clindermatol.2011.09.006. PubMed PMID: 22682183.

3. Ascioglu S, Rex JH, de Pauw B, *et al*. Defining opportunistic invasive fungal infections in immunocompromised patients with cancer and hematopoietic stem cell transplants: an international consensus. Clinical Infectious Diseases 2002;34:7–14.

4. Burmester A, Shelest E, Glockner G, Heddergott C, Schindler S, *et al*. Comparative and functional genomics provide insights into the pathogenicity of dermatophytic fungi. Genome Biol 2011;12: R7.

5. Chariyalertsak S Sirisanthana T, Saengwonloey O, *et al*. Clinical presentation and risk behaviors of AIDS patients in Thailand, 199+1998: regional variation and temporal trends. Clinical Infectious Diseases 2001;32: 955–962.

6. Chariyalertsak S, Supparatpinyo K, Sirisanthana T, *et al*. A controlled trial of itraconazole as primary prophylaxis for systemic fungal infections in patients with advanced human immunodeficiency virus infection in Thailand. Clinical Infectious Diseases 2002;34(2): 277–284.

7. Ghannoum M, Isham N, Sheehan D. Voriconazole susceptibilities of dermatophyte isolates obtained from a worldwide tinea capitis clinical trial. J Clin Microbiol 2006;44: 2579–2580.

8. Ghannoum MA, Wraith LA, Cai B, Nyirady J, Isham N. Susceptibility of dermatophyte isolates obtained from a large worldwide terbinafine tinea capitis clinical trial. Br J Dermatol 2008;159: 711–713.

9. Gupta AK, Cooper EA. Update in antifungal therapy of dermatophytosis. Mycopathologia 2008;166: 353–367.

10. Haddad NE, Powderly WG. The changing face of mycoses in patients with HIV/AIDS. AIDS 11, 2001;365–368,375–378.

11. Heyderman RS, Gangaidzo IT, Hakim JG, *et al*. Cryptococcal meningitis in human immunodeficiency virus-infected patients in Harare, Zimbabwe. Clinical Infectious Diseases 1998;26(2): 284–289.

12. Marr KA, Carter RA, Boeckh M, *et al*. Invasive aspergillosis in allogeneic stem cell transplant recipients: changes in epidemiology and risk factors. Blood 2002;100,4358–4366.

13. Marr KA, Carter RA, Crippa F, *et al*. Epidemiology and outcome of mould infections in hematopoietic stem cell transplant recipients. Clinical Infectious Diseases 2002;34:909–917.

14. McNeil MM, Nash SL, Hajjeh RA, *et al*. Trends in mortality due to invasive mycotic diseases in the United States, 1980–1997. Clinical Infectious Diseases 2001;33:641–647.

15. Mukherjee PK, Leidich SD, Isham N, Leitner I, Ryder NS, *et al*. Clinical *Trichophyton rubrum* strain exhibiting primary resistance to terbinafine. Antimicrob Agents Chemother 2003;47: 82–86.

16. Mwaba P, Mwansa J, Chintu C, *et al*. Clinical presentation, natural history, and cumulative death rates of 230 adults with primary cryptococcal meningitis in Zambian AIDS patients treated under local conditions. Postgraduate Medical Journal 2001;77:769–773.

17. Odds FC, Arai T, DiSalvo AF, *et al*. Nomenclature of fungal diseases: a report and recommendations from a subcommittee of the International Society for Human and Animal Mycology (ISHAM). Journal of Medical and Veterinary Mycology 1992;30:1–10.

18. Osborne CS, Leitner I, Favre B, Ryder NS. Amino acid substitution in *Trichophyton rubrum* squalene epoxidase associated with resistance to terbinafine. Antimicrob Agents Chemother 2005;49: 2840–2844.

19. Panackal AA, Hajjeh RA, Cetron MS, *et al*. Fungal infections among returning travellers. Clinical Infectious Diseases 2002;35:1088–1095.

20. White TC, Oliver BG, Graser Y, Henn MR, Generating and testing molecular hypotheses in the dermatophytes. Eukaryot Cell 2008;7: 1238–1245.

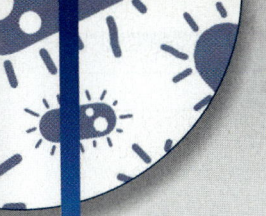

CHAPTER 2

Immunology and Pathogenesis of Dermatophytoses

Kabir Sardana

INTRODUCTION

The pathogenesis of dermatophyte infections is an interplay of four factors and it is important to understand the relationship between them specially in the era of recalcitrant infections.

The **4 factors** are the *fungi*, the *barrier* response, *host* factors and the *immune* response (Fig. 2.1). The most important aspect is the type of fungi and the host immune response and the role of the drug, specially if a systemic agent is used, is minimal. The cause of both recalcitrant infection and relapse is an interaction of the fungi and host immune response (Fig. 2.2).

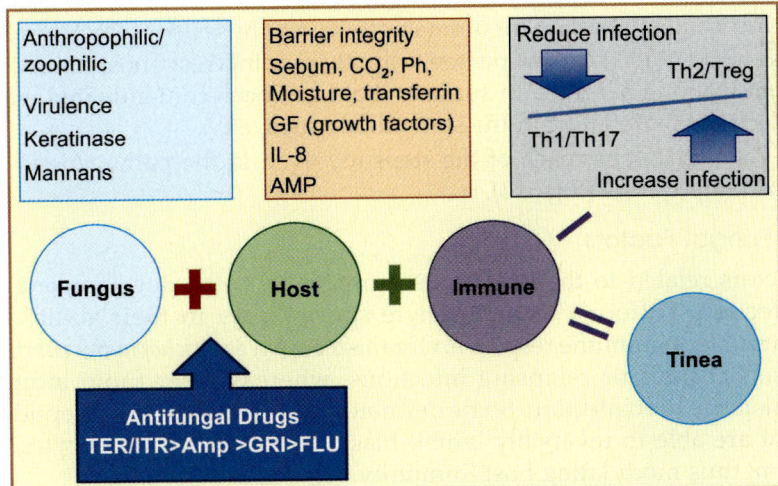

Fig. 2.1: Summary of factors determining an overt dermatophyte infection (GF = Growth factors, AMP = Antimicrobial peptides), TER = Terbinafine, ITR = Itraconazole, Amh = Amphotericin B, GRI = Griseofulvin, FLV = Fluconazole

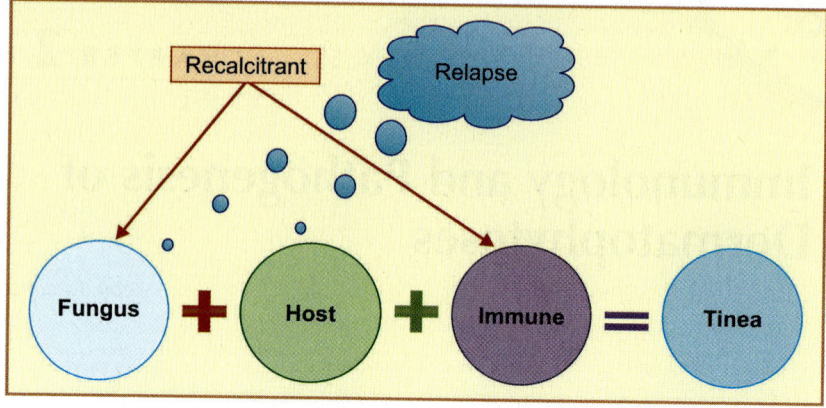

Fig. 2.2: Proposed factors for recalcitrance and relapse

The most prevalent dermatophytes are mainly those of the genera—Trichophyton, Microsporum and Epidermophyton, classified as anthropophilic, zoophilic and geophilic according to their primary habitat. The most common cause of persistent infection is the anthropophilic dermatophyte, *Trichophyton rubrum*, that can cause non-inflammatory chronic infections of the skin, one of the causes of the chronicity is the large number of cases caused by *T. rubrum*.

The pathogenic reservoir of *T. rubrum*, as an anthropophilic dermatophytes, is only found in the person himself or in his home. The infection pathways for dermatophytes are thus either direct (rarely, via skin contact from one person to another) or indirect (most common, from walking barefoot on surfaces that have been contaminated with infectious material from the skin, floors, rugs, etc.).

We will discuss each of the steps involved in the pathogenesis of dermatophytosis (Fig. 2.3).

1. Fungal Factors

Factors related to the fungus also contribute to the development of infection. Different dermatophyte species vary in their ability to stimulate an immune response: Organisms such as *Trichophyton rubrum* cause chronic or relapsing infections, whereas other fungi induce resistance to reinfection. Some dermatophytes produce glycopeptides that are able to reversibly inhibit blastogenesis of T lymphocytes *in vitro*, thus modulating host immunity.

It is important to emphasize that dermatophytes cause infection regardless of the patient's immune status. On rare occasions, individuals that are immunocompromised, develop infections caused by dermatophytes with invasion of the subcutaneous tissue.

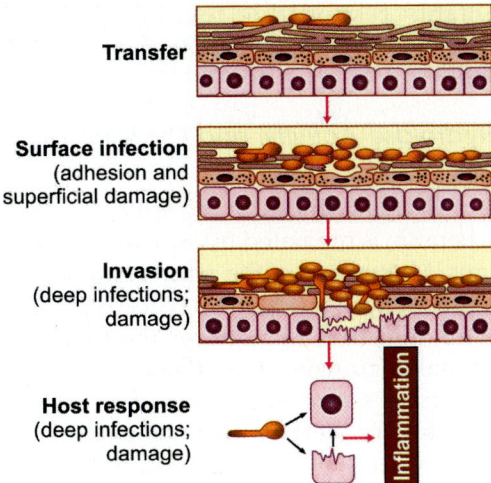

Fig. 2.3: Steps involved in dermatophytic infections (1) transfer to and colonization of host surfaces; (2) adhesion to and infection of the surface (moderate invasion, disruption of superficial layers); (3) penetration or deep infection (deeper invasion, severe damage induced); (4) reaction of host to invading pathogen and vice versa (this is crucial and includes the complex immune responses)

Dermatophyte infections induce specific humoral and cellular immune response, with protective response against dermatophytes being mediated primarily by delayed type hypersensitivity reaction, which is characterized by the action of macrophages as effector cells with increased activity of key cytokines of the **Th1 pole** (type 1 T helper lymphocytes) such as IL-12 (interleukin-12) and IFN-γ (interferon gamma). Lately an emphasis on the role of Th17 cells has been discovered and this is largely protective (Fig. 2.1).

Virulence Factors of Dermatophytes

Although various factors related to the potential host create the conditions for dermatophytosis (predisposition), dermatophyte virulence factors must also be present for a cutaneous infection to occur (Fig. 2.1). The target structure for infection and dermatophyte proliferation in the stratum corneum of the epidermis is the hard, firm cytokeratin found in the skin, hair, and nails. Dermatophytes degrade these complex proteins via *keratinase*. In a study that compared the keratolytic activity of *T. rubrum*, *T. interdigitale*, *M. canis*, and *M. gypseum* using spectrophotometry , *Trichophyton* spp. produced the highest keratinase activity. The high level of enzyme activity of *Trichophyton* spp. at normal body temperatures and pH levels of the skin is presumably responsible for the adaptation of certain dermatophytes to the surface of human skin. This is referred to as **"anthropozation"**.

Adherence, Hydrolase Activity, and Cysteine Dioxygenase of Dermatophytes

The adherence of dermatophytes to the epithelial tissue of the host, which contains keratin, is mediated by *mannan glycoproteins* in the cell wall of the fungus. Maturation of the arthroconidia produces hyphae, which are able to penetrate the deeper layers of the skin tissue. Other factors include the nutritive medium for the fungus, host-pathogen interactions (signals), transport proteins, synthesis of structural proteins in the fungus and secretion of proteolytic enzymes, predominantly hydrolase (keratinase, nuclease).

The hydrolase activity is inhibited by disulfide bridges, which link epidermal keratins. These disulfide bonds must be broken by cysteine dioxygenase to set the process of keratinolysis in motion. Keratin degradation is caused by keratinase, cysteine dioxygenase, and a sulfite efflux pump.

Recalcitrant Dermatophytosis

Chronic or relapsing infections with *T. rubrum* in immunocompetent individuals are related to the prevalence of immediate hypersensitivity mediated by IgE (immunoglobulin E) to the fungus, as well as high serum levels of IgE and IgG4 (immunoglobulin G4). Certain dermatophytes like *T. rubrum* produce substances, e.g. the *mannans* associated with glycoproteins that *diminish* the immune response, thus prevent complete eradication of the fungus. This is mediated via the following steps:

a. Anthropophilic fungi induce *immunosuppression* through toll-like receptor 2 (TLR2) mediated IL-10 release, and this leads to generation of CD4+ CD25+ T-regulatory cells with immunosuppressive potential.

b. Also *T. rubrum* has the ability to *suppress* the expression of *toll-like receptors* in keratinocytes and Langerhans' cells in dermis and epidermis necessary for stimulation of Th1-type cell response. Consequently, there would be increased Th2-type responses that are inadequate to fight fungal infections. This allows a chronic and extensive infection to set in.

c. Mannans derived from dermatophytes can *inhibit DC-SIGN-dependent* cell adesion to ICAM-3 of wild-type T cells, which reinforces the hypothesis that dermatophyte mannans could also avoid initial interactions between DC and wild-type T cells, thus blocking antigen presentation and activation of T cells, favoring the development of invasive or disseminated infections caused by dermatophytes.

The *clinical correlate* of this is the leathery, lichenified look that some patients have and is a surrogate clinical sign of chronicity.

2. Keratinocyte–Fungal Interaction

It is known that keratinocytes are the first cellular elements with which dermatophytes come into contact during infection and that they modulate the host immune response.

a. Cytokines/AMP

Upon exposure to dermatophytes or their antigens, these keratinocytes produce a wide range of cytokines, which include **IL-8** (potent neutrophil chemotactic factor) and the pro-inflammatory cytokine **TNF-α** (tumor necrosis factor-alpha), which together can destroy dermatophytes.

The various species of dermatophytes differ in their ability to induce secretion of proinflammatory cytokines in keratinocytes. Zoophilic species, for instance, are more effective in causing a greater degree of inflammation in the host's skin. Human keratinocytes also secrete *antimicrobial peptides* such as cathelicidins and defensins with potent antifungal activity. Several authors have shown that human defensin and cathelicidin IL-37 are fungistatic and fungicidal *in vitro* against *T. rubrum* and that their expression is increased *in vivo* in tinea corporis.

b. Fungal-Kc immune interaction (innate response)

Epidermal dendritic cells (DC), especially LC, are essential to initiate and modulate adaptive responses of the immune system against dermatophytes. They are usually equipped with receptors for pathogen-associated molecular patterns called pattern recognition receptors (PRRs). They interact with pathogen-associated molecular patterns (PAMPs) and damage-associated molecular patterns (DAMPs) that are present during fungal infections are recognized by pattern recognition receptors (PRRs) (Fig. 2.4).

These PRRs include *toll-like receptors* (TLRs), which have a central role in the activation of DC, and lectin and *lectin*-like receptors, specialized in recognizing pathogen structures associated with carbohydrates. An important example is DC-SIGN (CD209) [dendritic cell-specific intercellular adhesion molecule-3 (ICAM-3)-grabbing non-integrin], a type 2 transmembrane protein belonging to the C-type lectin family of the PRRs.

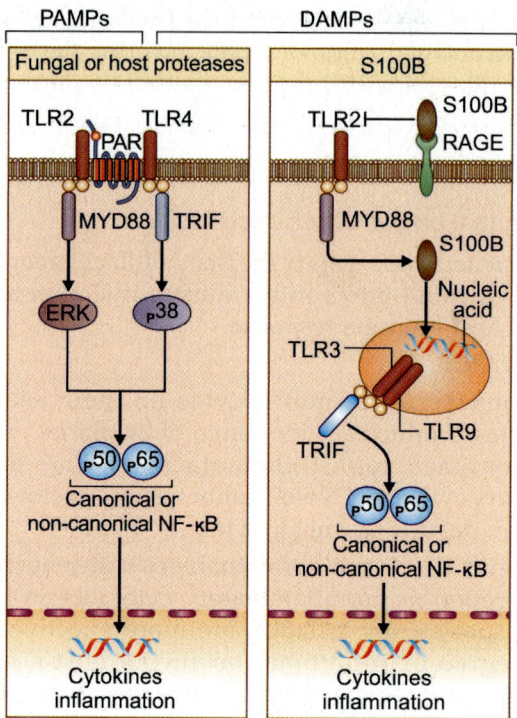

Fig. 2.4: Pathogen-associated molecular patterns (PAMPs) and damage-associated molecular patterns (DAMPs) that are present during fungal infections are recognized by pattern recognition receptors (PRRs). After TLR activation, protease-activated receptors (PARs), sense proteolytic virulence factors and tissue injury and contribute to fungal recognition through a dual-sensor system

The study of the role of PRRs in immune response to fungi could explain the chronicity. Several molecules have been described, including **Dectin-2**, a C-type lectin-like receptor expressed in most differentiated DC, such as LC, which is able to recognize and bind to *M. canis* and *T. rubrum* hyphae, determining the secretion of proinflammatory cytokines such as TNF-α. In contrast to this immunostimulatory effect, phagocytosis of *T. rubrum* conidia by macrophages induces secretion of **IL-10**, a cytokine with *anti-inflammatory properties*, while other factors related to protective immunity such as human leukocyte antigen class II (MHC-II), CD54 and CD80 lymphocytes (costimulatory molecules), nitric oxide and IL-12 are suppressed.

In addition to keratinocytes and DC, neutrophils are important cellular elements in innate immunity to dermatophytes, accumulating early—soon after the adherence of conidia to corneocytes—during germination. Neutrophils are believed to be, together with macrophages, the final effector cells in elimination of dermatophytosis, via Th1-dependent inflammatory response.

3. Acquired Immune Response

Humoral and Cellular Immunity

The relative contribution of specific humoral and cellular immunity against fungal infections has been controversial in the field of medical mycology. Cell-mediated immunity (CMI) has been shown to mediate protection against many fungi, an elaborate cascade has been described in Fig. 2.5.

Several studies suggested that the cellular immune response participates in modulating the disease by increasing epidermal proliferation and facilitating dermatophyte elimination.

The type of CMI is critical to define resistance or vulnerability to fungal infection (Fig. 2.5). Overall, **Th1**-type CMI is usually required for elimination of a fungal infection, while **Th2** response results in susceptibility to infection or leads to allergic responses (Fig. 2.1). Th1 cells produce predominantly cytokines such as IFN-γ, and promote phagocyte activation. In contrast, Th2 cells produce predominantly cytokines and tend to promote antibody production. Activation of cutaneous and/or circulating T cells by dermatophytes could induce a **Th2**-response that results in enhanced production of **IL-4**, **IL-5**, and **IL-13**. The first two cytokines can further lead to IgE production by B cells and eosinophil recruitment by VCAM-VLA-4 adhesion molecule pathway while IL-5 enhances eosinophil production from the bone marrow.

Recent work has focused on the role of the Th17 cell pathway in promoting Th1-type immune responses and restraining Th2-type responses, and also explain the immunological findings observed in patients with chronic mucocutaneous candidiasis and autosomal dominant hyper IgE syndrome.

In terms of effector functions, although the ability of **IL-17A** to mobilize neutrophils and induce the production of defensins greatly contributes to the prompt and efficient control of an infection at different body sites, conflicting results have been obtained regarding whether the IL-17A–IL-17RA pathway is essential or not during infection. This suggests that the activity of this pathway may depend on the stage and site of infection, and is probably influenced by environmental stimuli that induce cells to produce Th17 cell-associated cytokines, including IL-22.

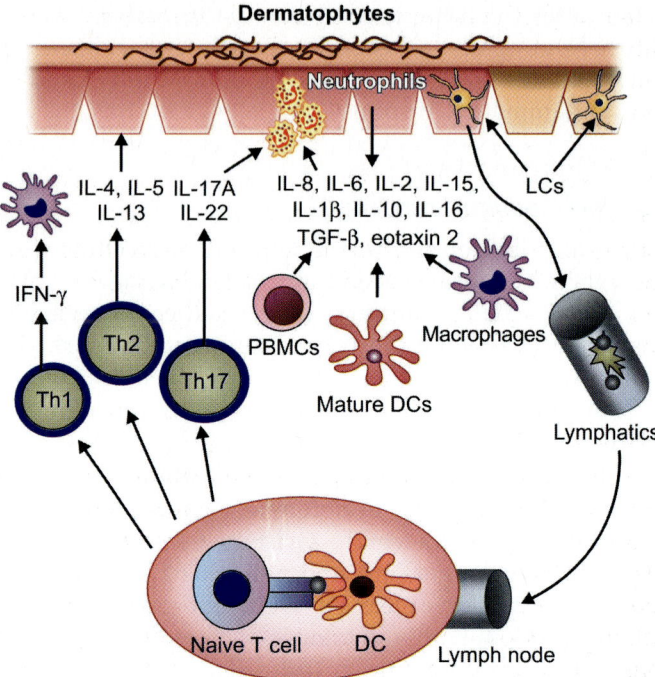

Fig. 2.5: Immune responses to dermatophytes. Anthropophilic dermatophytes such as *Trichophyton rubrum*, *Trichophyton schoenleinii* and *Trichophyton tonsurans* induce the production of interleukin (IL)-8, IL-6, IL-1β and eotaxin-2 in keratinocytes, peripheral blood mononuclear cells (PBMC) and THP-1 cells, macrophages and dendritic cells (DC), while zoophilic dermatophytes such as *Arthroderma benhamiae* induce a wide range of cytokines including IL-1β, IL-6, IL-8, IL-10, IL-2, IL-15, IL-16, transforming growth factor (TGF)-β, interferon (IFN)-γ (T-helper (Th)1), IL-17 (Th17), IL-4, IL-5 and IL-13 (Th2), leading to various pro-inflammatory processes such as neutrophil chemo attraction as well as macrophage and DC activation resulting in fungal killing and clearance

The mechanisms that link inflammation to chronic infection may involve a failure to restrain inflammation following IL-17A-dependent neutrophil recruitment, thereby preventing optimal protection and favouring fungal persistence. Thus, the Th17 cell pathway could be involved in the immunopathogenesis of chronic fungal diseases, in which persistent fungal antigens may promote immune dysregulation. This may occur in patients with autoimmune polyendocrine syndrome type 1 and in the mouse model of this disorder (autoimmune regulator (AIRE)-deficient mice), in which excessive Th17-type responses to fungi have been observed.

The debate between the relative merits of humoral and cellular immunity concluded that although CMI remains the main mechanism for defense but certain types of antibody responses can also provide protection.

Resolution of the disease is generally associated with the development of a *DTH*, while the *persistence* of the infection seems to be accompanied by the absence of this response and with a poor *in vitro* lymphoproliferation.

In conclusion, it is clear that the immune system works as a whole in harmony involving the combination of diverse components to the defence of the host organism. According to the circumstances, some parts contribute more than others, but they are all important for the overall protection.

Clinical Implications

It is obvious that the immunological interaction of the host immune response and the fungi determine the clinical sequelae. Thus a understanding of the variety of complex immune responses to *Trichophyton rubrum* is essential to the treating physician in developing therapeutic strategies for those individuals who suffer from a chronic manifestation of tinea infections. About a fifth of all *T. rubrum* skin infections will develop into a *chronic* state. *T. rubrum* colonizes the superficial layers of skin and causes common, but persistent infections such as "athlete's foot", onychomycosis in the nails, "jock itch" in the groin, and ringworm on any epidermal surface.

Often, acute manifestations of *T. rubrum* may be treated successfully with a topical antifungal. However, in the *chronic* form, *T. rubrum* can invade the deeper levels of the epidermis, suppressing an immune response, and prolonging symptoms such as mild to intense itch, scaly pattern on the skin, and plaques and lesions. This type of dermatophyte can have severe implications for those suffering from a chronic infection, which often does not respond to treatment. Exploring the mechanisms by which *T. rubrum* evades the initial host defense and manipulates the cellular immune response is vital to developing effective treatment modalities. A more successful treatment for *chronic dermatophytoses* would involve targeting the mechanisms of *T. rubrum* that deactivate the immune response, such as the ways in which it inhibits TLRs, and determining a way to restore the cell-mediated immune response, such as reactivating the phagocytic activity of the macrophages.

It is amply clear why this has become an issue in India as the wide spread use of topical steroids suppresses the very CMI which is crucial for resolution. This with the concomitant *T. rubrum* suppression is the cause for persistence of infection.

4. Host Factors

Susceptibility to dermatophytosis is variable. Individual susceptibility factors are still unclear and may be related to variations in the composition of sebum fatty acids, skin surface carbon dioxide tension, presence of moisture or presence of inhibitors for the growth of dermatophytes in sweat or serum, such as transferrin (Fig. 2.1).

It was experimentally observed that the main efferent arm of immune resistance to fungal infection is T lymphocytes, which is not influenced by administration of specific antibodies. Apparently, the kinetics of the immune response in humans would be similar. During infection, there is development of both delayed hypersensitivity skin reaction to trichophytin and blastogenic response of T lymphocytes with progression to healing, which relates chronicity to incomplete cellular immune responses.

Participation of each element of the immune response has been explored and gradually elucidated over time: Langerhans' cells (LC) act as antigen presenting cells; mononuclear phagocytes, especially polymorphonuclear neutrophils, lyse dermatophytes both intra and extracellularly via the oxidative pathway; and dermatophyte antigens have shown to be chemotactic to human leukocytes, activating the alternative pathway of the complement. However, with the exception of clinical cases of inflammatory tinea, neutrophils are not usually seen as part of the inflammatory infiltrate observed in histological sections under the microscope. This indicates that other mechanisms of fungal clearance must be involved in this process.

Other factors including skin fragility, ichthyosis, psoriasis, diabetes mellitus (DM), immunosuppression, clothing, etc. have been implicated.

CONCLUSIONS

It is obvious that the clinical picture of tinea infection is consequent to an intricate interplay of fungus/host interaction, which includes fungus species, host species, immmune response capacity and response modulation by the parasite, which exert influence on the degree of inflammatory reaction, define the clinical presentation and duration of the lesion.

It is obvious that the role of dermatophytes on the skin, either by new infection or relapse of a previous infection can lead to a clinical episode of tineas and this can be inhibited by the immune system and antifungal drugs. *Immune dysfunction* can reduce the immune response to these infections, and *drug resistance or tolerance* can overcome the action of the drugs. Resistance or tolerance to antifungal drugs is *implied* but is not documented in dermatophyte.

Thus, it is eminently obvious that it is the local immune suppression that is responsible for the recalcitrant infection we see in India. Contrary to my mycologist colleagues it is my belief that a rising MIC level does not mean resistance as that is consequent to the overuse of drugs and the fact that every conceivable antifungal cocktail has been tried in India and failed without a concomitant resistant MIC in the same proportion is a reason to believe that the answer lies elsewhere.

A re-look at the interplay between the host and the fungi (Fig. 2.1) may be the answer to this vexing problem in India.

Bibliography

1. Al HM, Fitzgerald SM Saoudian M Krishnaswamy. G Dermatology for the practicing allergist, tinea pedis and its complications. Clin Mol Allergy 2004; 2:5.

2. Almeida SR. Immunology of dermatophytosis. Mycopathologia 2008, 166: 277–283.

3. Bellocchio S, Bozza S, Montagnoli C, Perruccio K, Gaziano R, Pitzurra L, Romani L. Immunity to *Aspergillus fumigatus*, the basis for immunotherapy and vaccination. Med. Mycol 2005; 43(1): S181–188.

4. Calderon RA. Immunoregulation in dermatophytosis. Crit Rev Microbiol. 1989;16:339–368.

5. Criado PR, Oliveira CB, Dantas KC, Takiguti FA, Benini LV, Vasconcellos C. Superficial mycosis and the immune response elements. An Bras Dermatol 2011; 86:726–731.

6. Dahl MV. Suppression of immunity and inflammation by products produced by dermatophytes. J. Am. Acad. Dermatol 1993; 28: S19–23.

7. Grumbt M, Monod M, Yamada T, *et al*. Keratin degradation by dermatophytes relies on cysteine dioxygenase and a sulfite efflux pump. J Invest Dermatol 2013; 133: 155.

8. Hay RJ, Reid S, Talwet E, Macnamara K. Immune responses of patients with tinea imbricata. Brit J Dermatol 1983;108:581–589.

9. Hay RJ. Dermatophytosis and other superficial mycosis. In: Principles and practice of infectious diseases. 4th ed. New York: Churchill-Livingstone; 1995. p. 2375–2386.

10. Jensen JM, Pfeiffer S, Akaki T, Schröder JM, Kleine M, Neumann C, *et al*. Barrier function, epidermal differentiation, and human beta-defensin 2 expression in tinea corporis. J Invest Dermatol 2007;127:1720–1727.

11. Jones HE, Reinhardt JH, Rinaldi MG. Acquired immunity to dermatophytosis. Arch Dermatol 1974;109: 840–848.

12. Kasperova A, Kunert J, Raska M. The possible role of dermatophyte cysteine dioxygenase in keratin degradation. Med Mycol 2013; 51: 449–454.

13. King RD, Khan HA, Foye JC, Greenberg JH, Jones HE. Transferrin, iron, and dermatophytes. I. Serum dermatophyte inhibitory component definitively identified as unsaturated transferrin. J Lab Clin Med 1975;86:204–212.

14. López-García B, Lee PH, Gallo RL. Expression and potential function of cathelicidin antimicrobial peptides in dermatophytosis and tinea versicolor. J Antimicrob Chemother. 2006;57:877–882.

15. MacGregor JM, Hamilton A, Hay RJ. Possible mechanisms of immune modulation in chronic dermatophytosis—an *in vitro* study. Br J Dermatol 1992;127:233–238.

16. Mignon B, Tabart J, Baldo A, Mathy A, Losson B, Vermout S. Immunization and dermatophytes. Curr Opin Infect Dis 2008;21:134–140.

17. Mignon BR, Coignoul F, Leclipteux T, Focant C. Losson BJ. Histopathological pattern and humoral immune response to a crude exoantigen and purified keratinase of *Microsporum canis* in symptomatic and asymptomatic infected cats. Med. Mycol 1999; 37:1–9.

18. Nakamura Y, Kano R, Hasegawa A, Watanabe S. Interleukin-8 and tumor necrosis factor-alpha production in human epidermal keratinocytes induced by *Trichophyton mentagrophytes*. Clin Diagn Lab Immunol. 2002;9:935–937.

19. Netea MG, Sutmuller R, Hermann C, van der Graaf CA, van der Meer JW, van Krieken, JH, Hartung T, Adema G, Kullberg BJ. Toll-like receptor 2 suppresses immunity against *Candida albicans* through induction of IL-10 and regulatory T cells. J. Immunol 2004; 172: 3712–3718.

20. Saijo S, Ikeda S, Yamabe K, Kakuta S, Ishigame H, Akitsu A, et al. Dectin-2 recognition of mannans and induction of Th17 cell differentiation is essential for host defense against *Candida albicans*. Immunity 2010;32:681–691.

21. Sato K, Yang XL, Yudate T, Chung JS, Wu J, Luby-Phelps K, et al. Dectin-2 is a pattern recognition receptor for fungi that couples with the Fc receptor gamma chain to induce innate immune responses. J Biol Chem. 2006;281:38854–38866.

22. Sharma A, Chandra S, Sharma M. Difference in keratinase activity of dermatophytes at different environmental conditions is an attribute of adaptation to parasitism. Mycoses 2012; 55: 410–415. (JDDG)

23. Sugita K, Kabashima K, Atarashi K, Shimauchi T, Kobayashi M, Tokura Y. Innate immunity mediated by epidermal keratinocytes promotes acquired immunity involving Langerhans' cells and T cells in the skin. Clin ExpImmunol 2007;147:176–183.

24. Tani K, Adachi M, Nakamura Y, Kano R, Makimura K, Hasegawa A, et al. The effect of dermatophytes on cytokine production by human keratinocytes. Arch Dermatol Res 2007;299:381–387.

25. Traynor TR, Huffnagle GB. Role of chemokines in fungal infections. Med. Mycol 2001;39:41–50.

26. Willment JA, Brown GD. C-type lectin receptors in antifungal immunity. Trends Microbiol 2008;16:27–32.

27. Woodfolk JA, Platts-Mills TA. The immune response to dermatophytes. Res Immunol 1998;149:436–445.

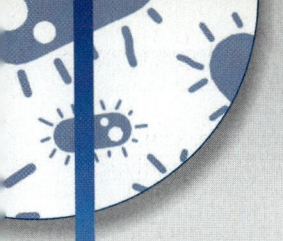

CHAPTER 3

Laboratory Diagnosis of Fungal Infections: A Primer

Autar K Miskeen, Priya Uppuluri

INTRODUCTION

In spite of their high prevalence, dermatomycoses are often misdiagnosed in general practice. Most cases of suspected dermatomycoses lead to the prescription of an antifungal drug on the basis of clinical signs alone. A favorable outcome from this treatment is then taken as a confirmation of the original diagnosis. However, such a practice frequently leads to a "hit or miss" diagnosis, causing the patients to undergo lengthy, unnecessary therapies that often exacerbate the existing problem. Since there is no urgency to initiate treatment at the first consultation for most benign dermatological conditions, confirmation of the clinical finding by a few simple tests could lead to more efficient and effective outcomes. Some diagnostic approaches that are considered as gold standards in diagnosis of fungal infections will be discussed in this chapter. Another burning issue deliberated, will be on the topic of the "supposed" antifungal drug resistance, and the emerging recalcitrant nature of certain class of dermatophytic fungi.

Superficial fungal infections of the nails, hair, epidermis, and mucous membranes are distributed worldwide, and cause varied degrees of morbidity. In recent times, a paradigm shift is noticed in the nature and extent of some conditions, like dermatophytosis and pityrosporosis. Recalcitrant presentations with extensive involvement of the skin have become common and worrisome events. Besides, atypical and incognito presentations further compound the problem of clinical diagnosis. The role of clinical laboratory investigations in mycology thus becomes all the more imperative.

The laboratory investigations ordered, for superficial infections would typically include: (a) A microscopic examination of the specimen (e.g. skin, hair and nails), by making a fresh KOH preparation, (b) selective cultures for growth and phenotypic identification of the

Mycology Tray

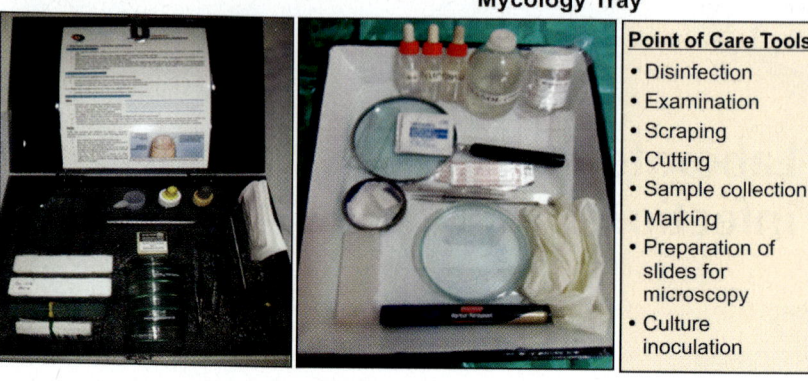

Point of Care Tools
• Disinfection
• Examination
• Scraping
• Cutting
• Sample collection
• Marking
• Preparation of slides for microscopy
• Culture inoculation

Fig. 3.1: Mycology tray that has a comprehensive set of components for collection of specimen by the patient's bedside

fungus, (c) newer molecular diagnostic procedures, and (d) *in vitro-*antifungal drug susceptibility tests.

The successful identification of the underlying etiological agent of infection depends tremendously on the quality and quantity of the specimen sent to the laboratory for testing. Specimen collection procedures are unique for each body site, and need to follow some carefully crafted guidelines. A clinical laboratory normally possesses a ready stock of materials, for collection/sampling of skin, hair or nail specimen. It is recommended that every busy diagnostic dermatology clinic keep a "Mycology tray" handy for specimen collection, transportation and perhaps even culture by the patients' bedside (Fig. 3.1).

SKIN

Fungi, if present, can be visualized as hyaline, septate, smooth/vesiculated, branching fungal mycelia or short filaments over a clear background of skin epithelial cells. Also, the presence of any arthroconidial spore forms, pigmented dematiaceous hyphae or budding yeasts may be noted, and recorded. Specimens from pityrosporosis and pityriasis versicolor show a presentation of spherical refractile meat-ball like large yeasts, and sphagetti-like hyphal filaments, mostly in vegetation.

In recent years we have been seeing a paradigm shift in the nature and extent of dermatophytosis. Extensive and recurrent involvement of glabrous skin has become a frequent occurrence. Further, clinical failure to treatment in several of our cases is common. Such a massive build up of fungal elements is indicative of an epidemiological transformation and adaptation of this group of pathogens. This aspect of a luxuriant growth of such fungi over skin is a definite contrast to the picture seen a few decades ago, when the load of fungal filaments was scarce. Here we present appearances of several of the fungi that we have diagnosed over the years, from skin specimen of patients referred to our laboratory by dermatologists around the country.

1. *Trichophyton rubrum* is the single most common dermatophyte species of the anthropophilic (human) type reported from India, and can be found in two different colony morphologies—var. downy, and var. granulare (Fig. 3.2).

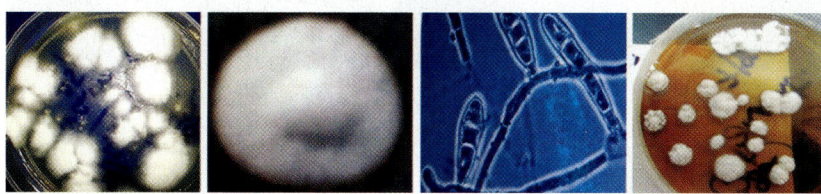

Fig. 3.2: *T. rubrum* var. downy and *T. rubrum* var. granulare

2. *T. mentagrophytes:* Detailed mycological studies carried out on 500 cases of dermatophytosis at our center have indicated a yet another significant aspect of the epidemiology of these keratinophilic fungi. The species showing preponderance in all cases in the present series is *Trichophyton mentagrophytes*. These isolates, growing rapidly in the primary culture (in five to seven days), appear as powdery and granular colonies,with whitish to creamy variants, abounding in macroconidial spore forms. We are, therefore, confronted with a surge in the "zoo/geo-philic" forms of these less parasitic, highly sporulating and rapidly growing strains of *T. mentagrophytes* (Fig. 3.3).

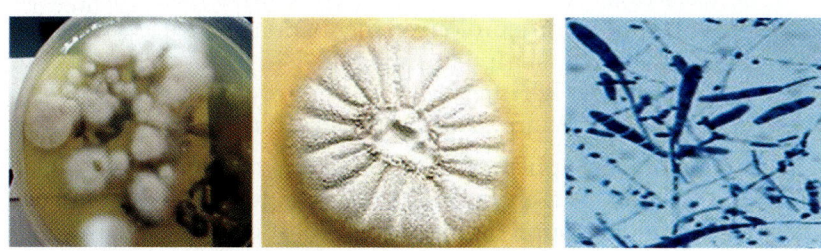

Fig. 3.3: *T. mentagrophytes*

3. *Epidermophyton floccosum.* Rapidly growing, khaki-brown, powdery colonies are produced, fanning out with a mycelial fringe. Large numbers of septate, conical macroconidia, in aggregates of three, are commonly observed (Fig. 3.4).

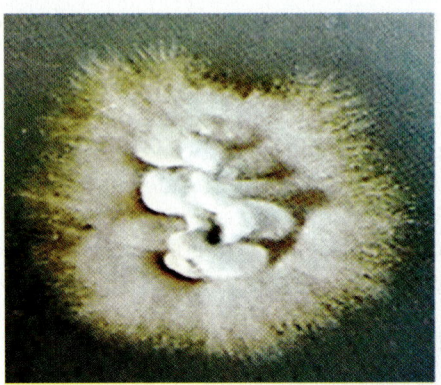
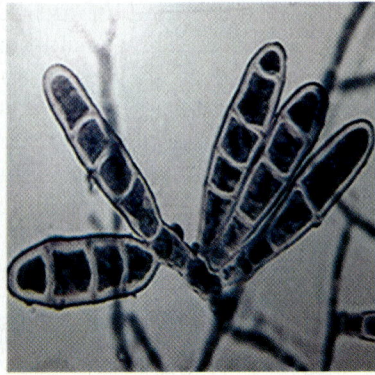

Fig. 3.4: *Epidermophyton floccosum*

4. *Microsporum canis.* Whitish to golden-yellow coloured fluffy and granular growth, rich in six or more celled spindle shaped, knob-ended, thick walled macroconidia. (most of the cases encountered in the present series were isolated from cases of zoophilic, incognito presentations with a history of animal (cat) contact (Fig. 3.5).

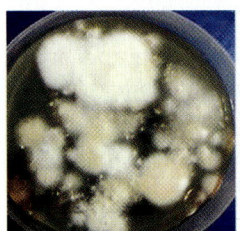
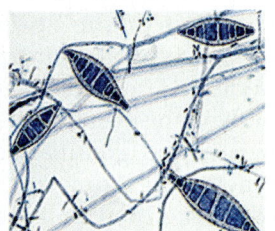
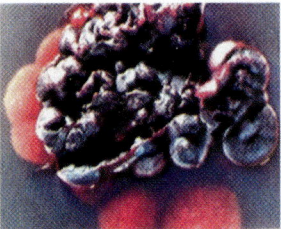

Fig. 3.5: *Microsporum canis* and *T. violaceum*

5. *T. violaceum.* A deep violet colored, convoluted, waxy slow growth appears on a prolonged incubation. All the isolates were from cases of scalp ringworm—grey patch type, and inflammatory kerions. Macro-/microconidia are scanty, chlamydoconidia are, however, noticeable.

Certain protocols apply when it comes to collection of specimen from infected site. These practices (as elaborated below) have been considered standard approaches, yielding best quality yields.

- First step entails gentle rubbing of the lesions with an isopropyl alcohol skin prep swab. For soggy, macerating or delicate intertriginous areas or while investigating the mucous membrane, glans/vulvovaginal/perianal surface, or the buccal mucosa, a cotton swab or a gauze-piece, soaked in sterile distilled water is employed.

- For each infected site to be examined, a glass slide is correspondingly labelled. Using disposable hand gloves, the skin is held with the left hand, and the skin lesions scrapped using a scalpel blade. This process is repeated, using few drops of water, to affect a suitable collection. Alternatively, a white clean sheet of paper is spread beside the patient, and the scales or keratinaceous dust collected over it. Specimen can now be transported to the lab.
- It is essential that an adequate number of scales from the skin scrapings are collected over a drop of filtered 10–20 per cent KOH solution, with or without gentle warming (depending on thickness of the scales) over a glass slide. Large square cover glass is put over the KOH-preparation, and left for 'digestion' for a few hours or overnight. Using a wet chamber such as a petri plate, containing a wet filter paper, enables keeping the slide mount/preparation fresh and prevents it from drying. A mycologist may also stain the specimen with a solution of Calcofluor dye, followed by examination under a fluorescent microscope. This procedure enhances observation of various morphological features of the fungi.
- When attempting a culture, for identifying the causative species or for performing the Antifungal Drug Susceptibility test, a part of the scrapped material is aseptically inoculated by stabbing it across the surface of selective fungal culture media, contained in petri plates.

Fungi, if present, can be visualized as hyaline, septate, smooth/ vesiculated, branching fungal mycelia or short filaments over a clear background of skin epithelial cells. Also, the presence of any arthroconidial spore forms, pigmented dematiaceous hyphae or budding yeasts may be noted, and recorded. Specimens from pityrosporosis and pityriasis versicolor, will show a presentation of spherical refractile meat-ball like large yeasts, and sphagetti-like hyphal filaments, mostly in clusters vegetations.

HAIR

It is the short, broken and rough hair stubs, observed in cases suspected of having ringworm of scalp (rather than the intact, fully grown hair) that give results positive for dermatophytosis. Such hair shows masses of dermatophytic-spores/arthroconidia besides fragmenting hyphal forms within the hair shaft (endothrix involvement), or on their outer surface (ectothrix involvement).

Endothrix: Tiny broken stubs of fragile hair show compact chains of rectangular hyaline arthroconidia and fragmented hyphal forms. The involved hair can be easily epilated with a pair of forceps, or scraped out with a scalpel blade. Entire hair may however be pulled out when examining for any parasitic involvement like pediculosis, other fungal involvement like Piedra or when looking for any suspected hair abnormality like trichorrhexis nodosa or monilethrix. Fresh wet KOH-mount preparations of hair need gentle handling because of their fragile and easily distortable nature.

White piedra: White piedra of the hair is reported with increasing frequency from India. Multiple firm nodules with whitish to greyish appearance envelope the hair. The nodules show plenty of arthroconidia and yeasts, embedded in cementation material. The most common causative agent of white piedra is the yeast-like, arthroconidia-bearing species *Trichosporon inkin* that grow as wrinkled, convoluted, creamy, tan, soft colonies that tend to furrow (Fig. 3.6).

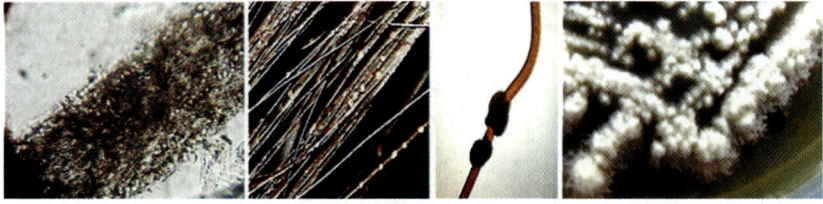

Fig. 3.6: Endothrix, white piedra and *T. inkin*

The most common species of dermatophytes associated with tinea capitis—both the quiet/grey-patch-types and the boggy, kerionic inflammatory types are *Trichophyton violaceum*. Among the other, less common species encountered are *T. tonsurans*, *T. schoenleinii*, *T. mentagrophytes* and *Microsporum canis*. For selective culture of these organisms, samples of hair stubs and scalp scrapings are inoculated into Sabouraud's dextrose agar (SDA) fortified with chloramphenicol and cycloheximide (Acti-dione).

Another infection, called the black piedra, of the hair is caused by the dematiaceous (brown or black coloured) mold-fungus, *Piedraia hortae*. The gritty whitish or black nodules noticed in piedra are gently pressed to visualize the presence and nature of the causative agent in fresh wet microscopic preparations. Bits of infected hair are also streaked across SDA medium, to allow the growth of the fungus.

NAILS

For an effective and substantive diagnosis of fungus involvement of nails, the basic pre-requisite is one of proper sampling of specimens of the affected areas. It is a hard and painstaking process, demanding a concerted effort at digging out subungual muck or keratinaceous dust from the depth of a nail, of any presentation.

Accurate diagnosis is crucial for successful treatment and requires identification of physical changes and positive laboratory analysis. Only 50% of nail problems are caused by onychomycosis, and clinical diagnosis by physical examination alone can be inaccurate. Psoriasis, chronic nail trauma, and other causes must also be considered.

Avulsed or clipped nails, suspected of a mycotic infection, are cleaned with isopropyl alcohol, and transported dry. A solitary nail involvement especially of the great toes, usually follows a history of trauma/ischemia of the nail. The causal agents in such stubborn, chronic, dystrophic nails are species of some of the common environmental saprophytic mold fungi, i.e. Acremonium, Aspergillus, Scopulariopsis, etc. (Figs 3.7 to 3.9). Multiple nail involvement is usually caused by dermatophytes, especially *T. rubrum*.

Acremonium

Nails infected with *Acremonium* spp., usually display a greyish yellow dystrophic great toe nail. The fungal hyphae often fragment into spore forms. Acremonium forms glabrous, velvety, white, pale grey or pale pink colonies. Reverse side: Uncolored or rose colored pigment. This fungus has characteristic fusiform conidial structure (Fig. 3.7).

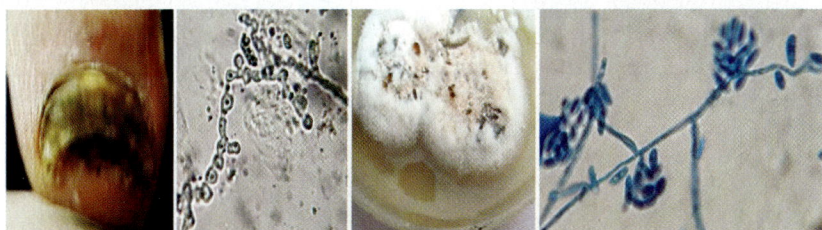

Fig. 3.7: Clinical morphology and colony characteristics of *Acremonium*

Aspergillus Spp.

- Lytic, white dystrophic great toe nail
- Tortuous, vesiculated, hyaline septate branching hyphae
- Large greenish yellow powdery growth (Fig. 3.8)

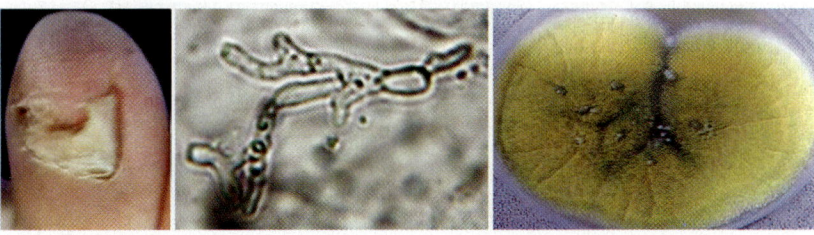

Fig. 3.8: Chronic morphology and microbiological findings in *Aspergillus* spp.

Mold: Scopulariopsis Spp.

- Beaked, greenish yellow great toe nails
- Pinkish velvety colonies
- Branching conidiophores with characteristic conidiospores (Fig. 3.9)

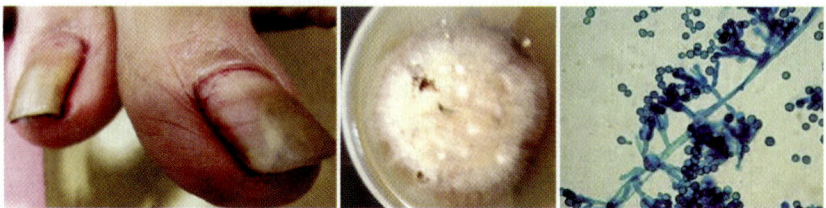

Fig. 3.9: Clinical morphology and microbiological features of *Scopulariopsis*

Fusarium Spp.

- Thick, raised, greyish yellow dystrophic nail
- Glaborous, white, feathery growth
- Clusters of sickle-shaped macroconidia (Fig. 3.10)

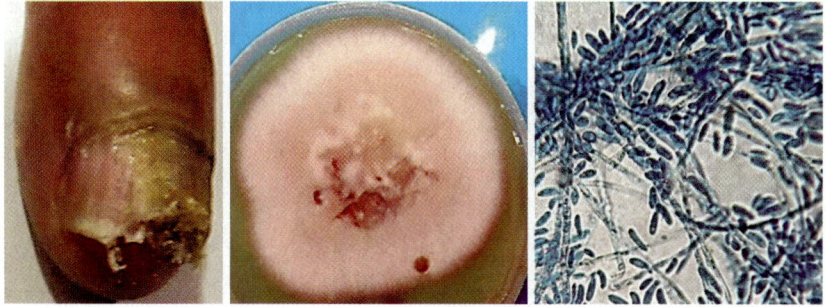

Fig. 3.10: Clinical and microbiological findings of *Fusarium* spp.

A point to note is that multiple nail involvement is usually caused by dermatophytes, especially *T. rubrum* (Fig. 3.11).

For collection of infected nail specimen, the following procedure needs to be followed.

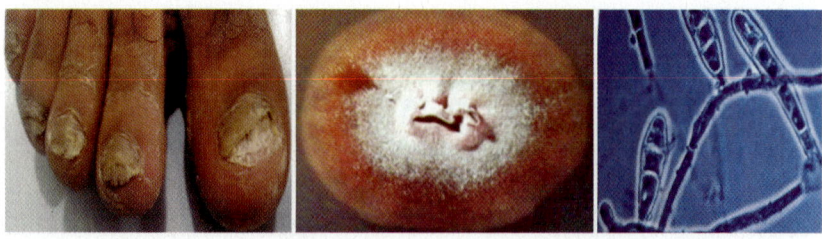

Fig. 3.11: Clinical and microbiological findings of *T. rubrum*

A cover glass—fresh wet preparation/mount of each labelled specimen of nail, i.e. scraped or avulsed bits, or deep scooped out sub-ungual keratinaceous powder, should be kept for sufficient time for "digestion"/dissolution in a 10 to 20% solution of KOH (filtered). It may be kept fresh for several hours or till overnight, by placing it in a petri plate over moist filter paper. Replenish any dried up or crystallised mounts, by introducing a few drops of the KOH solution under the cover glass. To further enhance a proper clearance and better dissolution of the keratin, the slide preparations may be gently warmed over a flame or a hot plate. The cover glass preparation should be gently pressed over a clean piece of filter paper, to blot out any excess of KOH, and to make the preparation even.

A microscopic examination under 10X and 40X helps appreciate the presence of any smooth, hyaline, septate, branching fungal hyphae. One should also look for the presence of any additional features, like vesiculated/tortuous forms, arthroconidial bodies and pseudohyphal filaments with budding yeasts (Fig. 3.12).

1. Stock KOH 10%, 20%; dissolve/keep to 'digest', warm
2. Scrape the undersurface (nails)
3. Make even mounts, recompensate with KOH–post 'digestion'
4. Observe with light microscope under 10X, 40X objective

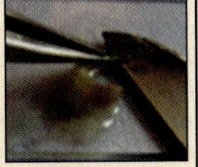

- Smooth, septate, hyaline, branching 'fungal' hyphae: **Dermatophytes (a)**
- Tortuous/vesiculated, often arthrospore-forming, thick, septate, hyaline or dematiaceous fungus forms: **Mold species (b)**
- Oval, budding yeasts with/without pseudohyphal filaments: **Candida spp. (c)**

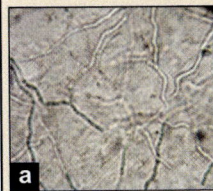 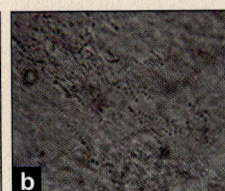 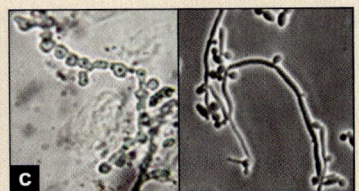

Fig. 3.12a to c: Microscopic observations

Despite the number of available treatments, not all patients with onychomycosis are cured. Numerous factors have been cited to explain the lack of response to therapy, such as nonadherence to treatment, incorrect diagnosis, or advanced disease. For those who appear to be cured, recurrent infection is a risk, with a number of factors increasing the chance of recurrence. Risk factors include concomitant disease, genetic factors, immunosuppression, incorrect dosing or duration of treatment, moisture, occlusive footwear, older age, poor hygiene, tinea pedis, and trauma. Recurrence can be caused by lack of mycotic cure or reinfection, and the reported rate of clinical recurrence of onychomycosis ranges from 10 to 53%, regardless of the treatment method used. Many patients tire of continued unsuccessful treatments or recurrences, and ultimately elect to undergo permanent nail removal.

ANTI-DERMATOPHYTIC SUSCEPTIBILITY TESTING

In the last two decades the incidence of infections caused by dermatophytes and other fungi has increased considerably. A standardized dermatophyte susceptibility testing technique encompasses the following: An ideal growth medium, a specific protocol with reference to the initial inoculum size, a specific incubation time, a specific incubation temperature, and an MIC endpoint determination which is applicable to all dermatophytes.

Several workers have carried our extensive *in vitro* tests, and standardized the procedures, besides determining the ranges of MICs for various common species of dermatophytes. Studies on drug susceptibility profiles and Minimum Inhibitory Concentrations have in some cases brought out the presence of "resistant" strains of dermatophytes. Break-points for determining susceptibility or resistance in dermatophytes have not yet been recommended by the Clinical and Laboratory Standards Institute (CLSI). However, based on various published reports by leading laboratories in the world, an MIC range for standard dermatophytic strains have been determined, as given in Table 3.1.

Table 3.1: MIC ranges for antifungal drugs against reference strains of dermatophytes

Organism	Purpose	Antifungal agent	MIC range (µg/ml)	Mode	% of MICs within range	Incubation times
T. mentagrophytes MRL 1957 ATCC MYA-4439	Reference	Ciclopirox	0.5–2	1.0	97.5	4 days
		Griseofulvin	0.12–0.5	0.25	96.3	
		Itraconazole	0.03–0.25	0.06	96.2	
		Posaconazole	0.03–0.25	0.06	95.2	
		Terbinafine	0.002–0.008	0.004	97.9	
		Voriconazole	0.03–0.25	0.06	95.2	
T. rubrum MRL 666 ATCC MYA-4438	Reference	Ciclopirox	0.5–2	1.0	97.5	4 days
		Fluconazole	0.5–4	1.0	95.2	
		Voriconazole	0.008–0.06	0.015	96.1	

Studies investigating the *in vitro* response of dermatophytes to antifungal agents have been few and far in between. The reason for this lag in research is the lack of proper technical expertise to perform antifungal susceptibility tests of fastidious fungi in the laboratory. Furthermore, no automated method exists. The rampant increase in cases of dermatophyte infections that are recalcitrant, stubborn and non-responsive to current regimens necessitates an identification of the response patterns of these filamentous fungi to these agents.

We have utilized the Broth micro-dilution procedures recommended by the CLSI for testing the filamentous fungi including dermatophytes and those associated with invasive and cutaneous infections (CLSI Document-M 38-A2). Test isolates of dermatophytes are grown on Oat Meal Agar to induce sporulation (conidiation). Standardized spore suspensions are inoculated into an RPMI medium-1640 (with glutamine, without bicarbonate, using phenol red as a pH indicator). Antifungal drugs are dissolved and diluted in dimethyl sulfoxide, and suspended in RPMI medium. A range of different concentrations of the test drugs, i.e. terbinafine, itraconazole and griseofulvin, from 0.001 µg/ml to 32 µg/ml is tested. The MIC is the lowest concentration of an antifungal agent that substantially inhibits growth of the organism, as detected visually. Growth controls and media controls are run in parallel with the test sample.

A total of 100 dermatophytic cultures were included in the study, a majority identified as *T. mentagrophytes* (53%) (Table 3.2).

Table 3.2: Analysis of dermatophytic culture reports

Sl. no.	Causative species (100 cases)	
	Dermatophyte species/VAR	**No. of isolates**
1.	*Trichophyton mentagrophytes* (var. granulare)	43
2.	*Trichophyton mentagrophytes* (var. downy) interdigitale	10
3.	*Trichophyton rubrum* (var. downy)	25
4.	*Trichophyton rubrum* (var. granulare)	17
5.	Others	5
	Total	100 cases

Out of these 100 positive cultures, 95 were subject to anti-dermatophytic susceptibility testing, and it was observed that ~90% of the cultures displayed elevated susceptibilities (at least twofold higher than the proposed MICs of between 0.001 and 0.03) to the "supposed" drug of choice, terbinafine.

(1) **Terbinafine:** Susceptible range: 0.001 to 0.03 µg/ml*						Total
MIC	Observed values					
	MIC					
ranges	0.001–0.03	0.03–0.064	0.064–0.128	>0.128	>0.256	
No. of isolates	10	38	21	17	9	95

Griseofulvin was found to be an effective drug against the dermatophytes. All cultures tested were susceptible to the drug which had MICs less than 2 µg/ml.

(2) **Griseofulvin:** Susceptibility range: 0.25–2.0 µg/ml*						Total
MIC	Observed values					
	MIC					
ranges	0.03–0.06	0.06–0.1	0.1–0.2	0.2–0.5	0.5–2.0	
No. of isolates	8	28	37	12	10	95

The third drug itraconazole was also found to be effective in eradicating the fungi. Most cultures were susceptible within the MIC range of <1 µg/ml. Only 5 out of the 95 cases were found to require higher concentration of the drug for inhibition, while the rest fell into the susceptibility range.

(3) **Itraconazole:** Susceptibility range: 0.05–1.0 µg/ml*						Total
MIC	Observed values					
	MIC					
ranges	0.05–0.25	0.25–0.5	0.5–1.0	>1	>2 (resistant)	
No. of isolates	5 cases	13	38	34	5 cases	95

Personal communications and discussions with world leaders in the field have emphasized upon the non-usage of the term "Resistant" for a strain of dermatophyte, pending the definition of "anti-fungal drug susceptibility break points of these organisms" by the CLSI-Clinical Laboratory Standards Instt, US. There are no interpretative

*Ghannoum MA, V Chaturvedi, A Espinel-Ingroff, MA Pfaller, MG Rinaldi, W Lee-Yang and DW Warnock. Intra- and interlaboratory study of a method for testing the antifungal susceptibilities of dermatophytes. J Clin. Microbiol. 2004:42:2977–2979.

breakpoints for terbinafine or any other anti-dermatophyte agents. Thus it is not possible to assign S, I or R. However, MIC of the drugs may be reported, and in fact should be routinely monitored for any increase in MIC50 or MIC90 against the fungal organism, over time.

CURRENT ADVANCES IN DIAGNOSTICS

For the successful treatment of onychomycosis as for other dermatophytoses, there is a need for accurate and rapid diagnosis. Culture has a low sensitivity (±75%) and is time consuming, particularly for slow growing dermatophytes. This is why a lot of recent work has focused on the detection of dermatophytes directly on sample material such as nails, hair and skin scrapings. Molecular tools offer the ability to rapidly diagnose dermatophytosis within 48 h. The power of these methods is increased by direct extraction from clinical specimens which allows time consuming culture to be bypassed. Many in-house methods and less frequently commercial PCR tests have been developed.

Molecular Tools for the Detection and Identification of Dermatophytes using DNA Extracted Directly from Infected Tissues

A modification of the PCR approach for biological material is the nested PCR in which conventional PCR is followed by another amplification of a smaller region inside the initial amplified fragment. Pan dermatophyte nested PCR was evaluated in 2007 by Garg et al. for the diagnosis of onychomycosis. Primers targeting the pan-dermatophyte specific sequence chitin synthase I (CHSI) were used and compared with KOH microscopy. This team concluded that pan dermatophyte nested PCR could be considered as the gold standard for the diagnosis of dermatomycosis in nails, as the method shows a higher sensitivity than KOH microscopy.

In 2007, Arabatzis et al. reported the development of a multiplex real-time PCR for the direct detection of dermatophytes in nail and skin clinical specimens. ITS1 and ITS2 regions were the two targeted regions. Real-time PCR detected and correctly identified the causal agent in specimens with cultures positive for *T. rubrum*, *T. interdigitale*, *M. audouinii* or *T. violaceum*, and also identified a dermatophyte species in an additional seven specimens that were negative on microscopy and culture. This real-time PCR method directed against ITS1 for use with skin, nails and hair was compared with convenional methods by Wisselink et al. The real-time PCR showed a sensitivity of 97%, representing a significant increase in the detection rate for dermatophytes in clinical samples compared with culture. In 2014, a multiplex PCR based on chitin synthase I and the ITS region was developed for detection and identification of *T. rubrum* and *T. mentagrophytes* in nail specimens. The sensitivity of the method was 97% in contrast to 81.1% for conventional methods. Specificity was also excellent.

There are several other molecular methods to identify the causative agent directly from a growing culture. Restriction fragment length polymorphism (RFLP) is an alternative method also used for dermatophyte identification. This method is based on the choice of several restriction enzymes that produce different fragment patterns after enzyme digestion according to species or strain.

Matrix-assisted laser desorption/ionization time-of-flight mass spectrometry (MALDI-TOF MS) for rapid identifications has raised considerable interest in the clinical microbiology community. This assay generates spectra, comparable to protein fingerprint signatures of microorganisms which can then be identified within minutes by comparing their spectra with those in a reference spectra database. For the past few years, MALDI-TOF MS has enhanced routine bacterial identification in the clinical microbiology laboratory. More recently, MALDI-TOF MS has been applied to the routine identification of yeasts and molds. However, several drawbacks of the technique exist. The major limitation of this method is the architecture of the references spectra database. Identification results are improved only when the spectra included in the reference database and those obtained from the sample to be identified are processed with the same culture and extraction protocol. The machine is extremely expensive, and needs access to a comprehensive database that add to the cost. The MALDI-TOF is a fairly new technique and its reliability for filamentous fungi is still under question. The major shortcoming of this method is also that unlike PCR, it cannot be performed directly on specimen rather only after cultures are grown. In fact, several factors such as the right age of culture, growth media, and proper specimen processing severely handicap MALDI-TOF accuracy. Besides, the causative organisms can in most cases be identified only to the genus level, and not species.

"Why is there a Recurrence of Fungal Infections, Despite Treatment?"

The investigations performed in our lab determined that most dermatophytes were sensitive to at least two (itraconazole and griseofulvin) out of the three drugs tested, while showing moderate levels of sensitivity to terbinafine. In the light of this study, the question still remains, "Why is there a recurrence of fungal infections, despite treatment?"

From a mycologists point of view, there may be several factors compounding failed treatments:

1. Topical formulations may get rid of a large population of infecting cells, but not a 100%. A small pocket of "persistor cells" that escape killing, survive and regrow, re-establishing a new infection. In fact, these cells may evolve with tougher, more drug resistant properties.
2. Some sites of infection may be inaccessible to drugs, such as nooks, crevices or deeper layers of nails/skin.
3. It is possible that some of the drugs used are fungistatic rather than fungicidic.
4. Presence of thick multilayer biofilms of fungi on soft tissues (yeast balanitis), that are inherently drug resistant.

From a clinician's point of view, there may be some more practical reasons for recalcitrance of infections:

a. Lack of persistence by the patient to prolonged treatment periods.
b. Some drug formulations not patient-friendly, hence poor compliance.
c. Low residence time of the drug onto the site of infection.
d. Violation of compliance to proper personal hygiene.

CONCLUSIONS

Molecular methods applied to the detection and identification of dermatophytes have recently become increasingly available driven by the fact that they ensure fast and accurate identification. However, these methods have not been introduced in many clinical laboratories. Sequencing methods targeting the ITS region are the most popular techniques used for definitive identification of a fungal strain. However, only reference laboratories and laboratories with a large PCR platform can use this tool. In the near future, many smaller laboratories will use PCR assays for the detection of dermatophytes directly on nail, skin and hair samples because more and more commercial kits are being validated. The use of such methods will reduce the turn-around time from that seen with culture-based identification methods, particularly when full automation is achieved, and their use will also increase because they are much more sensitive than culture-based methods and because skilled technicians in mycology are scarce. However, these molecular methods applied directly on the sample cannot replace microscopic and histopathological examination particularly to assess the involvement of contaminants/pathogens such as Fusarium, or other non-dermatophyte molds, and also because a microscopic examination provides a faster result than any PCR assay.

Bibliography

1. Arabatzis M1, Bruijnesteijn van Coppenraet LE, Kuijper EJ, de Hoog GS, Lavrijsen AP, Templeton K, van der Raaij-Helmer EM, Velegraki A, Gräser Y, Summerbell RC. Diagnosis of common dermatophyte infections by a novel multiplex real-time polymerase chain reaction detection/identification scheme. Br J Dermatol 2007 Oct;157(4):681–689.

2. Badali H, Mohammadi R, Mashedi O, de Hoog GS, Meis JF. In vitro susceptibility patterns of clinically important Trichophyton and Epidermophyton species against nine antifungal drugs. Mycoses 2015 May;58(5):303–307.

3. Baghi N, Shokohi T, Badali H, Makimura K, Rezaei-Matehkolaei A, Abdollahi M, Didehdar M, Haghani I, Abastabar M. In vitro activity of new azoles luliconazole and lanoconazole compared with ten other antifungal drugs against clinical dermatophyte isolates. Med Mycol 2016 Apr 26.

4. Bhatia VK, Sharma PC. Determination of minimum inhibitory concentrations of itraconazole, terbinafine and ketoconazole against dermatophyte species by broth microdilution method. Indian J Med Microbiol 2015 Oct-Dec;33(4):533–537.

5. Bindu V, Pavithran K. Clinico-Mycological study of dermatophytosis in Calicut. Indian J Dermatol Venereol Leprol 2002;68:259–261.

6. C. J. Jessup, J. Warner, N. Isham, I. Hasan, and M. A. Ghannoum. Antifungal Susceptibility Testing of Dermatophytes: Establishing a Medium for Inducing Conidial Growth and Evaluation of Susceptibility of Clinical Isolates. J ClinMicrobiol 2000 Jan; 38(1): 341–344.

7. Dhib I, Fathallah A, Yaacoub A, HadjSlama F, Said MB, Zemni. R. Multiplex PCR assay for the detection of common dermatophyte nail infections. Mycoses 2014;57:19–26

8. Dhiman N, Hall L, Wohlfiel SL, Buckwalter SP, Wengenack NL. Performance and cost analysis of matrix-assisted laser desorption ionization-time of flight mass spectrometry for routine identification of yeast. J ClinMicrobiol 2011;49:1614–1616.

9. Elewski BE, Charif MA. Prevalence of onychomycosis in patients attending a dermatology clinic in north-eastern Ohio for other conditions. Arch Dermatol1997;133:1172–1173.

10. Espinel-Ingroff A, Fothergill A, Ghannoum M, Manavathu E, Ostrosky-Zeichner L, Pfaller MA, Rinaldi MG, Schell W, Walsh TJ. Quality control and reference guidelines for CLSI broth microdilution method (M38-A document) for susceptibility testing of anidulafungin against molds. J Clin Microbiol 2007 Jul;45(7):2180–2182.

11. Faergemann J, Baran R. Epidemiology, clinical presentation and diagnosis of onychomycosis. Br J Dermatol 2003;149(suppl 65):1–4.

12. Garg J, Tilak R, Singh S, Gulati AK, Garg A, Prakash P, Nath G. Evaluation of pan-dermatophyte nested PCR in diagnosis of onychomycosis. J Clin Microbiol 2007 Oct;45(10):3443–3445.

13. Havlickova B, Czaika VA, Friedrich M. Epidemiological trends in skin mycoses worldwide. Mycoses 2008;51:2–15.

14. Huda MM, Chakraborty N, Sharma Bordoloi JN. A clinicomycological study of superficial mycoses in upper Assam. Indian J Dermatol Venereol Leprol 1995;61:329–332.

15. Kanbe T. Molecular approaches in the diagnosis of dermatophytosis. Mycopathologia 2008 Nov-Dec;166(5–6):307–317.

16. Kuokkanen K, Alava S. Fluconazole in the treatment of onychomycosis caused by dermatophytes. J Dermatol Treat 1993;3:115–117.

17. Kurade SM, Amladi SA, Miskeen AK. Skinscraping and a potassium hydroxide mount. Indian J Dermatol Venereol Leprol. 2006 May-Jun;72(3):238–241.

18. Marie-Pierre Hayette, Rosalie Sacheli. Dermatophytosis, Trends in Epidemiology and Diagnostic Approach. Current Fungal Infection Reports September 2015; (9)3:164–179.

19. Norris HA, Elewski BE, Ghannoum MA. Optimal growth conditions for the determination of the antifungal susceptibility of three species of dermatophytes with the use of a microdilution method. J Am Acad Dermatol 1999;40(6, part 2):S9–13.11.

20. Oberai C, Miskeen AK. Superficial fungal infections, In: IADVL Textbook and Atlas of Dermatology, Edited by Valia RG, Valia AR, Siddappa K, Bhalani Publishing House Bombay 1994;173–212.

21. Scher RK. Onychomycosis is more than a cosmetic problem. Br J Dermatol1994;130: 15.

22. Schmidt V, Jarosch A, März P, et al. Rapid identification of bacteria in positive blood culture by matrix-assisted laser desorption ionization time-of-flight mass spectrometry. Eur J Clin Microbiol Infect Dis 2012;31:311–317.

23. Seng P, Drancourt M, Gouriet F, et al. Ongoing revolution in bacteriology: routine identification of bacteria by matrix-assisted laser desorption ionization time-of-flight mass spectrometry. Clin Infect Dis 2009;49:543–551.

24. Tendolkar U, Shinde A, Baveja S, Dhurat R, Phiske M. Trichosporon inkin and Trichosporon mucoides as unusual causes of whitepiedra of scalphair. Indian J Dermatol Venereol Leprol 2014 Jul-Aug;80(4):324–327.

25. Viswanath V, Kriplani D, Miskeen AK, Patel B, Torsekar RG. White piedra of scalphair by Trichosporon inkin. Indian J Dermatol Venereol Leprol 2011 Sep-Oct;77(5):591–593.

26. Weitzman I, Summerbell RC. The dermatophytes. ClinMicrobiol Rev. 1995;8:240–259.

27. Westerberg DP, Voyack MJ. Onychomycosis: Current trends in diagnosis and treatment. Am Fam Physician 2013 Dec 1;88(11):762–770.

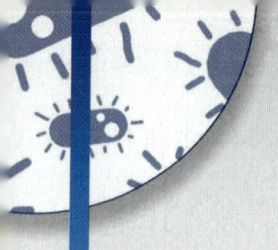

CHAPTER 4

Microbiological Aspects of Dermatophytes: Clinical Relevance

Shukla Das, SN Bhattacharya

INTRODUCTION

Infections caused by pathogenic fungi are widely recognized as emerging threats to human and animal health. Some of the fungal species may cause infections, others may remain as harmless colonizers.

Dermatophytosis is the most common superficial skin infection in the world, affecting millions of people annually worldwide, commonly referred to as ringworm or "tinea" infections and named with reference to the area of the infected body part, e.g. tinea capitis, tinea pedis, tinea unguium, etc. Dermatophytes are a group of highly specialized keratinolytic fungi that invade the keratinized tissue, have the unique ability to infect immunocompetent people and are associated with considerable morbidity and socioeconomic trauma. Despite significant understanding of the causative pathogen, the mechanistic details of interaction between host skin and the causative dermatophyte agents and the resultant pathogenesis, is poorly understood. Consequently effective therapeutics, specific to dermatophytes are limited. Recent emerging reports of drug resistance are further compounding the problems of effective treatment and clearance of the fungal pathogen.

Dermatophytic Agents

The common dermatophytes causing human infections belong to the genera Trichophyton, Microsporum and Epidermophyton. They infect the skin, hair and nails of humans and animals. Onychomycosis is one of the major clinical manifestations of dermatophytosis, showing reported prevalence as high as (27.06%) in Himachal Pradesh, (32.6 and 23.07%) in Central India, (29.54%) in Aurangabad and (66%) in West Bengal. Hot and humid climate of the country may be the plausible explanation for the high frequency of this clinical expression of dermatophytosis in our country and its ability to adapt to the hard keratin of nail. Common species like *Trichophyton rubrum*, *Trichophyton mentagrophytes* and *Trichophyton tonsurans* have been reported as causes of these nail infections. The epidemiology of tinea capitis varies in different geographical areas throughout the world and in any given location; the predominant etiological species may change with time. In the course of evolution, dermatophytes have developed host specificity, due to difference in the composition of host keratins and have been categorized in three ecological groups as geophiles (soil), anthropophiles (man) and zoophiles (animals). *T. violaceum*, *T. rubrum* and *T. mentagrophyte* are the common species identified as agents of tinea capitis, in the Indian subcontinent.

Taxonomy and Nomenclature

Strain typing by phenotypic methods is practically difficult, since the dermatophytes on subculture show morphological variations among the isolates. Although on molecular based analyses, the identification of dermatophytes has become possible, but due to fluctuation in the taxonomy, these techniques overcome limitations experienced by the routine conventional methods and aid in the rapid identification of specific dermatophytes. Species identification may not alter clinical treatment but dermatophyte identification is necessary for epidemiological concerns.

Knowledge about the local epidemiology plays a vital role in infection control and community health management. For instance, *T. rubrum*, considered to be the most ancient asexual filamentous fungus, has been classified and grouped under *Trichophyton rubrum* complex, based on molecular taxonomy which also includes two strains of *T. rubrum* and *T. violaceum*. The most preferred current method for taxonomic classification is MLST (multi locus sequence typing) which enabled the identification of the African-Asiatic variant of *T. rubrum*, referred to *T. raubitshekii*, characterized by positive urease activity unlike the other *T. rubrum* variants. On the other hand, the sequencing results, categorized *T. mentagrophyte* type I and type II to anthropophillic *T. interdigitale* strains, while type III is identical with zoophilic *T. interdigitale*, and type IV is *A. benhamiae* strain. These results indicate the need to re-evaluate the boundaries of Trichophyton species, using better molecular tools.

Based on what is known today, from molecular biological analysis, *T. mentagrophytes spp.* is now only used to refer to the *anthropophilic* varieties of *T. mentagrophytes*, and several *zoophilic* strains, previously classified as var. mentagrophytes or var. granulosum, are not genetically distinguishable from *T. interdigitale* and are thus now collectively known as *T. interdigitale* species. This new classification may initially appear confusing in clinical practice, given infection sites—tinea capitis or tinea corporis—yet the practitioner should be aware of it. Knowledge of different species play an important role in cases of reinfection related to dermatophytosis, whether it has occurred with the same dermatophyte species, a variant or a different species producing similar type of lesions. Other molecular methods have been developed to discriminate the various species and strains such as restriction fragment length polymorphism (RFLP), arbitrary primed polymerase chain reaction (AP-PCR), random amplified polymorphic DNA (RAPD) analysis and sequence analysis of the internal transcribed spacer (ITS) region.

EPIDEMIOLOGICAL BOTTLENECKS

Dermatophytes are among the few fungi causing communicable disease, acquired from infected animals, birds or, from fomites. The analysis of *T. rubrum* genomics reveals recent gene gain and loss events within the dermatophytes, and suggest candidates for role in infection and host specialization, which could help guide the development of new therapies. These species-specific adaptations could be important in host immune system interaction or survival in the environment. For instance, the dermatophyte structure most commonly associated with contagion, is the oblong to rounded, persistent "spore," "arthroconidium," or "chlamydospore", found within or attached to the exterior of infected hairs and within skin scales. These structures, particularly in certain species, may persist for years in the environment and are highly heat resistant, particularly when embedded in hair or skin scales. In some anthropophilic species arthroconidia have a tendency to adhere *in vitro*, to corneocytes derived from particular body sites. It is possible that they may dissociate from skin cells in the environment and come in contact with new potential hosts as disseminated arthroconidia. Their persistence in the environment may lead to recurrent outbreaks of dermatophytosis in individuals and in institutions. Within the anthropophiles, polymorphous morphological variation is common and numerous atypical and variant types are recognized, probably indicating further genetic drift.

Several anthropophilic species have well-defined areas of endemicity while others, such as *T. rubrum* and *T. tonsurans*, are newly cosmopolitan, but appear to have had a more restricted distribution in the past, having been transported widely as a result of human migration (the anthropophiles travel with their human hosts).

Clinical Identification and Epidemiology of Dermatophytes

Recognition of dermatophyte taxa is clinically relevant. The need for species identification of dermatophytes in clinical settings is often related to epidemiological concerns. Especially relevant is the identification of dermatophytes that (i) may have animal carriers; (ii) are linked to recurrent institutional or family outbreaks, such as *T. tonsurans* and *Trichophyton violaceum*; (iii) may cause rapidly progressing epidemics, such as *M. audouinii* and *T. tonsurans*; and (iv) are geographically endemic, reflecting exposure during travel or residence in the area of endemicity, or contact with a person with such a history.

Epidemiology is important in infection control and public health issues related to the different types of dermatophytosis. Clinical classification of dermatophytosis is according to site: Tinea capitis, tinea pedis, tinea manuum, tinea unguium (or onychomycosis), tinea barbae, tinea cruris and tinea corporis. Tinea capitis, in general is a condition most commonly seen in children; the predominant agents are *T. tonsurans* and *Microsporum canis*. The former is usually acquired from infected humans or their fomites and has a progressive course of disease, often leading to long-term carriers with subclinical scalp infection and, may intermittently shed viable inoculum for decades. In symptomatic adults, *T. tonsurans* is more frequently seen as an agent of tinea corporis or, as tinea manuum and onychomycosis. Similar patterns of age and body site preferences are found in other more geographically concentrated agents of endothrix and tinea capitis as *T. violaceum*. It is the predominant agent of tinea capitis in India and in some parts of Europe, and South America. *M. canis* is usually acquired from infected cats or dogs, although limited human-to-human transfer leading to outbreaks can occur. Zoophilic and geophilic dermatophytes, in general, tend to form lesions that are more inflammatory than those formed by anthropophilic dermatophytes but, are also more likely to resolve spontaneously as seen with *M. canis*, *E. floccosum*, as compared to *T. mentagrophytes* var. interdigitale show a common pattern of association with tinea corporis, tinea cruris, and tinea pedis. In addition, *T. rubrum* and *T. mentagrophytes* are associated with tinea manuum and onychomycosis. Although the ecological and host factors involved in developing symptomatic infection are poorly understood but common risk factors include foot dampness and abrasion, combined with likely exposure to high fungal inoculums in swimming pools and showers.

HOST IMMUNE RESPONSE

Dermatophyte colonization is characteristically limited to the dead keratinized tissue of the stratum corneum and results in either a mild or intense inflammatory reaction. Although the cornified layers of the skin lack a specific immune system to recognize this infection and rid itself of it, nevertheless, both humoral and cell-mediated reactions and specific and non-specific host defense mechanisms respond actively and eventually eliminate the fungus, preventing invasion into the deeper viable tissue. There are two major classes of dermatophyte antigens: Glycopeptides and keratinases. The glycopeptides preferentially stimulates cell-mediated immunity (CMI), whereas the polysaccharide portion stimulates humoral immunity. Keratinases, produced by the dermatophytes, enable skin invasion, and elicit delayed-type hypersensitivity (DTH) responses. Although the host develops a variety of antibodies to dermatophyte infection (i.e. IgM, IgG, IgA, and IgE), they apparently do not help eliminate the infection since the highest level of antibodies is found in those patients with chronic infection and raised IgE, which mediates immediate hypersensitivity, and appears to play no effective role in the defense process.

Rather, the development of CMI, which is correlated with DTH, is usually associated with clinical cure and clearing of the stratum corneum of the offending dermatophyte. In contrast, the lack of CMI or defective CMI prevents an effective response and predisposes the host to chronic or recurrent dermatophyte infections. Experimentally infected volunteers, deliberately infected with *T. mentagrophytes*, who developed CMI associated with intense inflammation which was accompanied by T-cell-mediated DTH to the trichophytin skin test (glycoprotein skin test antigen), all achieved a mycologic cure. A protective immunologic memory was indicated by the rapid inflammatory response and elimination of the fungus on reinoculation and a continued positive trichophytin test. These individuals, however, had a normal response to other skin test antigens, indicating a selective or induced immune deficit, that was found in 10 to 20% of the population in temperate climates. An association between chronic dermatophytosis and (asthma or allergic rhinitis) atopics is well recognized.

Approximately 80 to 93% of chronic or recurrent dermatophyte infections are estimated to be caused by *T. rubrum*; these patients often fail to express a DTH reaction to trichophytin, when injected intradermally. Infections by *T. rubrum*, often elicit less of an inflammatory response and are less likely to elicit an intense DTH response than infections caused by geophilic or zoophilic dermatophytes, which characteristically evoke an intense inflammatory reaction. Dermatophyte infections are readily treatable but immunocompromised patients can experience severe disseminated disease. Enhanced proliferation/turnover of the skin, in response to the inflammation, is a probable mechanism that removes the fungus from the skin, by an eventual increase in epidermal desquamation. *T. rubrum* also produces mannan, a glycoprotein component of the fungal cell wall, that diminishes the immune response, especially in atopic or other persons, susceptible to the mannan-induced suppression of CMI.

In India, in the past few years, tinea corporis and cruris have been associated with predominance of *T. mentagrophyte*, a changing trend in geographical distribution of these agents, suggesting their selective property of anthrophilic adaptation and underlying host/environmental factors allowing their persistence in the environment.

LABORATORY DIAGNOSIS

Sampling of Clinical Material

Under Wood's lamp (an ultraviolet light which emits UV-light at 360 nm), hair may first be examined in a darkened room before sampling. Hair infected by some species of Microsporum, particularly *M. canis*, even when no clinical symptoms are apparent, emit a greenish yellow fluorescence. Medication, artificial fibres and natural secretions can also obscure true fluorescence. Direct microscopy of a KOH mount is essential to make a primary diagnosis. With a false negative in 5 to 15% of cases in ordinary practice, it is still a highly efficient screening technique. Scrapings and hairs may be mounted for direct examination in 10% KOH or NaOH, mixed with 5% glycerol, heated (e.g. for 1 h at 51°C) to emulsify lipids, and examined under 400X for fungal structures.

Alternatively 20% KOH–36% dimethyl sulfoxide, and calcofluor white technique or Congo red staining method, may be used. Culture is a valuable adjunct to direct microscopy and is essential at least in all nail infections and in any infection to be treated by systemic medication. In all cases, a medium selective against most non-dermatophytic moulds and bacteria, is used as a primary isolation medium. Dermatophytes from infected materials can be isolated using SDA, containing penicillin/gentamicin or chloramphenicol and actidione, incubated at 25–30°C. The incubation period generally varies from 1 to 4 weeks on SDA medium.

Sequence for the Identification of Dermatophytes in Pure Culture

Procedure

1. Examine the colony for color of the surface and reverse, topography, texture, and rate of growth.
2. Prepare teased mounts and search for identifying microscopic morphology, for presence, appearance, and arrangement of macroconidia and microconidia. If results are inconclusive, proceed to step 3.
3. Prepare and examine slide culture for characteristic morphology. Consider special medium if sporulation is absent (potato glucose agar, Sabouraud glucose agar plus 3–5% NaCl, or lactrimel agar).
4. Perform as many of the physiological tests listed below as necessary for identification:
   a. Urease test.
   b. Nutritional requirement if a *Trichophyton* spp. is suspected
   c. Growth on rice grains if a *Microsporum* spp. is suspected
   d. *In vitro* hair perforation
   e. Temperature tolerance and/or optimum temperature for growth.

Although there are no serological kits commercially available, to specifically detect and identify antibodies to dermatophytes, studies of dermatophyte antigens by monoclonal antibodies highlight the potential use of such reagents in the immunoidentification of dermatophytes.

Molecular Biology

The traditional taxonomy of the dermatophytes is based, essentially on gross and microscopic morphology, with minor emphasis on physiology and nutrition. However, identification of species from amongst isolates has been complicated by the overlapping characteristics, variability, and pleomorphism. A variety of taxonomic methods have been developed to bypass the traditional methods of identification, and to determine relationships between the various species. These include disc electrophoresis of culture filtrate proteins, pyrolysis-gas-liquid chromatography to study fatty acids, polyacrylamide gradient gel electrophoresis of total cell protein extracts for zymogram patterns, and isoelectric focusing of somatic extracts thin-layer polyacrylamide gels.

Dermatophyte Virulence Factors

Understanding the phenomena of pleomorphism in dermatophytes was made possible by the discovery of sexual reproduction, and the subsequent application of classical genetic analysis to the progeny of sexual crosses. Pleomorphism amongst the dermatophytes can be observed and studied through the spontaneous appearance of white fluffy tufts of aerial mycelium, on the surface of colonies, which results in the loss of characteristic pigmentation and conidiation.Weitzman analyzed that this phenomenon resulted from single chromosomal gene mutation seen in mutants showing diminished conidiation and/ or a conidial mutant capable of reproducing sexually. The clinical relevance of such morphological transition(s) however is not yet clear.

The locus for virulence is independent of colonial morphology, but it is related to growth rate. All cultures with a normal growth rate are virulent, whereas those with a lower growth rate are considered avirulent. Secreted proteases have been suggested to be important virulence factors of dermatophytes (Jousson et al, 2004; Monod 2008) and are found to be enriched in dermatophyte genomes. The secreted proteome or the 'secretome' of *T. rubrum* strain number IGIBSBL-CI1 (Petersen et al, 2011), predicted 575 secreted proteins. For instance, one of the major predicted virulence enzymes being subtilases (belonging to SB clan of MEROPS, comprising of 16 members), as the most abundant amongst the secreted protease family.

DRUG RESISTANCE IN DERMATOPHYTES

Dermatophytes belong to a small category of disease causing organisms and are phylogenetically related to each other. They have a generous susceptibility to drugs, except for certain species like *T. verruccosum* or *T. mentagrophyte* (var. *granulosum*), which have a reduced susceptibility to the common antifungals. Discounting the minor differences in susceptibility, identification of individual species remains important because dermatophytosis in the community and its outcomes, is largely determined by epidemiological circumstances that determine the chances of reinfection and persistence in the environment. Therapeutic outcome also can vary with respect to the dermatophyte species. *T. tonsurans* invades the hair shaft which retains drugs incorporated into the shaft through the root when administered during hair growth, so efficacy is better than *M. canis* where the arthoconidia on the scalp surface have more limited contact with the antifungals which can more readily be eluted. It is important to distinguish non-dermatophyte mould (NDM) from dermatophytes as agents of onychomycosis, as NDM often do not respond to conventional anti-dermatophyte drugs. The genesis of resistance to the antifungal drug is a phenomenon similar to other pathogens in the microbial world, but presently, the magnitude of the problem does not seem to be as critical as in bacteria.

Drug resistance is defined as failure in elimination of the agent from the host, despite administering recommended appropriate dosages for the appropriate period. Inadequate dosing often results in encouraging the growth of resistant strains. Intrinsic resistance is defined as inherent property of the fungus and primary resistance is the presence or acquisition of resistance by the organism without any prior exposure to the drug.

Acquired or secondary resistance is due to selective pressure, exerted by specific drug, leading to mutation or adaptation, allowing the survival of the organism. These mutants may persist even in absence of the drug, and get adapted to humans. Evolution of drug resistance is not a sudden phenomena, the resistant phenotype is not always sharply defined as it may co-exist along with the drug sensitive ones. Overall drug resistance can be due to any one or more of the following mechanisms:

i. Alteration in drug target;
ii. Altered sterol synthesis;
iii. Efflux pump upregulation;
iv. Overexpression of target.

It is important to understand that dermatophytes causing infection have adapted to the host environment, hence host factors play an important role in the clearing of the fungus. Moreover, there are only a limited number of antifungal agents available and the phylogenetic proximity of fungi to eukaryotes ensures that the potential drug targets available that are specific only to fungus and not to the host, are few. The strategy adopted by dermatophytes to express excessive amounts of proteases while under stress, gives it an advantage that sometimes enables survival even in presence of drugs. In a recent study it was observed that *T. rubrum* genome has 8265 protein coding genes and of these, 575 secretory proteins are major virulence factors (expresses serine proteases in abundance). Therefore, existing specific antifungal drugs, inhibition of these secretory enzymes and blockade of fungal metabolic pathways with specific fungal calcium channel blockers, are avenues that can be explored as alternative or adjunct therapeutic measures.

Common antifungal agents approved currently for the treatment of dermatophytosis belong to two major types, namely (i) ergosterol (fungal) synthesis blockers/inhibitors (such as (a) allylamines, (b) azoles and imidazoles, (c) morpholines) and (ii) other mechanism of fungal inhibition (such as (a) griseofulvin, (b) polyenes, (c) cyclopirox olamine, (d) tolnaftate, etc.). Though oral antifungal (such as itraconazole, fluconazole, and terbinafine) have been the current choice of treatment for extensive and widespread dermatophytoses, prevalence of clinical therapeutic failure and/or recurrence on cessation of therapy has risen in the past few years.

To evaluate drug resistance in dermatophytes, it is recommended to perform broth dilution susceptibility testing method, to measure MIC (i.e. the minimum inhibitory concentration of the drug which inhibits the growth of the fungus *in vitro*). *In vitro* susceptibility testing for dermatophytes as per CSLI M38 A2 guidelines are tedious and require technical expertise. The endpoint determination as reduction in growth by 80% (inhibition) by itraconazole, griseofulvin, voriconazole, amorolfine, ciclopirox and, for terbinafine, a 100% growth inhibition, as compared to growth control, is indicative of susceptible strains. Drugs that can be subjected to MIC testing are fluconazole, voriconazole, clotrimazole, sertaconazole, ketoconazole, terbinafine, amorolfine, ciclopirox and griseofulvin. Briefly, the microdilution trays are inoculated with different dilutions of the drugs, RPMI1640 medium and MOPS, incubated at 35°C to determine the MIC. Each microdilution is given a numerical score as: 4+ (no reduction in growth); 3 + (75% growth reduction); 2+ (50% growth reduction); 1+ (25% or absence of growth or slight growth).

The current status of antifungal resistance (identified as raised MICs) among dermatophytes (unpublished) is noted as 20% for fluconazole, 5% for itraconazole and terbinafine each and 17% for griseofulvin. The *in vitro* susceptibility pattern and *in vivo* response to the drug, often may not match as microconidia from culture have different cell wall composition as compared to arthoconidia existing in the patients. Also various other factors, like the pharmacokinetics and pharmacodynamics, can influence the clinical outcomes and may not always correlate with the *in vitro* drug sensitivity results.

A half of the patients, reporting with clinical resistance, have a strong family history of the condition exisiting in the close contacts. The IgE pattern amongst these patients are also suggestive of atopy. About 10% of the dermatophytosis patients are diabetic, resulting in delayed cures. It is established that resistant strains exist either in the environment or in humans serving as reservoirs (as asymptomatic carriers). Sometimes, formation of dermatophytomas are associated with biofilm formation in recalcitrant nail infections. Molecular detection of drug resistance is important for enabling the monitoring of the susceptibility pattern of the circulating strains of the dermatophytes in the community, however, its important to remember that acquisition of drug resistance in dermatophytes is a complex phenomenon.

The most common site of anti-dermatophyte drug action is the ergosterol synthesis pathway, by most antifungals except ciclopirox, flucytocine, caspofungin, griseofulvin. It is documented that under the influence of certain azoles (ketoconazole, itraconazole) a selective upregulation of Erg (ergosterol) gene occurs which may lead to dampened response of dermatophytosis caused by an otherwise *in vitro* susceptible strain. The fungistatic drugs are more prone to induce resistance mutation(s) as compared to the fungicidal drugs.

It needs to be noted that though dermatophyte drug resistance is now percieved to have become a menace and has shown a rising trend, the situation is not as alarming as seen in the spread of bacterial resistance. The absence of mechanisms in dermatophytes to transfer drug resistance (such as those seen in bacteria) like transposons, mobile elements, plasmids, etc. restricts the widespread dissemination of resistant strains of dermatophytes.

It is important for the clinicians to remember that drug *compliance* and adequate *dosage* as per the weight of patient, are two crucial factors which lead to adequate threshold levels of the drug required for the inhibition of the fungal agent. Under sub-MIC levels, activation of efflux pump and multiplication of arthoconidia will result in uninhibited proliferation of the fungus. Synergistic action of azole and allylamines as combinations can be explored as alternative therapy, in patients with relapses.

CONCLUSIONS

The current rise in cases of dermatophytosis and relapses observed, in a high percentage of the affected population, is indicative of emergence of drug resistance in dermatophytes apart from an increasing population of susceptible hosts. Molecular identification and antifungal susceptibility testing may become necessary in cases with clinical failure or poor responders to systemic therapy. With close monitoring of such cases and with regular follow-up of patients, a surveillance network of clinicians and microbiologists would enable us to have a better understanding of the host pathogen interactions. The ultimate challenge would be to boost cell-mediated immunity as a strategy by developing fungal vaccine(s) to produce sterilizing immunity and protection against fungal reactivation.

Bibliography

1. Anzawa K, Kawasaki, Mochizuki T, Ishizaki H. Successful mating of *Trichophyton rubrum* with *Arthroderma simii*. J Med Mycol, 2008, 49:311–318.
2. Burkhart CN, Burkhart CG, Gupta AK. Dermatophytoma: recalcitrance to treatment because of existence of fungal biofilm. J Am Acad Dermatol 2002;47:629–631.

3. Burmester A, Shelest E, Glöckner G, *et al.* Comparative and functional genomics provide insights into the pathogenicity of dermatophytic fungi. Genome Biol 2011-12-1-r7.

4. Degreef H. Clinical forms of dermatophytosis (ringworm infection). Mycopathologia 2008; 166(5–6):257–265.

5. Graser V, Scott J, Summerbell R. The new species concept in dermatophytes a polyphasic approach. Mycopathologia, DOI 10.1007/s11046–008–9099.

6. Khosravi AR, Hojjatollah S, Mansouri P. Immediate hypersensitivity and serum IgE antibody responses in patients with dermatophytosis. Asia Pac J Allergy Immunol 2012; 30 (1):40–47.

7. Latka C, Dey SS, Mahajan S, Prabu R, Jangir PK, Gupta C, Das S, Ramachandran VG, Bhattacharya SN, Pandey R, Sharma R. Genome sequence of a clinical isolate of dermatophyte, *Trichophyton rubrum* from India. FEMS microbiology letters 2015 Apr 1;362(8):fnv039.

8. M38-A2 I Reference Method for Broth Dilution Antifungal Susceptibility Testing of Filamentous Fungi, 2nd Edition.

9. Martinez-Rossi NM, Peres NT, Rossi A. Antifungal resistance mechanisms in dermatophytes. Mycopathologia 2008 Nov 1;166(5–6):369–383.

10. Mukherjee PK, Leidich SD, Isham N, Leitner I, Ryder NS, Ghannoum MA. Clinical *Trichophyton rubrum* Strain 12 Exhibiting Primary Resistance to Terbinafine. Antimicrob Agents & Chemother 2003; (47):182–186.

11. Rawlings ND, Barrett AJ, Bateman A. MEROPS the database of proteolytic enzymes, their substrates and inhibitors Nucleic Acids Res 2012 Jan; 40 (Database issue): D343–350.

12. Sarma S, Capoor MR, Deb M, Ramesh V Aggarwal. Epidemiologic and clinicomycologic profile of onychomycosis from north India. Int J Dermatol 2008; 47(6):584–587.

13. Sawada Y, Nakamura M, Kabashima-Kubo R, Shimauchi T, Kobayashi M, Tokura Y. Defective epidermal innate immunity and resultant superficial dermatophytosis in adult T-cell leukemia/lymphoma. Clin Cancer Res 2012; 18(14):3772–3779.

14. Summerbell RC, Haugland R, Li A, Gupta AK. Ribosomal RNA gene internal transcribed spacer 1 and 2 sequences of asexual, anthropophilic dermatophytes related to *Trichophyton rubrum*. J Clin Microbiol 1999; 37:4005–4011.

15. Vandeputte P, Ferrari S, Coste AT. Antifungal resistance and new strategies to control fungal infections. International Journal of Microbiology 2011 Dec 1;2012.

16. Weitzman I, Summerbell RC. The dermatophytes. Clin Microbiol Rev 1995; 8:240–259.

17. Woodfolk JA. Allergy and dermatophytes. Clin Microbiol Rev 2005;18(1): 30–43.

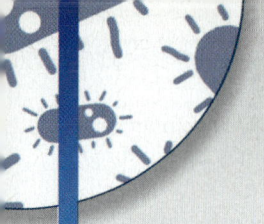

CHAPTER 5

Superficial Fungal Infections

Khushbu Mahajan, Sukriti Sharma,
Kabir Sardana, Aastha Gupta

A. DERMATOPHYTOSES

Dermatophytosis denotes an infection caused by dermatophytes. Dermatophytes are a unique group of fungi capable of infecting nonviable keratinized cutaneous structures including stratum corneum, nails, and hair. (Arthrospores can survive in human scales for **12 months**.)

In this category, dermatophytosis of skin constitutes the most common type, while there can be dermatophytosis of hair and hair follicles or onychomycosis or tinea unguium.

The term tinea is best used for dermatophytoses and is modified according to the anatomic site (Fig. 5.1) of infection, e.g. tinea pedis (of feet). "Tinea" versicolor is referred to as pityriasis versicolor except in the United States; it is not a dermatophytosis but rather an infection caused by the yeast Malassezia. Tinea nigra is caused by a pigmented or dematiaceous fungus, not a dermatophyte.

Classification of Dermatophyte Species
- **Anthropophilic:** Person-to-person transmission by fomites and by direct contact.
- **Zoophilic:** Animal-to-human by direct contact or by fomites.
- **Geophilic:** Environmental.

Classification of Dermatophytosis
In vivo, dermatophytes grow only on or within keratinized structures and, as such, can be classified in the following types:
- Epidermal dermatophytosis. Tinea faciei, tinea corporis, tinea cruris, tinea mannum, tinea pedis.
- Dermatophytoses of nail apparatus. Tinea unguium (caused by dermatophytes in toenails, and/or fingernails) and onychomycosis

TINEA

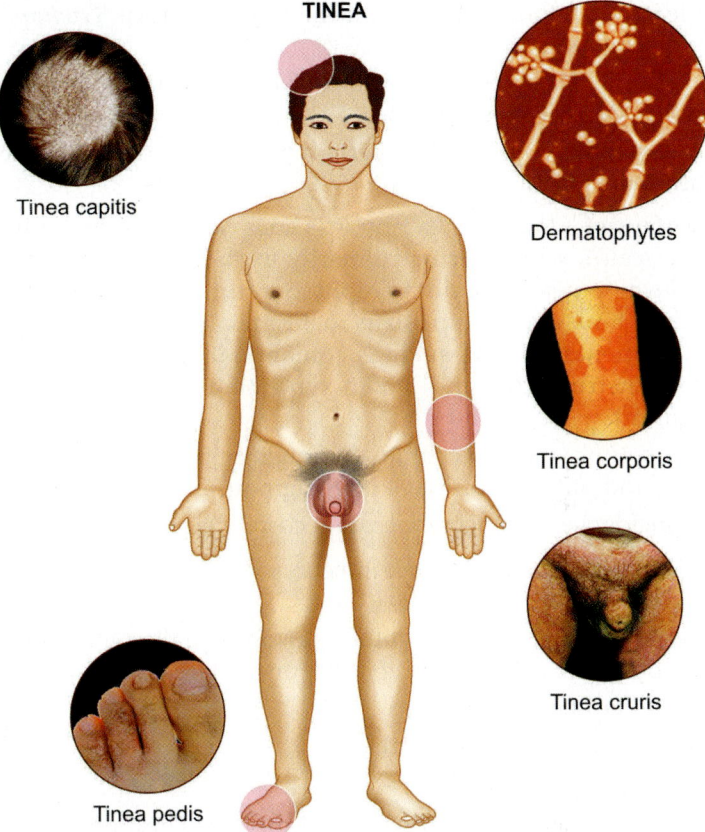

Tinea capitis

Dermatophytes

Tinea corporis

Tinea cruris

Tinea pedis

Fig. 5.1: An artistic depiction of various sites of tinea infections

(more inclusive term, including nail infections caused by dermatophytes, yeasts, and molds).

- Dermatophytoses of hair and hair follicle: Dermatophytic folliculitis, Majocchi granuloma, tinea capitis, tinea barbae.

Epidemiology and Etiology

Human travel and migration, coupled with advances in antifungal therapy, have brought about changes in the geographic distribution of dermatophytes. Other important epidemiologic factors include socioeconomic status, occupation, air conditioning and the use of footwear.

1. **Etiology:** There are there three genera of dermatophytes, *Trichophyton, Microsporum, Epidermophyton.*

   Trichophyton rubrum is the most common cause of epidermal dermatophytosis and onychomycosis in industrialized nations, while in India, the most common emerging species is ***Trichophyton mentagrophytes***.

Trichophyton tonsurans: It is the most common cause of tinea capitis in North America and Europe.

T. concentricum is endemic to certain parts of the South Pacific and South America.

2. **Age of onset** One major exception is tinea capitis (dermatophytosis of the scalp), which occurs primarily in children. Risk factors for the development of a dermatophyte infection during childhood include household exposure to tinea capitis or tinea pedis; environmental factors such as contaminated hats, brushes and barber instruments, and Down syndrome (especially for tinea unguium).

   Dermatophytoses occur most frequently in postpubertal hosts. Young and older adults have intertriginous infections.

   (The incidence of onychomycosis is correlated directly with age).

3. **Transmission:** Dermatophyte infections can be acquired from three sources:
   a. Most commonly from **another person** [usually by fomites, less so by direct skin-to-skin contact (tinea gladiatorum)]
   b. From **animals**.
   c. Least commonly from **soil**.

4. **Predisposing factors**
   a. *Atopic diathesis:* Predisposes to cell-mediated immune deficiency for *T. rubrum*.
   b. *Topical immunosuppression by application of glucocorticoids: Tinea incognito.* This may be the most common type in India as numerous OTC steroid combinations are available without prescription and most commonly used combinations of steroids contain superpotent steroids. If such an agent is essential, it is advisable to use a milder steroid, like clobetasone butyrate than potent steroids like betamethasone valerate.
   c. *Systemic immunosuppression:* Patients have a higher incidence and more intractable dermatophytoses; follicular abscesses and granulomas may occur (Majocchi granuloma).

Pathogenesis

The pathogenesis of dermatophytosis has three main aspects which determine its course. This includes, the host response, barrier function and the fungi.

The frequent case of relapse which is mistaken for resistance is due to the various ambient local factors. Microbiological resistance, is a wrong term as *in vitro* resistance is rare, and is probably a clinical resistance due to the various factors that determine the interplay of the fungal species and the host immune response. Thus the meaningless changing of drugs or combination of drugs may have a little use, specially if one appreciates that it is the host immune response that determines ultimate clinical response. Only a checker board pattern of *in vitro* analysis can determine the efficacy of combination therapy of various antifungals or prolonging the duration of antifungals or even combine and add oral azoles to therapy, as that is not a solution when microbiological resistance is not an issue.

The steps in pathogenesis are given below.

Invasion of the Epidermis

Starts with adherence between arthroconidia and keratinocytes, followed by penetration through and between cells and the development of a host response.

Adherence

On the stratum corneum, the first phase of dermatophyte invasion involves the adherence of infectious arthroconidia to keratinocytes. *In vitro*, this process is completed within about 2 hr of contact, at which stage germination and penetration of the keratinocyte occurs. The germination of arthroconidia and hyphal prolongation that follows adherence proceeds radially.

Penetration

Dermatophytes are keratinophilic. They produce a variety of proteolytic enzymes, which can work in acidic, alkaline or neutral environment. Keratinase activity in certain dermatophytes is inducible by low-molecular-weight peptides released from the epidermis by the action of other fungal proteinases. Other enzymes such as sulphur transporters and serum metalloproteases are also involved.

T. rubrum rarely invades hair but frequently invades nail; *Epidermophyton floccosum* never invades hair and only occasionally invades nail.

Dermatophytes (e.g. *T. rubrum*) that initiate a little inflammatory response are better able to establish chronic infection. Organisms such as *Microsporum canis* cause an acute infection associated with a brisk inflammatory response and spontaneous resolution.

Mannans in the cell walls of dermatophytes have immuno-inhibitory effects. In *T. rubrum*, the mannans may also decrease epidermal proliferation, thereby decreasing the likelihood of the fungus being sloughed off prior to invasion. This mechanism is thought to contribute to the chronicity of infections caused by *T. rubrum*. Also *Trichophyton* spp. produces the highest keratinase activity. The high level of enzyme activity of *Trichophyton* spp. at normal body temperatures and pH levels of the skin is presumably responsible for their adaptation to the surface of human skin. This is referred to as "anthropozation".

Local factors that favour dermatophyte infection include sweating, occlusion, occupational exposure, geographic location and high humidity (tropical or semitropical climates). In India, a common cause for persistence is the type of clothing. We have moved from cotton to denim, the latter being a preferred cloth of the Western world, suited for their cold climate. In our climate this prevents evaporation of sweat and thus does not let the skin "breathe". In our practice almost all such patients have recurrences. Another observation is that the use of leather shoes predisposes to tinea pedis. It is usually seen that a villager, who usually works barefoot does not have tinea pedis, though the well heeled, usually have tinea pedis and commonly onychomycosis!

The severity of clinical disease is also affected by several host factors. Sebum has an inhibitory effect on dermatophytes, and disease activity may be related to the number and activity of sebaceous glands in a particular body region. Broken or macerated skin encourage dermatophyte invasion, and increased susceptibility may be inherited or related to the competency of the immune system. Other host factors that facilitate dermatophyte infections include atopy, topical and systemic glucocorticoids, ichthyosis and collagen vascular disease. Once dermatophytes have invaded and begun to proliferate in the skin, several mechanisms aid in limiting the infection to keratinized tissue. These include the preference of dermatophytes for the cooler temperature at the skin's surface, serum factors that inhibit dermatophyte growth (e.g. β-globulins, ferritin and other metal chelators) and the host immune system. Cell-mediated immunity and antimicrobial activity of polymorphonuclear leukocytes restrict dermatophyte pathogenicity.

Thus, the clinical presentation of dermatophytoses depends on several factors: Site of infection, immunologic response of the host, and species of fungus.

Diagnostics of Fungal Infection

Diagnostics in dermatomycology are based primarily on microscopic and cultural detection. The sampling methods are enlisted in Table 5.1.

Table 5.1: Diagnostic sampling		
Type of dermatomycosis	*Instrument used for sampling*	*Procedure*
Tinea corporis	Scalpel, curette	Skin scrapings from (inflammatory) lesional borders
Tinea pedis inter-digitalis et plantaris	Sample swab for skin scales, curette, scalpel	Vigorous rubbing with a swab or take scrapings using curette. Scalpel: Skin scraping from dry, hyperkeratotic areas of the sole.
Tinea unguium (onychomycosis)	Scalpel, curette, (scissors), fraise	Disinfection with ethanol (70%) or some other cutaneous disinfectant (optional).
		Shortening nails with scissors; disposing of whole nail pieces; thereafter, tangential removal of the nail plate. Small and medium-sized, crumbly, partially thready subungual nail clippings at the transition between diseased and healthy tissue represent the optimal material for mycologic evaluation.
Tinea capitis	Epilation tweezers, scalpel	1. Shortening hairs with scissors down to roughly 3–5 mm in length; disposing of cut hairs; harvesting approximately 10–20 hair roots using epilation tweezers.
		2. Skin scrapings using a scalpel
		3. Taking a swab from pustules or abscesses
		4. *Brush method:* Repeated combing of hair with a sterile head massage brush (alternatively toothbrush), followed by direct inoculation onto culture medium (agar plate)—this method especially superor in anthrophilic cases and in screening

1. *Microscopic Preparations*

- The KOH (potassium hydroxide) examination using 20% KOH represents the simplest method to microscopically detect fungi, however, it has insufficient diagnostic sensitivity, especially in case of onychomycosis (40–68%). Positive scrapings are characterized by presence of refractile, long, smooth, undulating, branching, and septate hyphal filaments with or without arthroconidiospores. False negative results are seen in 15% cases.
- Tetraethyl ammonium hydroxide (TEAH) may be used alternatively.
- Fluorescent staining with optical brighteners (diaminostilbene) is the most sensitive method to microscopically detect fungi in skin scales, nail clippings, hair roots, hair. These substances bind to chitin, the main cell wall component of fungi. Currently available stains are Blankophor® or Calcofluor®.

2. *Culture*

As fungi are heterotrophic microorganisms, culture media should contain organic nutrients required for growth and reproduction of fungi which include a carbon source (glucose), a nitrogen source (peptone, meat extract), water, vitamins and antibiotics. Sabouraud dextrose agar (SDA, 4% peptone, 1% glucose, agar, water) is the most commonly used isolation media for dermatophytosis and serves as the medium on which most morphologic descriptions are based. Modified SDA, with addition of gentamicin, chloramphenicol and cycloheximide is more selective for dermatophytes as chroramphenicol inhibits the growth of saprophytic fungus. Dermatophyte test medium is an alternative to isolation media and contains pH indicator phenol red. It is incubated at room temperature for 5–14 days.

Cultures are incubated at a temperature of 26–32°C, optimally at 28°C, for 3–4 weeks and visually checked for fungal growth twice weekly. Most dermatophytes can grow at 37°C, yet, because of their adaptation to human skin surface temperature, they do however grow better at lower temperatures. If a slow-growing dermatophyte is suspected, e.g. T. verrucosum or T. violaceum, the incubation period should be extended to at least 4–6 weeks. Dermatophytes utilize the protein resulting in excess ammonium ion and alkaline environment which turns the medium from yellow to bright red.

T. interdigitale (*T. mentagrophytes*) does not develop any pigment reminiscent of *T. rubrum*. This important differential feature of the two most common dermatophytes cannot be assessed on a dye-containing agar. Therefore, Sabouraud 2% or 4% glucose agar is still the best option. By contrast, culture media exhibiting a chemically induced color change (Taplin agar) are inadequate, as they mask the pathogens' natural pigment.

The differentiation of dermatophytes, yeasts, and molds is predicated on macroscopic (upper and bottom side of colonies as well as pigmentation) and microscopic characteristics (formation of macro and microconidia, respectively other growth forms) as well as biochemical properties (for example, urea hydrolysis on Christensen urea agar).

3. Antifungal Susceptibility Resting

i. *Microdilution method:* The broth microdilution assay for antifungal susceptibility testing of dermatophytes has been previously developed as a modification of the Clinical and Laboratory Standards Institute M38-A2 standard method. The final concentration of terbinafine and itraconazole used is 0.06–32.0 µg/ml and for fluconazole, 0.13–64.0 µg/ml. A standardized inoculum is prepared by counting the microconidia microscopically. Cultures are grown on SDA slants for 7 days at 35°C to produce conidia. Sterile normal saline (85%) is added to the agar slant, and the cultures are gently swabbed with a cotton-tipped applicator to dislodge the conidia from the hyphal mat. The suspension is transferred to a sterile centrifuge tube, and the volume is adjusted to 5 ml with sterile normal saline. The resulting suspension is counted on a hemacytometer and is diluted in RPMI 1640 medium to the desired concentration. Microdilution plates are set up in accordance with the reference method. The microdilution plates are incubated at 35°C and read visually after 4 days of incubation. The minimum inhibitory concentration is defined as the concentration at which the growth of the organism will be inhibited by 80% when compared with the growth in the control well.

ii. *Minimum fungicidal concentration (MFC) determination:* For determination of the MFC, 100 µl aliquots are removed from the assay wells showing no visible growth at the end of incubation and streaked onto SDA plates. The plates are incubated at 30°C for 7 days. The MFC is defined as the lowest drug concentration at which no visible fungal growth or colonies developed.

4. Histology

In tinea corporis, fungal hyphae are found in the stratum corneum, the epidermis shows marked spongiosis with neutrophils and intracorneal pustule formation. Special stains most commonly used are periodic acid-Schiff and Gomori methanamine silver which help to highlight hyphae.

In follicle-associated fungal dermatophytosis, epidermis shows hyperkeratosis and parakeratosis with serum lakes, pustule-like accumulation of neutrophils, and a cystically dilated follicular ostium. There is also psoriasiform epithelial hyperplasia with moderate spongiosis. Upper dermal and perifollicular lymphocytes and neutrophils with exocytosis into the epidermis and the follicular ostium may be seen.

The histologic detection of fungi in fungal nail infections displays a high sensitivity. Specificity, however, is low because it does not identify the fungal genus or species. Particularly in those cases where neither microscopy nor cultures come back positive for fungi, histologic analysis of nail material facilitates the correct diagnosis. However, care should be taken to avoid false positive interpretation of secondary mycotic growth, e.g. in nail psoriasis, as fungal nail infection.

5. *Dermoscopy*

The comma hairs, which are slightly curved fractured hair shafts and corkscrew hair have been described as the dermoscopic marker of tinea capitis. Broken and dystrophic hairs are also seen. However, in tinea corporis, the involvement of vellus hair as seen on dermoscopy is an indication for systemic therapy.

6. *Molecular Biology*

These methods increase the sensitivity and specificity of mycologic diagnostics.

Uniplex PCR: Nucleic acid amplification techniques (NAAT) use primers to recognize specific gene regions of individual dermatophyte species for specific pathogen detection in clinical samples *in vitro*. The primers either use a specific sequence of the topoisomerase II gene, or (a sequence of the internal transcribed spacer (ITS) region) for individual dermatophytes. The uniplex PCR ELISA test separately identifies different species and also shortens the time to diagnosis (24 hours).

Multiplex PCR: It enables simultaneous amplification of 21 dermatomycotic pathogens with subsequent DNA detection by means of agarose gel electrophoresis.

Real time PCR for dermatophyte DNA detection: Although quite complex, it represents a comparatively fast, highly specific and sensitive molecular method for the amplification and simultaneous quantification of DNA. Real time PCR, too, allows for the detection of multiple pathogens, albeit consecutively, not simultaneously.

Newer methods: MALDI-TOF (matrix-assisted laser desorption ionization-time of flight) mass spectrometry (MS)—it enables simultaneous identification of up to 64 dermatophyte strains, with results coming back within minutes. Although the test's specificity-based on protein mass fingerprint or mass spectrum is high, the plausibility of identified species should still always be verified.

To summarize, clinical diagnosis of cutaneous dermatophytic infection should always be supplemented by mycologic confirmation. While traditional methods like direct demonstration of fungus by KOH offer a reasonably sensitive and inexpensive option, newer noninvasive methods such as dermoscopy have additional advantage of ease of use, ability to detect involvement of vellus hair and thus, influence the choice of treatment (topical versus systemic). Fungal culture and antifungal testing are costlier and more specialized investigations, but such infrastructure needs should be set up at most centers, especially in the present scenario of rising prevalence of nonresponsive dermatophytosis. Other methods such as PCR and reflectance confocal microscopy are still used primarily for research purposes.

Clinical Features

Before we discuss the main types we will focus on two separate entities.

Trichophyton Rubrum Syndrome

(Syn: Chronic dermatophytosis syndrome, generalized chronically persistent rubrophytia, tinea corporis generalisata).

Trichophyton rubrum syndrome represents a chronic and generalized dermatophytosis. Predisposing factors include previously administered topical or systemic corticosteroid therapy, Down syndrome, HIV infection, diabetes mellitus and Cushing's disease.

Criteria

- At least four body sites are affected: feet (plantar), hands (palmar), nails, as well as one other site. The *inguinal* region which is a common site of tinea, is explicitly *excluded*.
- Microscopic fungal detection (KOH or Blankophor®) from all four sites.
- Cultural detection of *T. rubrum* from at least three out of the four sites.

It still remains unclear whether *T. rubrum* syndrome represents a distinct nosologic entity.

Dermatophytid Reaction

This is a non-infective cutaneous infection representing an allergic response to a distant focus of dermatophyte infection.

It is now clear that the essential criteria required for the diagnosis of an id reaction to a dermatophyte infection are the following:

1. Proven dermatophyte infection, which usually becomes highly inflamed before the appearance of the secondary rash.
2. A distant eruption, which is demonstrably free of ringworm fungus.
3. Spontaneous disappearance of the rash when the ringworm infection settles, with or without treatment.

Even with these criteria, id reactions may be overdiagnosed. An additional criterion has been recommended: The morphology of the id eruption should match one of the well-recognized types.

Clinical Features

The main id reactions include:

1. A widespread eruption of small **follicular papules** grouped or diffusely scattered. The eruption is symmetrical, usually pronounced on the trunk, but in severe cases extending down the limbs, even at times covering the face. Sometimes the follicular papules are topped by horny spines. The common cause of this type of id reaction is a scalp kerion, typically caused by *T. verrucosum*.
2. A **pompholyx-like** id affecting the web spaces and palmar surfaces of the fingers, the palms and sometimes the dorsal surfaces of the hands. This eruption is characteristically associated with an acutely inflammatory tinea pedis, which may have arisen spontaneously or as a result of inappropriate treatment (Fig. 5.2).

The palmar and web space skin may be covered with papules or vesicles and bullae or pustules may also occur. Clinically, this is indistinguishable from a constitutional eczema of the pompholyx variety.

Of the many other suggested morphologies for id reactions, **erythema nodosum** seems the most acceptable. The **erythema multiforme**, **erythema annulare** and **urticaria** may, on occasion, be manifestations of an allergic reaction to a ringworm infection.

TINEA CAPITIS

Definition

Tinea capitis describes infection of the scalp and hair with a dermatophyte.

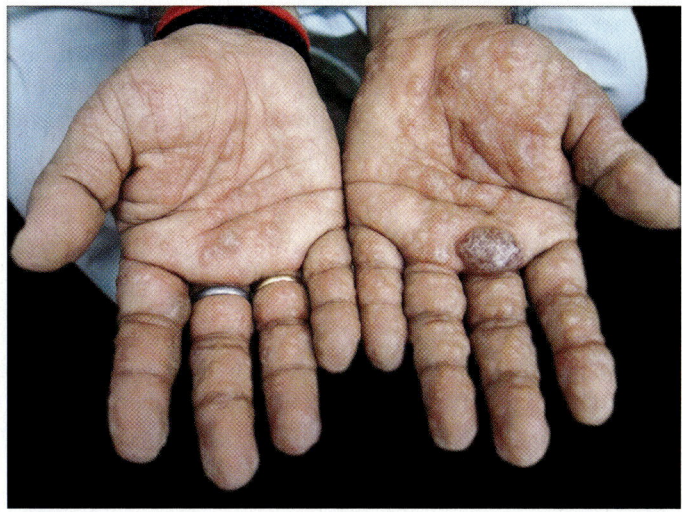

Fig. 5.2: A pompholyx id consequent to tinea pedis infection

Organism

Several *Trichophyton* spp. and *Microsporum* spp.

Zoophilic *M. canis* (cats and dogs) is commonly seen in those who have pets.

Anthropophilic *T. violaceum* is one of the major culprit and this species can be contagious and endemic.

T. tonsurans is increasing in prevalence, especially in North America.

Predisposing Factors

Large family size, crowding, and low socioeconomic status increase the chance of infection. Infectious fungal particles that have fallen from the infected person may remain viable for months.

Tinea capitis can be transmitted by infected persons, fallen hairs, animals, fomites (e.g. clothing, bedding, hairbrushes, combs, hats) and furniture.

Zoophilic dermatophytes are acquired from contact with pets or wild animals. Sources of *M. canis* infection are cats, dogs and guinea pigs. The animals may harbor the pathogen in their fur (colonization) even if clinical symptoms are not visible. *Microsporum gypseum* infection comes from contaminated soil.

Asymptomatic scalp carriage of dermatophytes by classmates and adults is probably an important factor contributing to disease transmission and reinfection. The asymptomatic carriage persists for an indefinite period. In superficial tinea capitis caused by anthropophilic dermatophytes, the alopecia areata-like lesions on the scalp are mostly dry, more or less erythematous, hyperkeratotic, and scaly. Some children are merely pathogen carriers. *T. tonsurans*, but also *M. audouinii*, frequently give rise to discrete pityriasis capitis. If left untreated, these individuals play a significant role in the transmission of tinea capitis among the population. In some cases, *T. tonsurans* causes recalcitrant and protracted dermatomycoses.

Pathogenesis

The fungus grows down through the keratin layer into the hair follicle and gains entry into the hair in the lower intrafollicular zone, just below the point where the cuticle of the hair shaft is formed. Because of the cuticle, the fungi cannot cross over from the perifollicular stratum corneum into the hair but must penetrate deep into the hair follicle to circumvent the cuticle. This may explain why topical antifungal agents are ineffective for treating tinea capitis. The fungi then invade the keratinized, outer root sheath; enter the inner cortex; and digest the keratin contained inside the hair shaft. The growth of hyphae occurs within the hair shaft above the zone of keratinization and keeps pace with the growth of hair (Fig. 5.3). Distal to this zone of active growth,

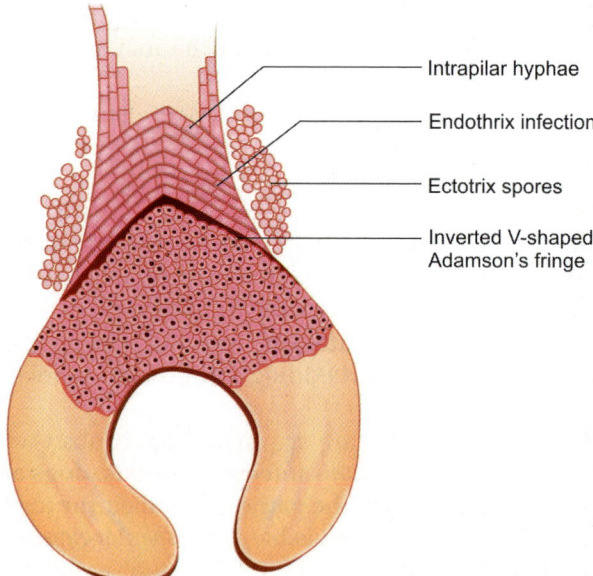

Intrapilar hyphae

Endothrix infection

Ectotrix spores

Inverted V-shaped Adamson's fringe

Fig. 5.3: A depiction of the two types of invasion of the hyphae in tinea capitis, i.e. ectothrix and endothrix. (**Note:** The endothrix infection does not spread beyond the Adamson fringe)

arthrospores are formed within or on the surface of the hair, depending on the species of dermatophytes. Hyphae grow inside and fragment into short segments called arthrospores.

The arthrospores remain inside the hair shaft in the endothrix pattern. In the ectothrix type, they dislodge, obscure and penetrate the surface cuticle on the hair shaft surface, and form a sheath of closely packed spheres.

Different clinical presentations arise from the various causative organisms. For example, *T. tonsurans* causes an endothrix infection, which classically results in "black dot" tinea capitis due to hair breakage near the scalp. In contrast, *M. audouinii* is an ectothrix form of tinea capitis that typically presents with dry, scaly patches of alopecia ("gray patch" tinea capitis). The pathogenicity of the culprit organism is not the only factor in determining the severity of disease; the host immune response to the organism plays an important role as well. Tinea capitis can range from a non-inflammatory scaling that resembles seborrheic dermatitis (especially *T. tonsurans*) to a severe pustular eruption with alopecia, known as a kerion.

Clinical Features

a. *Noninflammatory infection (gray patch)/gray patch tinea capitis:* Partial alopecia, often circular in shape, showing numerous broken-off hairs, dull gray from their coating of arthrospores. Fine scaling is seen with fairly sharp margin (Fig. 5.4). Hair shaft becomes brittle, breaking off at or slightly above scalp. It is mostly caused by

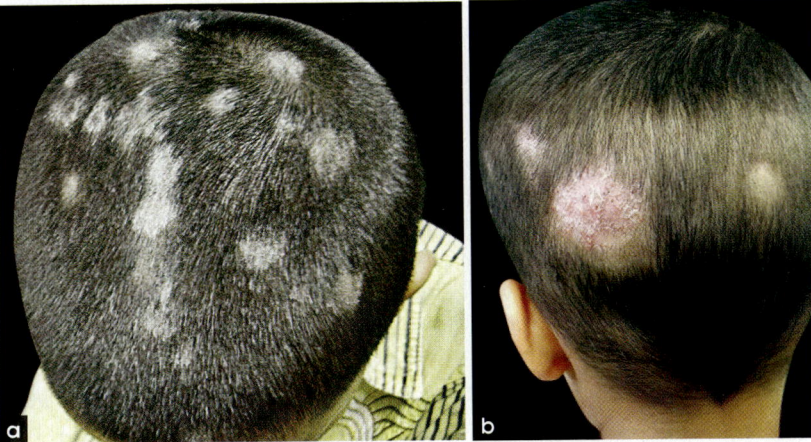

Fig. 5.4a and b: (a) A case of gray patch tinea capitis (b) a 6-year-old boy with patchy circular alopecia and fine scaling suggestive of gray patch tinea capitis. The fine scales represent the fungal arthrospores

M. audonii variant, which is differentiated on Wood's lamp by showing green fluorescence, the exception to this rule is *M. ferrugineum*.

b. *Trichophyton tonsurans infection*

   i. *Noninflammatory black dot pattern* (Fig. 5.5e). In the black dot (swollen hair) pattern, there are well-demarcated areas of hair loss, with hairs broken off at the follicular orifice, giving the characteristic appearance of black dots if the patient's hair is black. Red hairs will produce a "red dot" pattern. This is the most distinctive pattern. Large areas of alopecia are present without inflammation. There is a mild-to-moderate amount of scalp scale. Occipital adenopathy may be present. Lack of inflammation may be explained by the fact that cell-mediated immunity to Trichophyton antigen skin tests is negative.

   ii. *Inflammatory tinea capitis.* There can be various presentations (Fig. 5.5a to d) though mostly we focus on kerion. There are one or multiple inflamed, boggy, tender areas of alopecia with pustules on and/or in surrounding skin. Rarely, there are discharging sinuses and presence of mycetoma like grains on the surface. Fever, occipital adenopathy, leukocytosis, and a diffuse morbilliform rash may occur. Most patients with this infection pattern have a positive skin test to the Trichophyton antigen, suggesting that the patient's immune response may be responsible for intense inflammation. Approximately 35% of patients infected with *T. tonsurans* have this pattern. Potassium hydroxide wet mounts and fungal cultures are often negative because of destruction of fungal structures by inflammation, and treatment may have to be initiated based on clinical appearance.

   iii. *Seborrheic dermatitis type.* This type is common and the most difficult to diagnose because it resembles dandruff. There is diffuse or patchy, fine, white, adherent scale on the scalp (Fig. 5.6). Close examination shows tiny, perifolicular pustules and/or hair stubs that have broken at the level of the scalp: the black dot pattern. Less commonly, there is patchy or diffuse hair loss. Adenopathy is often present. Culture is often necessary to make the diagnosis because only 29% of affected patients have a positive potassium hydroxide examination and it also helps to identify secondary bacterial contamination, requiring antibiotics.

c. Favus caused by *Trichophyton schoenleinii*—this variety is rarely seen these days. The classic picture of tinea capitis caused by this organism is characterized by the presence of yellowish, cup-shaped crusts known as scutula. Each scutulum develops round a hair, which pierces it centrally.

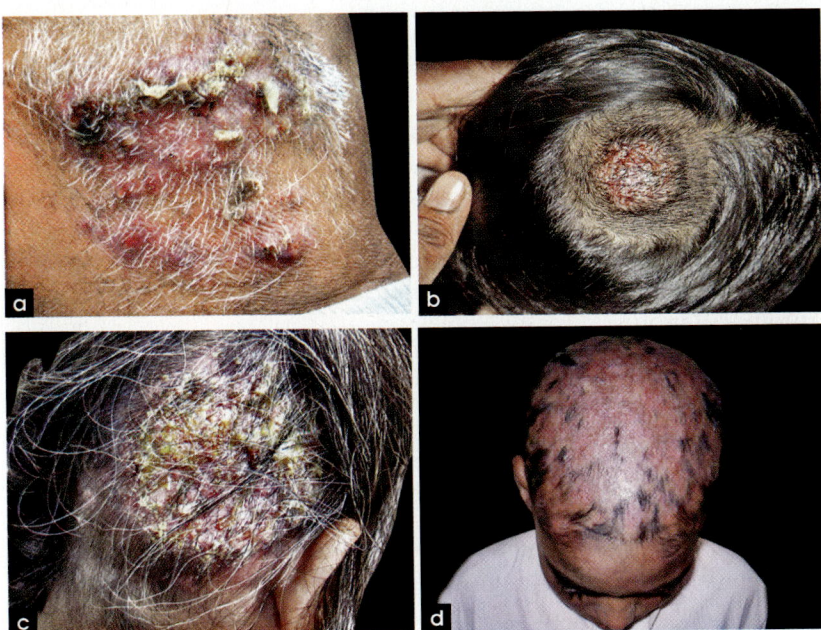

Fig. 5.5a to d: (a) A case of inflammatory tinea capitis in an adult patient who was treated with antibiotics and after an unsuccessful course was diagnosed as tinea capitis and treated successfully with griseofulvin; (b) inflamed, boggy, tender areas of alopecia in a case of kerion; (c) an inflammatory tinea capitis in a lady working in a cowshed , a case of zoophilic tinea capitis; (d) agminate folliculitis: A rare case with pustules all over the scalp with alopecia diagnosed and treated as a case of bacterial folliculitis

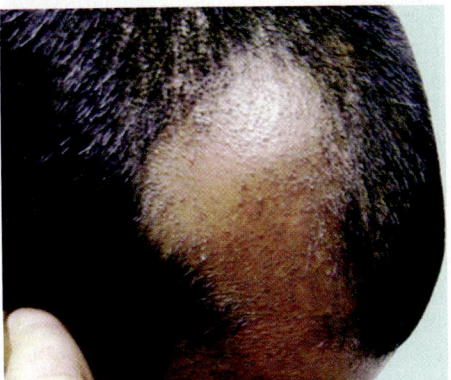

Fig. 5.5e: A case of "Black dot" tinea capitis, which was being treated as a case of alopecia areata. Pointer to diagnosis is black swollen areas of hair shaft seen in the alopecic patch

Tinea Capitis in Adults

Unlike children, adults are very rarely affected by tinea capitis. Due to the atypical clinical picture, other disorders are often initially diagnosed such as alopecia areata, scarring alopecia, pyoderms, seborrhoeic capitis, psoriasis, folliculitis decalvans, etc. resulting in anti-inflammatory topical corticosteroid therapy. Histology usually helps. Trichoscopy occasionally shows so-called "corkscrew hairs" in adult tinea capitis. *T. rubrum* is the most likely pathogen in the majority of cases of adult tinea capitis, similar to tinea incognito as a result of autoinoculation.

Infections of the Eyebrows

Infections of the eyebrows by dermatophytes are also included under tinea capitis. Due to their slow growth, such infections have proven to be recalcitrant and require prolonged treatment.

Secondary Bacterial Infection in Tinea Capitis

Secondary bacterial infections may potentially occur in tinea capitis, occasionally leading to misdiagnosis and subsequent topical and systemic antibiotic therapy. Some cases even result in unnecessary

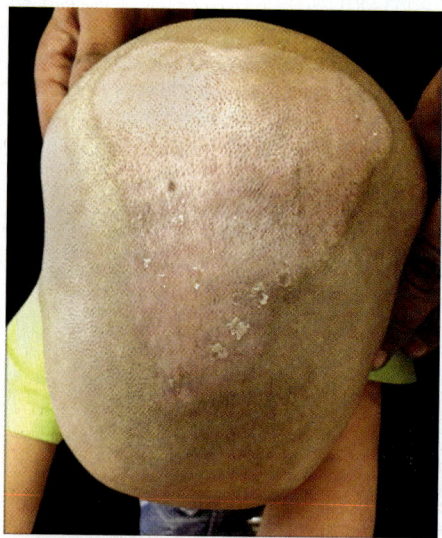

Fig. 5.6: Seborrheic dermatitis type of tinea capitis. Here the scales are more adherent to the scalp. Since seborrheic dermatitis is uncommon in children, it is useful to consider tinea capitis in such cases and get a culture done to confirm the diagnosis, if possible, as a KOH mount is usually negative in this variant

surgical procedures like incision and abscess drainage. As conventional mycologic diagnostics in slow-growing dermatophytes, e.g. *T. verrucosum*, are initially negative, other causal pathogens, first and foremost *Staphylococcus aureus*, are frequently considered. However, these bacteria are simply a sign of secondary infection in tinea capitis (profunda). Secondary infections by LA-MRSA (livestock-associated methicillin-resistant *Staphylococcus aureus*) may give rise to considerable diagnostic and therapeutic problems in cases of purulent, abscess-forming tinea capitis caused by *T. verrucosum*.

Treatment

A treatment ladder is depicted below.

Treatment ladder

First line
- Terbinafine: <20 kg, 62.5 mg; 20–40 kg, 125 mg; >40 kg, 250 mg. All given daily for 4 weeks
- Itraconazole 2–4 mg/kg/day for 4–6 weeks
- Griseofulvin 10 mg/kg for 6 weeks (20 mg/kg considered in some *T. tonsurans* and *T. schoenleinii* infections)

Second line
Itraconazole 5 mg/kg in weekly pulses for 2–3 rounds.

Topical

Topical treatment alone is not recommended for the management of tinea capitis. Local treatment with a topical antifungal with a fungicidal mechanism of action such as ciclopiroxolamine or terbinafine cream, may reduce the risk of infecting other people and shortens the duration of systemic treatment. The hair should be washed two times weekly using an antifungal shampoo (povidone-iodine, selenium disulfide).

Oral

All systemic antifungals are more effective in the presence of endothrix infection (e.g. Trichophyton spp.) than in patients with ectothrix disease (e.g. *M. canis*). Current data suggest that *M. canis* infections might respond better to itraconazole.

1. Griseofulvin

Side effects include nausea and rashes in 8 to 15% of cases. The drug is contraindicated in pregnancy and the manufacturers caution against men fathering a child for 6 months after therapy.

Advantages: Licensed; inexpensive; syrup formulation is more palatable; suspension allows accurate dosage adjustments in children; and extensive experience.

Disadvantages: Prolonged treatment required. Contraindicated in lupus erythematosus, porphyria, and severe liver disease.

Drug interactions: Warfarin, cyclosporine, and the oral contraceptive pill.

2. Terbinafine

Side effects include gastrointestinal disturbances and rashes in 5% and 3% of cases, respectively. Gastrointestinal symptoms subside with continuing therapy.

Advantages: Fungicidal, so shorter therapy required (cf. griseofulvin), therefore, increased compliance more likely.

Disadvantages: No suspension formulation, less effective against Microsporum species.

Drug interactions: Plasma concentrations are reduced by rifampicin and increased by cimetidine.

3. Itraconazole

Both fungistatic and fungicidal activity depending on the concentration of drug in the tissues. Nausea and vomiting can occur; abnormalities in liver functions occur in more than 1% of patients.

Advantages: Pulsed shorter treatment regimens are possible.

Disadvantages: Potential drug interactions.

Drug interactions: Enhanced toxicity of anticoagulants (warfarin), antihistamines (terfenadine and astemizole), antipsychotics (sertindole), anxiolytics (midazolam), digoxin, cisapride, cyclosporine, and simvastatin (increased risk of myopathy). Reduced efficacy of itraconazole with concomitant use of H_2-blockers, phenytoin, and rifampicin.

4. Fluconazole

Use has mainly been limited by side effects.

Side effects: Nausea and vomiting, but liver function test abnormalities are also reported.

Additional Measures

1. *Exclusion from school:* Although there is a risk of transmission of infection from patients to unaffected classmates, for practical reasons children should be allowed to return to school once they have started receiving appropriate systemic and adjuvant topical therapy.

2. *Familial screening:* Index cases resulting from the anthropophilic *T. tonsurans* are highly infectious. Family members and other close contacts should be screened (both for tinea capitis and for tinea corporis) and appropriate mycologic samples taken preferably using the brush technique, even in the absence of clinical signs.

3. *Cleansing of fomites: T. tonsurans* spores may remain viable on furniture, combs, and brushes. Scrupulous cleaning of all possibly contaminated objects helps to prevent reinfection. For all anthropophilic species these should be cleansed with disinfectant. Simple bleach or Milton sterilizing fluid can be used.

4. Careful removal of crusts in kerion is advised.

5. *Steroids:* The use of corticosteroids (both oral and topical) for inflammatory varieties (e.g. kerions and severe id reactions) is controversial, but may help to reduce itching and general discomfort. Although in the past, steroids have been thought to minimize the risk of permanent alopecia secondary to scarring, current evidence does not suggest any reduction in clearance time compared with griseofulvin alone.

6. *Cutting the hair or shaving the head:* It may significantly shorten the duration of treatment with a systemic antifungal. Shaving the affected areas of the scalp significantly reduces the infectious load. Shaving should be performed at the beginning of systemic treatment and again 3 to 4 weeks later. Shaving the hair once each week may significantly shorten treatment.

Treatment Failures

Some individuals are not cured. The following are reasons why this occurs:

1. Lack of compliance with the long courses of treatment
2. Suboptimal absorption of the drug
3. Relative insensitivity of the organism
4. Reinfection

T. tonsurans and *Microsporum* spp. are typical culprits in persistently positive cases. If fungi can still be isolated at the end of treatment, but the clinical signs have improved, the authors recommend continuing the original treatment for another month.

If there has been no clinical response and signs persist at the end of the treatment period, then the options include the following:

1. Increase the dose or duration of the original drug: both griseofulvin (in dosages up to 25 mg/kg for 8–10 weeks) and terbinafine have

been used successfully and safely at higher dosages or for longer courses to clear resistant infections.

2. Change to an alternative antifungal (e.g. switch from griseofulvin to terbinafine or itraconazole).

Carriers

The optimal management of symptom-free carriers (i.e. individuals without overt clinical infection, but who are culture positive) is unclear. In those with a heavy growth/high spore count on brush culture, systemic antifungal therapy may be justified because these individuals are likely to develop an overt clinical infection, are a significant reservoir of infection, and are unlikely to respond to topical therapy alone. Alternatively, they may represent a missed overt clinical infection. For those with light growth/low spore counts on brush culture, use shampoos containing 1–2.5% selenium sulfide, 1–2% zinc pyrithione, povidone-iodine, or ketoconazole 2% to inhibit the growth of fungi. They may be useful as adjunctive therapy to control spore loads in infected children and asymptomatic carriers. These agents are lathered, massaged well, and left on the scalp for 5 minutes. They are used two to three times each week during the course of treatment or longer.

TINEA FACIEI

It is characterized by erythematous, centrifugally growing, discretely scaly lesions with prominent borders, frequently on the cheeks, but also on the eyelids and sometimes in the submandibular region (Fig. 5.7). Mildly pruritic (or even non-pruritic), scaly facial lesions with accentuated borders should therefore always prompt a mycologic workup to rule out tinea faciei.

Differential diagnostic considerations include impetigo, atopic dermatitis, contact dermatitis, discoid lupus erythematosus, and herpes zoster. In children, zoophilic dermatophytes—zoophilic strains of *T. interdigitale* as well as *M. canis* and Trichophyton species of *Arthroderma benhamiae*—are the primary pathogens in tinea faciei.

Treatment

In localized cases, if promptly diagnosed, topical therapy seems to work well, especially with tolnaftate or one of the imidazoles. Where delay has occurred before the diagnosis is established, and especially when steroid therapy has modified the condition, terbinafine or itraconazole is generally preferred. Most cases will clear in 3 or 4 weeks, certainly in 6 weeks, but long standing infections may occasionally need longer periods of treatment.

Table 5.2: Treatment of tinea capitis

Drug	Dosage	Suspension,* capsule, tablet	Duration for Trichophyton (T), Microsporum (M) infections	Comments
Griseofulvin	10–25 mg/kg/day (micro-size) or 15 mg/kg/day (ultramicronized)	25 mg/ml 125 mg tablets 250 mg tablets 333 mg tablets 500 mg tablets Take with fatty foods	(T) 6–8 weeks or longer until cultures are negative (M) 8–12 weeks or longer until fungal cultures are negative	Treatment of choice, long experience of safety, no laboratory monitoring terbinafine for 4 weeks and griseofulvin for 8 weeks showed similar efficiency
Terbinafine	<20 kg: 62.5 mg daily 21–40 kg: 125 mg daily >40 kg: 250 mg daily	250 mg tablet	(T) 4 weeks (M) Efficacy in pediatric Microsporum infections is disputed	Shortest duration of therapy Drug interactions are few Liver function tests baseline and repeat if therapy is continued for >4 weeks
Itraconazole	5 mg/kg/day 3 mg/kg/day (oral suspension)* Capsule: simplified dosing 10–20 kg: 100 mg every other day 21–30 kg: 100 mg daily 31–40 kg: 100 and 200 mg On alternate days	100 mg tablet or oral suspension Note: Oral solution is better absorbed Take with a main meal	(T) 4 weeks, fungal monitoring, another 2 weeks of treatment if tests are positive (M) 6 weeks, fungal monitoring, another 2 weeks of treatment if test is positive	Cytochrome P-450 drug interactions Liver function tests baseline and if therapy is continued for >4 weeks

Contd.

Table 5.2: Treatment of tinea capitis (Contd.)

Drug	Dosage	Suspension,* capsule, tablet	Duration for Trichophyton (T), Microsporum (M) infections	Comments
	41–50 kg: 200 mg daily >50 kg: 200–300 mg daily			No significant difference in cure between itraconazole for 2 weeks compared with griseofulvin for 6 weeks No difference between itraconazole and terbinafine for treatment periods lasting 2–3 weeks
Fluconazole	Dose range studies still ongoing, 6 mg/kg body weight daily; alternatively, 6–8 mg/kg body weight once weekly	50 mg, 100 mg, and 200 mg tablets or oral suspension	(T) 3–4 weeks daily regiment 4–8 weeks weekly regimen (M) 6–8 weeks or longer	Cytochrome P-450/drug interactions Liver function tests baseline and if therapy is continued for >4 weeks Similar cure rates between 2 and 4 weeks of fluconazole with 6 weeks of griseofulvin

*Not available in India.

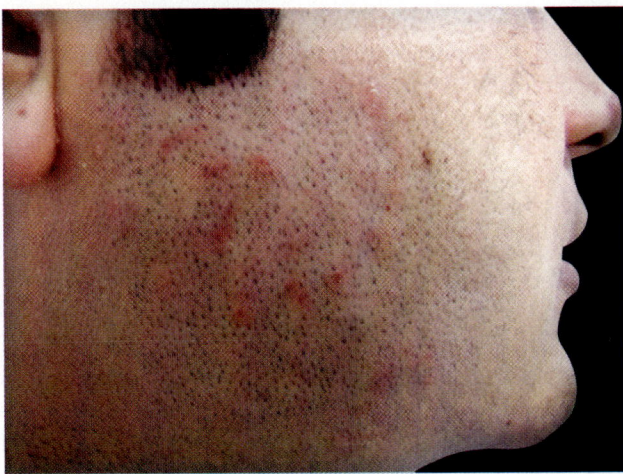

Fig. 5.7: A case of tinea faciei with discrete scaly lesions on lateral aspect of cheek extending to submandibular region

TINEA BARBAE

Definition

Tinea barbae is a dermatophytic infection that is limited to the coarse hair-bearing beard and moustache areas in men (while tinea of upper lip and chin area in female is classified as tinea faciei). Infection usually occurs after minor trauma such as from shaving.

Organism

Hair may be painlessly removed at almost any stage of the infection and examined for hyphae. Zoophilic *Trichophyton mentagrophytes* and *T. verrucosum* are the most common pathogens. *T. verrucosum* infection is acquired from the hide of dairy cattle and causes a severe pustular eruption on the face and neck. Many patients are dairy farmers.

Infection with *Microsporum canis* or *T. rubrum* is uncommon. In certain geographic regions, other anthropophilic dermatophytes (*T. schoenleinii, T. violaceum* and *T. megninii*) are endemic and cause tinea barbae. Disease is often acquired from animals. In the past, a common cause of infection was contaminated razors in barber shops. With the increased use of disposable razors and disinfectants, however, the incidence of tinea due to this source has dramatically reduced.

Fungal infection of the beard area (tinea barbae) should be considered when inflammation occurs in this area. Bacterial folliculitis and inflammation secondary to ingrown hairs (pseudofolliculitis) are common. However, it is not unusual to see patients who have finally been diagnosed as having tinea after failing to respond to several courses of antibiotics. A positive culture for Staphylococcus does not rule out tinea, in which purulent lesions may be infected secondarily with bacteria.

Clinical Features

Because zoophilic organisms are the most common culprit and due to the large number of terminal hair follicles in the affected areas, the clinical presentation tends to be severe, with intense inflammation and multiple follicular pustules. Abscesses, sinus tracts, bacterial superinfection and even kerion-like boggy plaques can develop. Like tinea capitis, the hairs are almost always infected and easily and painlessly removed and the lesions are less painful compared to a boil. The hair in bacterial folliculitis resists removal and if removed cause pain.

Cases may be associated with topical steroid therapy, pet contact, and contact with the hide of dairy cattle or horses. Lesions are usually unilateral and are found on the chin, neck, and maxillary or submaxillary areas. Upper lip involvement is usually seen as scattered, discrete, follicular pustules; kerion formation rarely occurs.

Superficial infection. This is superficial, less inflammatory, and similar to tinea corporis; *T. rubrum* is usually the causative agent in this variant (Fig. 5.8).

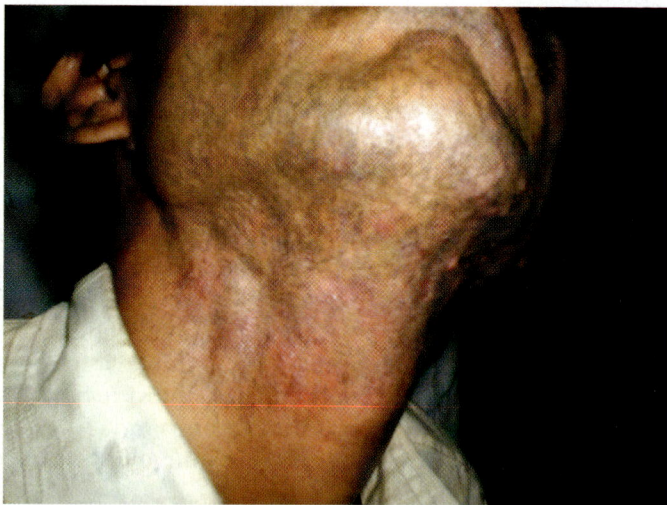

Fig. 5.8: A superficial pattern of tinea barbae in a 23-year-old male. Lesions resemble that of tinea corporis and *Trichophyton rubrum* is the usual culprit

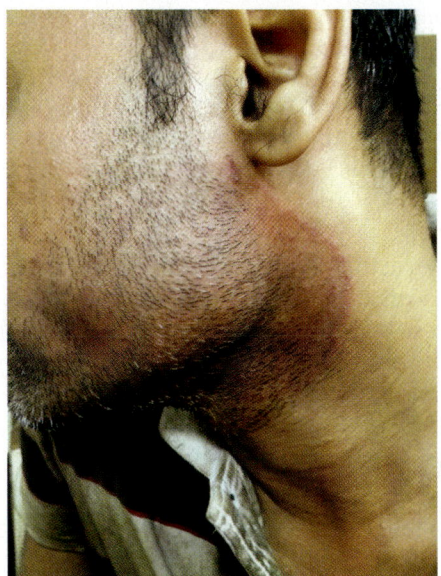

Fig. 5.9: A deep variant of tinea barbae with multiple follicular lesions with itching and little pain

Deep follicular infection. This pattern clinically resembles bacterial folliculitis except that it is slower to evolve and is usually restricted to one area of the beard. Bacterial folliculitis spreads rapidly over wide areas after shaving. Tinea begins insidiously with a small group of follicular pustules (Fig. 5.9). The process becomes confluent in time with the development of a boggy, erythematous, tumor-like abscess covered with dense, superficial crust similar to that of fungal kerions seen in tinea capitis.

Treatment

Beard infections usually respond satisfactorily to itraconazole or terbinafine, sometimes in combination with topical therapy over a period of 4–6 weeks. Fairly long-term follow-up is recommended, and late recurrences undoubtedly occur.

Infection control: Cases of tinea barbae are likely to continue to occur sporadically until more satisfactory means of controlling ringworm in cattle are found. Early diagnosis and prompt treatment of the individual patient and the encouragement of high standards of hygiene in the livestock industry are essential. A vaccine against *T. verrucosum* in cattle has resulted in a reduced incidence of infection, not only in cows but also among their human contacts, in some countries in eastern Europe.

TINEA CORPORIS

Definition

Infection of the skin of the trunk, legs and arms (glabrous skin) with a dermatophyte. It is seen worldwide, but more prevalent in tropical and subtropical regions.

Organism

Any dermatophyte can potentially cause tinea corporis, but *T. rubrum* is the most common pathogen worldwide, followed by *T. mentagrophytes* while the reverse is trending in India at present.

It is caused by many *Trichophyton* spp., *Microsporum* spp. and *Epidermophyton floccosum*.

Tinea corporis caused by *T. tonsurans* is sometimes seen in children with tinea capitis and their close contacts.

- Often zoophilic, occasionally geophilic organisms.
- Infection frequently contracted from a household pet (*M. canis* from cats and dogs most frequent).
- May follow infection of another body site.
- Person to person transmission may occur in contact sports.
- *T. verrucosum* from cattle in rural areas.

Clinical Features

Tinea corporis may affect any body site, but infections with zoophilic species are more likely to occur on exposed parts such as the face, neck and arms (Fig. 5.10) and they tend to follow an acute course and

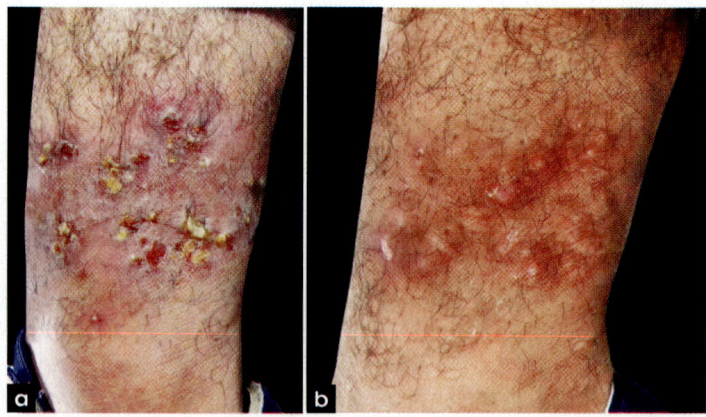

Fig. 5.10a and b: (a) A zoophilic tinea corporis infection caused by *Trichophyton verrucosum*, in a patient who was a farmer and had been given repeated courses of antibiotics; (b) After a course of itraconazole 200 mg for 14 days, the lesions responded significantly

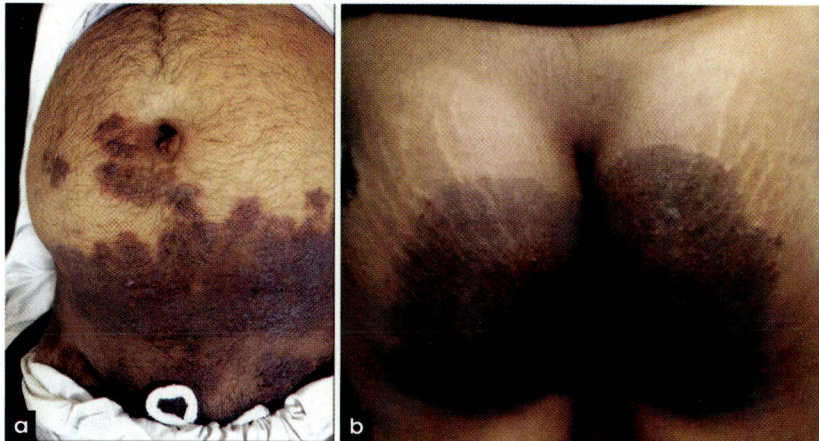

Fig. 5.11a and b: Tinea corporis presenting as hyperpigmented lichenified plaques with raised margins, highly suggestive of *T. rubrum* infection. The presentation points to chances of chronicity of infection and thus a need for longer duration of antifungal therapy in such patients

also show more inflammation, with the lesion becoming indurated and pustular, while anthropophilic species have a milder, more chronic course and have a thickend lichenified look (Fig. 5.11).

Patients may complain of mild pruritus. The clinical manifestations are variable, depending on the species of fungus involved and the extent of progression, but in typical cases, round scaling lesions which are dry, erythematous and clearly circumscribed are seen. As with most dermatophyte infections, the extent of inflammation depends on the causative pathogen and the immune response of the host. Also, because hair follicles serve as reservoirs for infection, body areas with more hair follicles may be more resistant to treatment.

The fungus is more active at the margin of the lesions and hence this is more erythematous than the middle, which tends to heal earlier. As the first ring of advancing infection continues to spread outwards, it may become surrounded by one or more concentric rings or arcuate patterns (Fig. 5.12). Adjacent lesions may fuse producing gyrate patterns. The lesions of tinea corporis are often more extensive but less obvious in immunosuppressed individuals.

Clinical variants of tinea corporis include tinea profunda, Majocchi's granuloma and tinea imbricata.

1. *Tinea profunda* results from an excessive inflammatory response to a dermatophyte (analogous to a kerion on the scalp) (Fig. 5.13). It may have a granulomatous or verrucous appearance and be

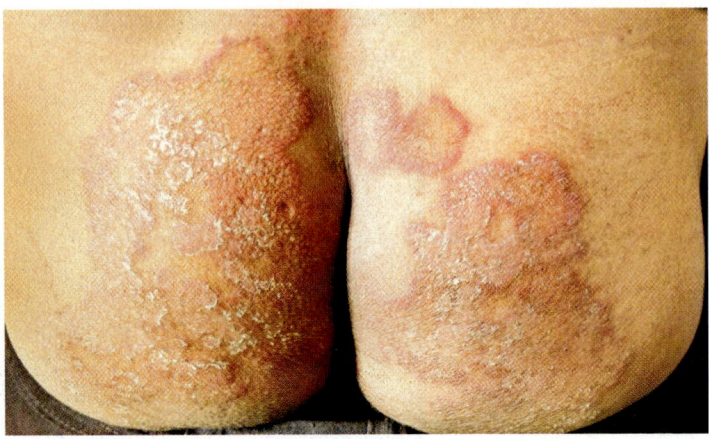

Fig. 5.12: A classical case of tinea corporis showing erythematous raised scaly advancing margins with central clearing showing increased activity of the fungus at the margins, active host immune response clears the fungus from the centre

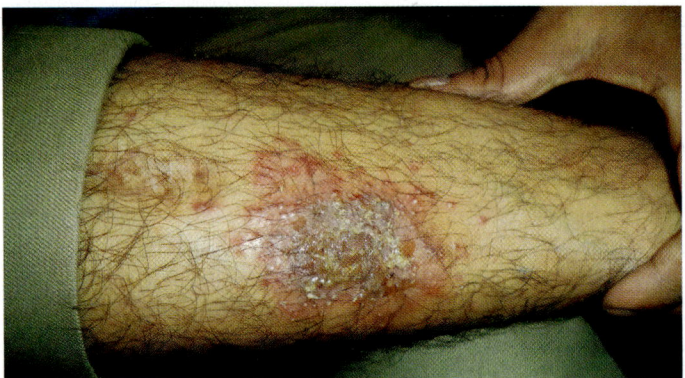

Fig. 5.13: An inflammatory tinea corporis with aggregated pustules (a case of tinea profunda)

mistaken for cutaneous tuberculosis, a dimorphic fungal infection or squamous cell carcinoma.

2. *Deep inflammatory lesions.* Zoophilic fungi such as *Trichophyton verrucosum* (barn itch) from cattle may produce a very inflammatory skin infection. The round, intensely inflamed lesion has a uniformly elevated, red, boggy, pustular surface. The pustules are follicular and represent deep penetration of the fungus into the hair follicle. (Fig. 5.10). Secondary bacterial infection can occur.

3. A distinctive form of inflammatory tinea called Majocchi's granuloma, caused by *T. rubrum* and other species, was originally

described as occurring on the lower legs of women who shave, but it is also seen at other sites in men and children. The primary lesion is a follicular papulopustule or inflammatory nodule (Fig. 5.14a). Intracutaneous and subcutaneous granulomatous nodules arise from these initial inflammatory tinea infections. Superficial dermatophytosis with subsequent deep infiltration of mycelia along hair follicles results in their rupture leading to a granulomatous follicle-associated inflammatory reaction. It particularly affects immunosuppressed patients, e.g. following a cardiac transplant. In most cases of Majocchi granuloma, *T. rubrum* is the causal pathogen, but other dermatophytes have also been described, e.g. *T. tonsurans* as pathogen of tinea corporis gladiatorum clinically presenting as Majocchi granuloma.

It has been described in patients on steroid therapy, specially rheumatology cases. Thus Majocchi variant is commonly seen in India due to the rampant topical steroid abuse. Also the use of topical corticosteroids may mask the diagnosis by altering the presenting features while the infection persists and is one of the commonest causes of persistent tinea infections. It presents with erythematous plaques or patches that reveal scattered papules (Fig. 5.14b), papulonodules (Fig. 5.14c), or pustules (Fig. 5.14d) studding the surface. If observed early in the course of the process, a hair may be noted in the center of the papular or pustular lesions.

4. *Tinea imbricata* (Tokelau) resulting from *T. concentricum*, an anthropophilic dermatophyte found in Southern Asia. The infection begins as a scaly ring; centrifugal spread follows, but within the area of central clearing a second wave of scaling soon arises (Fig. 5.15). The process is repeated to give numerous concentric rings and the whole body may become affected are prolonged clinical cause. Pruritus is intense and may lead to lichenification. Lesions may heal with hypopigmentation.

Treatment

The treatment protocol is summarized below:

The mild localised superficial lesions of tinea corporis respond to the antifungal creams after 2 weeks of twice-a-day application, but treatment should be continued for at least 1 week after resolution of the infection.

Extensive superficial lesions or those with papules respond more predictably to oral therapy.

Duration of therapy may vary depending on the clinical type. Thus, in cases of suspected steroid use, a duration of 4–6 weeks is advised.

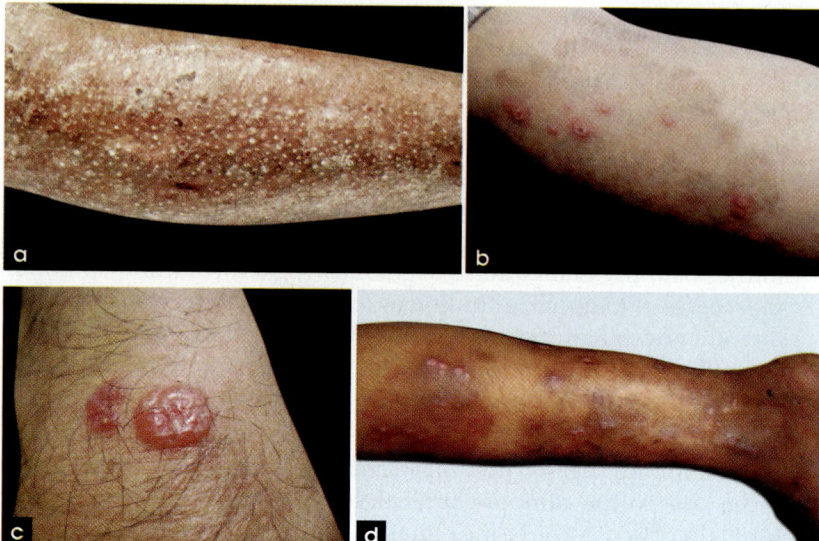

Fig. 5.14a to d: (a) A distinctive form of inflammatory tinea called Majocchi's granuloma, caused by *T. rubrum* and other species, with follicular papulopustules that are variably itchy; (b) A case of tinea where the use of OTC steroids have cleared the eruption but has led to a follicular invasion leading to papules; (c) A single papulonodule that responded to itraconazole 100 mg for 3 weeks; (d) A case of Majocchi granuloma that was treated as a case of MRSA, note the annular outline and the papulonodules in the periphery

Widespread disease

First line
1. Terbinafine 250 mg daily for 2 to 3 weeks
2. Itraconazole 100 mg daily for 2 to 4 weeks

Second line
1. Griseofulvin, 1 gram once daily for 4 weeks
2. Itraconazole 200 mg daily for 7 days
   or
   100 mg twice daily immediately after meals on days 1 and 8 or on days 1 and 2 may also be effective.
3. Fluconazole 50 to 100 mg daily or 150 mg once weekly for 2 to 4 weeks

Localized disease, recent onset
· Topical terbinafine twice daily for 2 weeks
  or
· Topical azole once or twice daily for 2–4 weeks

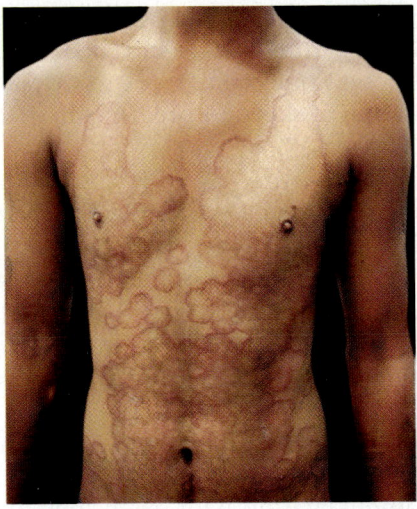

Fig. 5.15: A case of tinea imbricata. The classical presentation as seen here is of numerous concentric rings consequent to the formation of a second wave of ring within the zone of clearing as the centrifugal spread occurs. Such patients will have a long duration of disease and lesions might heal with hypopigmentation

Deep inflammatory lesions (Fig. 5.14) require 1 to 3 or more months of oral therapy. Bacterial superinfection is treated with the appropriate oral antibiotics. In case of highly inflammatory tinea (e.g. tinea verrucosum), the intense inflammatory response destroys the organisms and oral antifungals may not be required. As with tinea capitis kerion infections, a short course of prednisone may be considered for such patients.

TINEA MANUUM (TINEA OF THE HAND)
Definition
Tinea of the palmar aspect of the hand (tinea manuum).

Organism
Most common causative anthropophilic dermatophytes are *Trichophyton mentagrophytes* var. *interdigitale*, *T. rubrum* and *Epidermophyton floccosum*. Two non-dermatophyte fungi that cause "tinea manuum" are *Scytalidium dimidiatum* and *S. hyalinum*.

Most common causative zoophilic dermatophytes are *Microsporum canis* (cats and dogs), *T. verrucosum* (cattle), *T. mentagrophytes* var. *mentagrophytes* (rodents) and *T. erinacae* (hedgehogs). Occasionally infections can be seen due to geophilic *M. gypseum* and *M. fulvum*.

Acquired by contact with infected person, animal, soil or fomites, or by autoinoculation from another infected body site. Profuse sweating and eczema predisposes to infection. Wearing of wrist watches and rings also causes maceration of skin and predisposition to tinea.

Clinical Features

Usually unilateral, predominantly affecting right hand. It is commonly associated with tinea pedis.

- *Two forms:* Dyshidrotic (eczematoid) and hyperkeratotic:
  1. *Dyshidrotic:* Annular or segmental vesicles with scaling borders containing clear, viscous fluid on palms, palmar aspect of fingers and sides of the hand, characterized by intense pruritus and burning.
  2. *Hyperkeratotic:* Adjacent vesicles desquamate to form an erythematous, scaling lesion with a circular or irregular thick, white, squamous margin with extensions towards the centre. Chronic cases may cover the entire palm and fingers with fissuring in the palmar creases (Fig. 5.16).

Treatment

Treatment is the same as that for tinea pedis and, as with the soles, a high recurrence rate can be expected for palm infection.

Preventive measures include use of separate towels for hands and feet as the prevalence of *T. pedis* is directly related to that of *T. manuum.*

Treatment with imidazole or allylamine is often effective. Chronic ringworm infections of the palm are not easily cleared, and oral therapy is always needed. Itraconazole and terbinafine are both effective in this condition. Most cases clear with 2–4 weeks of treatment although it may be advisable to review the results a few months after the end of treatment. With griseofulvin, longer periods of treatment are necessary. Many patients will require 3 months of therapy and may even relapse after that. The treatment protocols used are:

1. Itraconazole 200–400 mg/day for 1 week
2. Terbinafine 250 mg/day for 2–6 weeks.

TINEA CRURIS

Definition

Infection of the skin of the groin and pubic region with a dermatophyte.

Tinea of the groin (tinea cruris, "jock itch" or dhobie's itch) occurs often in the summer months after sweating or wearing wet clothing and in the winter months after wearing several layers of clothing.

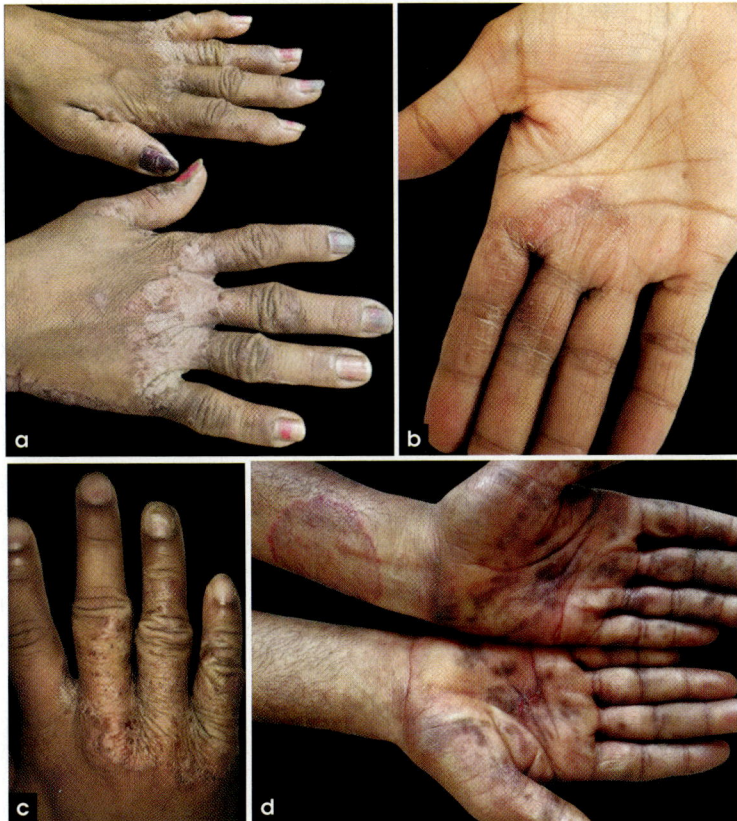

Fig. 5.16a to d: Tinea manuum. (a) Inflammatory tinea corporis on dorsa of hands of a 30-year-old female. Always examine nails and palms in such a case to look for presence of fungus there. Also note that lesions on dorsa of hands are included in corporis and not manuum. (b) A case of tinea manuum present on palmar aspect of right hand characterized by an erythematous scaly plaque with prominent borders. Sometimes vesicles may be seen on the margins of lesion which eventually desquamate to leave behind scaling. (c) A case of tinea manuum with concomitant involvement of nails and dorsa of hands. Always examine nails in any case of tinea manuum as if concominant tinea ungium is present patient should be prescribed longer treatment course as for tinea ungium. (d) An unusual case of tinea manuum presenting with hyperkeratotic bilateral symmetrical scaly plaques. It could be mistaken for a form of hand dermatitis but the concomitant presence of tinea corporis on forearm (as seen in picture) and a history of nonresponse to topical steroid therapy are important pointers to diagnosis. Thus, though asymmetry is a feature of tinea, sometimes bilateral lesions may be present

Predisposing Factors

The presence of a warm, moist environment, autoinfection from foot to groin, sharing of towels and sports clothings and wearing jeans in hot climate.

Men are affected much more frequently than women; children rarely develop tinea of the groin. Itching worsens as moisture accumulates and macerates this intertriginous area.

Organism

Anthropophilic dermatophytes: Epidermophyton floccosum and *Trichophyton rubrum* are most common. The infection is often transferred from another infected body site.

Clinical Features

The duration of infection depends on the causative pathogen. Infections with *T. rubrum* and many other anthropophilic species tend to be chronic (sometimes even leathery and lichenified) (Fig. 5.17a) and tend to extend to buttocks, lower abdomen and trunk, while the zoophilic form of *T. mentagrophytes* (var. *mentagrophytes*) and *T. interdigitale* often cause acute infections with a prominent inflammatory component (with or without pustules) and vesiculations.

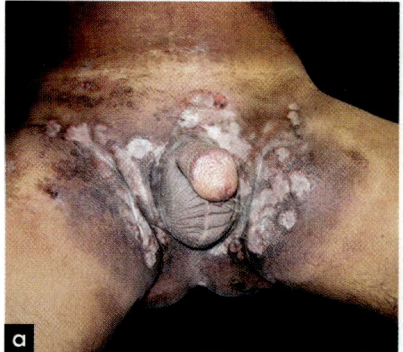 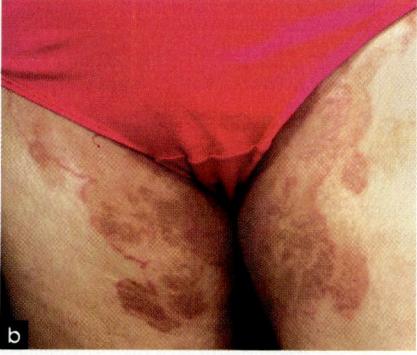

Fig. 5.17a and b: (a) A case of recalcitrant tinea cruris in a patient . Note the lichenified look and the sparing of the scrotum. This "look" is classic of *T. rubrum* infections and these infections are chronic in nature as the organism tends to subvert the Th1 response and the increased Th2 response leads to persistence of infection. The scratching instigated by the Th2 response causes the lichenified look. (b) A case of tinea cruris presenting with an erythematous plaque with red-brown less scaly centre. Red papules at the margins and within the plaque are suggestive of dermal nodules seen in chronic infection with *T. rubrum*

The lesions are mostly unilateral and begin in the crural fold. A half-moon-shaped plaque forms with well-defined scaling border, and sometimes a vesicular border advances out of the crural fold onto the thigh (Fig. 5.17b). The skin within the border turns red-brown, is less scaly, and may develop red papules. Acute inflammation may appear after a person has worn occlusive clothing for an extended period. The infection occasionally migrates to the buttock and gluteal cleft area.

Differential Diagnosis

1. *Candidosis:* Involvement of the scrotum is unusual—unlike Candida reactions, in which it is common
   - More common in women
   - Does not have a distinct raised margin.
   - White pustules are found which ruptures to form frayed, peeling edge
   - Numerous, small satellite lesions
2. Intertrigo
3. Erythrasma
4. Flexural psoriasis
5. Seborrheic dermatitis—other site involvement
6. Atopic eczema—shows lichenification
7. Others—contact dermatitis, Hailey-Hailey disease and flexural Darrier's disease.

Treatment

Topical

Lesions may appear to respond quickly, but creams should be applied twice a day for at least 10 days. The fungicidal allylamines (naftifine and terbinafine) and butenafine (allylamine derivative) allow a shorter duration of treatment compared with fungistatic azoles (clotrimazole, econazole, etoconazole, oxiconazole, miconazole, and sulconazole).

Moist intertriginous lesions may be contaminated with dermatophytes, other fungi, or bacteria. Antifungal creams with activity against Candida and dermatophytes (e.g. miconazole) are useful. Any residual inflammation from the intertrigo is treated with a group V through VII topical steroid twice a day for a specified length of time (e.g. 5 to 10 days). Absorbent powders, not necessarily medicated (e.g. Z-Sorb), help to control moisture but should not be applied until the inflammation is gone.

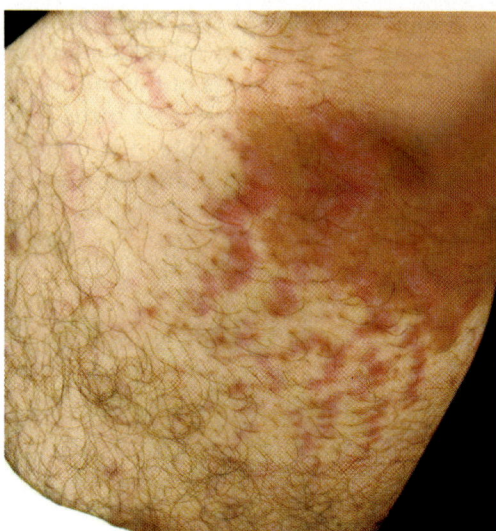

Fig. 5.18: A case of tinea cruris who was applying 'Dipsalic' for 3 weeks. Note the striae, consequent to this use and the lax implementation of the Schedule 'H' labeling of topical steroids in India

A topical steroid antifungal cream combination (betamethasone dipropionate/clotrimazole) may be used for initial treatment if lesions are red, inflamed, and itchy. A pure antifungal cream should be used once symptoms are controlled. Prolonged use of this steroid/antifungal preparation may not cure the infection and may cause striae at this site (Fig. 5.18).

Measures to prevent recurrences of tinea cruris include wearing loose clothing, drying thoroughly after bathing, using topical powders, weight reduction (if obese), laundering contaminated clothing and linens, and treating concomitant tinea.

Systemic therapy is often necessary.

1. Tinea cruris is effectively treated by 50 to 100 mg of fluconazole daily or 150 mg once weekly for 2 to 3 weeks.
2. Itraconazole 100 mg twice daily immediately after meals on days 1 and 8 or on days 1 and 2 may be effective. The standard treatments are itraconazole 100 mg daily for 2 weeks or 200 mg daily for 7 days.
3. Terbinafine 250 mg daily for 1 to 2 weeks. Griseofulvin 500 mg daily for 4 to 6 weeks is also effective.

As has been mentioned previously, a longer duration may be needed (up to 4–6 weeks), but higher dose (200 mg BD) for a longer duration (6 weeks) is strictly off label as itraconazole does *not* follow a linear dose PK kinetics, hence higher doses are of a little use. As the drug has a time dependent kinetics twice a day itraconazole makes more pharmacological sense, converse to the industries exhortations in their visual aids!

TINEA INCOGNITO

Definition

Tinea modified by use of corticosteroids (systemic or topical).

Clinical Features

Fungal infections treated with topical steroids often lose some of their characteristic features. Topical steroids decrease inflammation and give the false impression that the rash is improving while the fungus flourishes secondary to cortisone-induced immunologic changes. Treatment is stopped, the rash returns, and memory of the good initial response prompts reuse of the steroid cream, but by this time the rash has changed.

Tinea incognito, recently also termed tinea atypica, displays many overlapping features with the *T. rubrum* syndrome. There has been a worldwide increase in tinea incognito. On one hand, this may be attributed to an actual increase in the number of patients prone to contract extensive tinea corporis. On the other hand, however, it has to be critically noted that abandonment of a targeted mycologic workup mirrors the lack of differential diagnostic consideration of dermatomycosis in the first place. In India, however, rampant steroid use is the main cause.

The various *atypical* morphologies include (Fig. 5.19):
1. Scaling at the margins may be absent.
2. Diffuse erythema, diffuse scale, scattered pustules or papules, and brown hyperpigmentation (bruise-like) may result.
3. A well-defined border may not be present and localized process may have expanded greatly.

The intensity of itching is variable. Tinea incognito is most often seen on the groin, on the face, and on the dorsal aspect of the hand. Tinea infections of the hands are often misdiagnosed as eczema and treated with topical steroids. Hyphae are easily demonstrated, especially a few days after discontinuing use of the steroid cream when scaling reappears.

Treatment

Whatever site is affected, it is often best to treat steroid-modified ringworm with oral therapy, allowing a few applications of topical

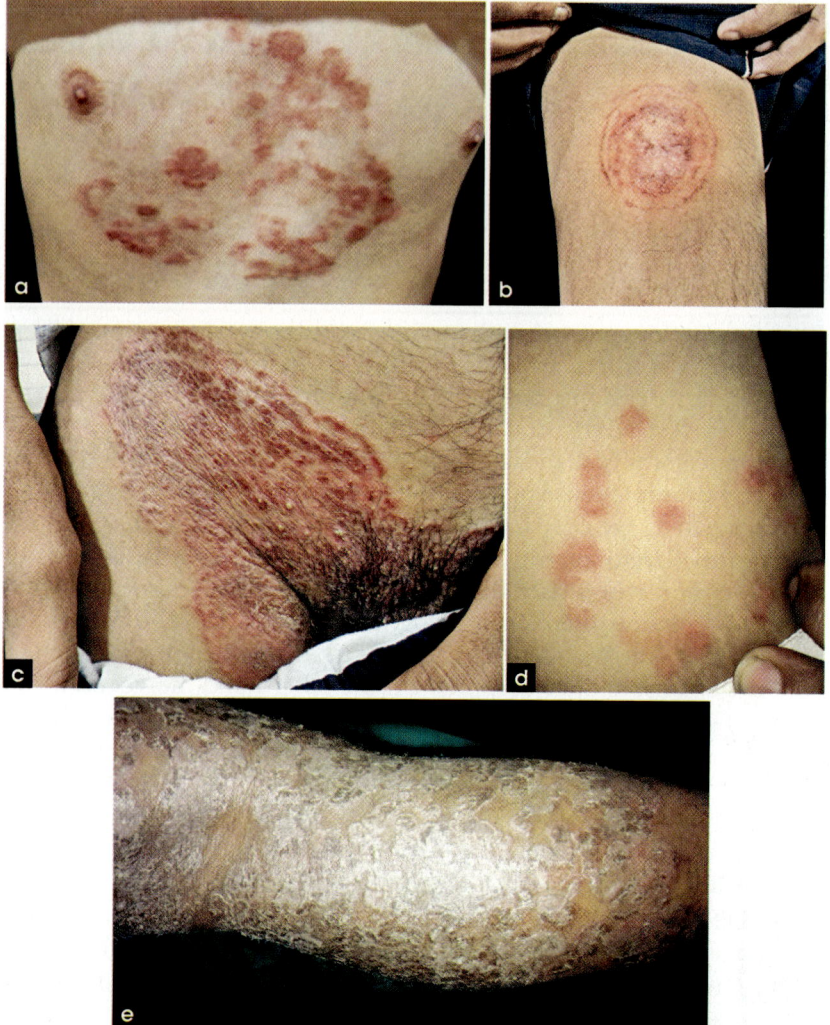

Fig. 5.19a to e: Tinea incognito. These represent various spectrums of steroid modified tinea which is the cause of most so-called "resistant" cases. (a) Multiple rings with little itching; (b) A case of tinea with multiple rings and follicular lesions which is a classic manifestation of tinea incognito with a Majocchi granuloma. (c and d) Cases with steroid abuse leading to red papules and pustules. (e) Diffuse scaly plaque—a case of atypical tinea corporis

steroid to continue until the terbinafine or itraconazole has begun to take effect. It is wise to use 1% hydrocortisone cream or at least a weaker steroid than that originally prescribed, and also to warn the patient about a possible rebound in spite of these measures. Follow-up to ensure steroid cream has been stopped and cure infection is mandatory. Systemic antifungal therapy may be indicated due to deep involvement of the hair apparatus. A standard dose but prolonged duration (6 weeks) is the dictum.

TINEA PEDIS

Definition

Dermatophyte infection of the feet.

The occurrence of tinea pedis seems to be inevitable in immunologically predisposed individuals regardless of elaborate precautions taken to avoid the infecting organism. Locker-room floors contain fungal elements, and the use of communal baths may create an ideal condition for repeated exposure to infected material. White socks do nothing to prevent tinea pedis. Once established, the individual becomes a carrier and is more susceptible to recurrences.

This condition is more common in adults than children and is found around the worldwide, affecting both sexes. The lack of sebaceous glands and the moist environment created by occlusive shoes are important factors in the development of tinea pedis.

Organism

Trichophyton rubrum is the most common cause. *Epidermophyton floccosum* and *T. mentagrophytes* var. *interdigitale* are also seen. It is often

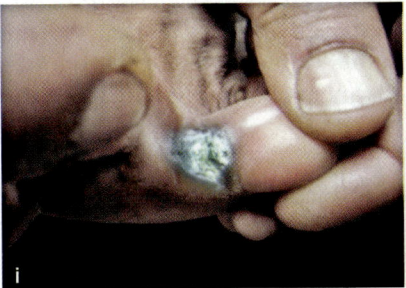 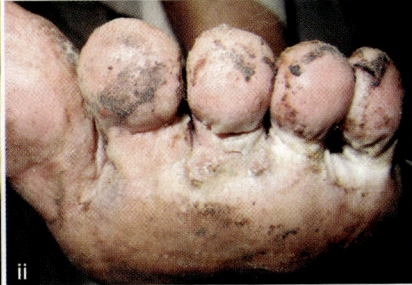

Fig. 5.20a: (i) Tinea pedis (toe web infection). Note the macerated look that involves the toe web. Note that such sites require an antibiotic course apart from an antifungal. Most of these are ignored and we have seen admissions of recurrent cellulitis where the route of entry was the toe web untreated for its fungal etiology. (ii) In some cases of tinea pedis a mild dermatophyte infection (dermatophytosis simplex) can induce damage to the stratum corneum, which allows overgrowth of resident bacteria and maceration, itching, and often malodor at the site (dermatophytosis complex)

contracted by walking barefoot on contaminated floors. Extensive sweating and occlusive footwear predispose to the condition. Infection with the moulds *Scytalidium dimidiatum* (*Hendersonula toruloidea*) and *S. hyalinum* is clinically indistinguishable. Occasionally, Candida spp. has been implicated (interdigital type).

Clinical Features

Three types are recognized:

- Acute or chronic interdigital infection: Itching, peeling, maceration and fissuring of toe webs (Fig. 5.20a and b)

  Tight fitting shoes compress the toes, creating a warm, moist environment in the toe webs; this environment is suitable for fungal growth. The web between the fourth and fifth toes is most commonly involved, but all webs may be infected. As allured to earlier this is rarely seen in farmers and labourers who walk barefoot but is seen in urban dwellers who wear shoes, usually all the time!

  The web can become dry, scaly, and fissured or white, macerated, and soggy. Itching is most intense when the shoes and socks are removed. The bacterial flora is unchanged when the tinea infected webs demonstrate scale and peeling without maceration. Overgrowth of the resident bacterial population determines the severity of interdigital toe web infection. The macerated pattern of infection occurs from an interaction of bacteria and fungus. The prevalence of *Staphylococcus aureus*, Gram-negative bacteria, *Corynebacterium minutissimum*, *Staphylococcus epidermidis*, and *Micrococcus sedentarius* increases. Extension out of the web space onto the plantar surface or the dorsum of the foot is common and occurs with the typical, chronic, ringworm type of scaly, advancing border or with an acute, vesicular eruption.

- *Chronic hyperkeratotic* (*moccasin or dry type*): Fine, white scaling limited to heels, soles and lateral borders of feet is plantar seen in hyperkeratotic or moccasin-type tinea pedis and is a particularly chronic form of tinea that is resistant to treatment (Fig. 5.20c). The entire sole is usually infected and covered with a fine, silvery white scale. The hands may be similarly infected. It is rare to see both palms and soles infected simultaneously; rather, the pattern is infection of two feet and one hand or of two hands and one foot. *Trichophyton rubrum* is the usual pathogen. This pattern of infection is difficult to eradicate. *T. rubrum* produces substances that diminish the immune response and inhibit stratum corneum turnover.

- *Vesicular (inflammatory) infection:* Vesicle formation occurs on soles, instep and interdigital cleft. A highly inflammatory fungal infection

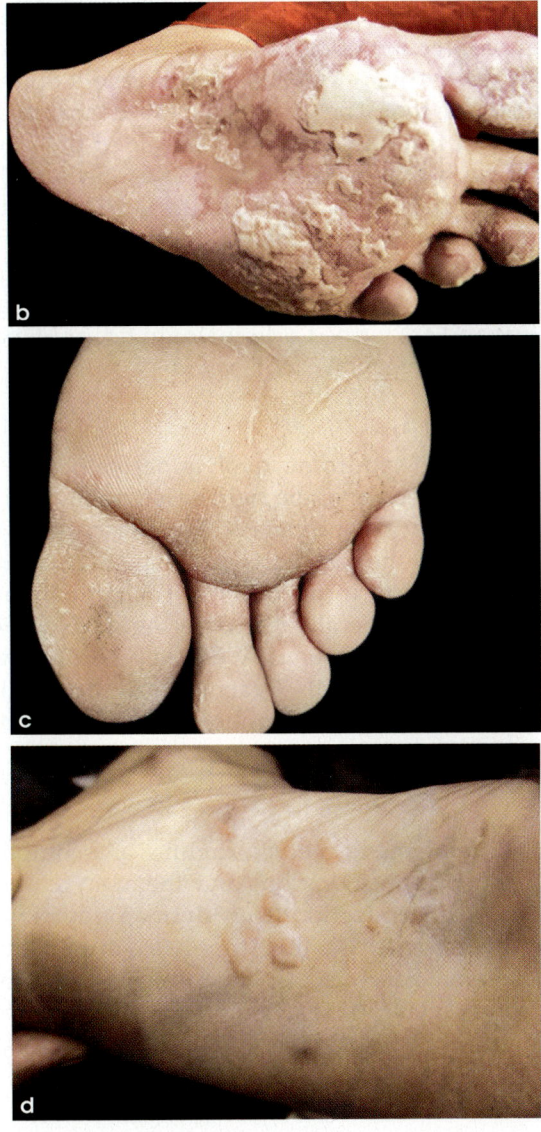

5.20b to d: (b) A macerated tinea pedis in a military jawan, desirous of a well-deserved medical rest. Patients usually have hyperhidrosis and can be given oxybutynin 2.5 mg twice a day apart from the antifungal drug. (c) The entire plantar surface is covered by diffuse white scale (Mocassin-type). (d) A case with recurrent relatively asymptomatic bullae, which worsened on sweating, an initial diagnosis of EB 'weber cockayne' was kept, but the biopsy revealed an hyphae and the patient responded to terbinafine may occur, particularly in people who wear occlusive shoes. This acute form of infection often originates from a more chronic web infection. A few or many vesicles evolve rapidly on the sole or on the dorsum of the foot. The vesicles may fuse into bullae or remain as collections of fluid under the thick scale of the sole and never rupture through the surface (Fig. 5.20d). Secondary bacterial infection occurs commonly in eroded areas after bullae rupture. A second wave of vesicles may follow shortly in the same areas or at distant sites such as the arms, chest, and along the sides of the fingers. These itchy sterile vesicles represent an allergic response to the fungus and are termed a dermatophytid, or id reaction. They subside when the infection is controlled.

Two Feet-One Hand Syndrome

The two feet-one hand syndrome involves dermatophyte infection of both feet and tinea infection of the right or left palm. Nail infection of the hands and feet may also be present. Most cases occur in men. The same organism infects the feet, hand, and nails. *Trichophyton rubrum* is the causative organism in most cases. The development of tinea pedis/onychomycosis generally precedes the development of tinea of the hand. Tinea manuum usually develops in the hand used to excoriate the feet or pick toenails. Patients whose occupation involves a high intensity of hands usage are more likely to develop the disease at an earlier age.

Complications

Each type has different associated morbidities and complications that can affect diagnostic considerations and therapeutic options. These include bacterial superinfection (the "dermatophytosis complex"), dermatophytid reactions, cellulitis (especially in patients who have venous hypertension, harvested saphenous veins and chronic edema), and even osteomyelitis leading to amputation in diabetics.

Treatment

Systemic

First line
1. Terbinafine 250 mg daily for 2 weeks
2. Itraconazole 400 mg daily for 1–2 weeks

Second line
1. Itraconazole 200 mg twice a day for 1 week
2. Pulse doses of fluconazole 150 mg orally once weekly

Topical

1. Terbinafine 1% cream applied twice daily for 1 week results in a high cure rate in interdigital tinea pedis. In one series, terbinafine gave progressive mycologic improvement; at 5 weeks after treatment, 88% of the patients were clear of infection. Effective short-course therapy with potent fungicidal drugs such as terbinafine may avoid treatment failure caused by noncompliance with fungistatic agents, such as clotrimazole, that require 4 weeks of treatment. In a gel preparation the active substance is rapidly transported into the skin, dries quickly after application, and is continuously released from the formed film over a period of up to four days. During this time, there is a 'depot effect' in the stratum corneum due to the lipophilicity of terbinafine. After a single application, terbinafine is detectable in the stratum corneum in fungicidal concentrations for up to 13 days.

2. Butenafine applied twice daily for 1 week is also highly effective in treating interdigital tinea pedis.

3. Econazole nitrate has activity against several bacterial species associated with severely macerated interdigital web spaces.

4. Sertaconazole nitrate 2% cream applied only once daily for four weeks also proved to be rapidly and adequately effective. Pruritus was significantly reduced after only two weeks of treatment.

It must be noted as many non-dermatophyte species cause tinea pedis, thus an azole may be preferred over terbinafine (Table 5.3).

The duration of therapy may need to be prolonged and though an off label advise, it can be extended to 4–6 weeks.

A summary of the organisms causing the various types of fungal infections and the treatment is given in Table 5.3.

Hyperkeratotic, moccasin-type tinea of the plantar surface responds slowly to conventional therapy. Oral terbinafine 125 mg daily for 4 weeks produced sustained cure rates of 95%. Griseofulvin 250 to 500 mg twice a day for 6 weeks resulted in a 27 to 35% cure rate. Speaking from our own experience, plantar hyperkeratotic tinea pedis can definitively be cured only by systemic antimycotic therapy. The current therapeutic regimen includes terbinafine 250 mg daily for two weeks, or alternatively itraconazole 200 mg daily for four weeks.

Acute vesicular tinea pedis responds to wet soaks applied for 30 minutes several times each day. Oral antifungal drugs control the acute infection. Secondary bacterial infection is treated with oral antibiotics. A vesicular id reaction sometimes occurs at distant sites

Table 5.3: Overview of etiology and treatment of tinea pedis

Moccasin	Dermatophyte *Trichophyton rubrum* *Epidermophyton Floccosum* Non-dermatophytes *Scytalidium hyalinum* *S. dimidiatum*	Topical antifungal plus product with urea or lactic acid Azoles are preferred if non-dermatophytes are the cause
Interdigital	Dermatophyte *T. mentagrophytes* *Trichophyton rubrum* *Epidermophyton floccosum* Non-dermatophytes *Scytalidium hyalinum* *S. dimidiatum* *Candida* spp. *Fusarium* spp.	Antibiotics Terbinafine/Azoles
Inflammatory	*T. mentagrophytes* (var. *mentagrophytes*)	Topical antifungals

during an inflammatory foot infection. Wet dressings, group V topical steroids, and, occasionally, prednisone 20 mg twice a day for 8 to 10 days are required for control of id reactions.

Anti-inflammatory Treatment of Tinea Pedis

Some antimycotics such as *bifonazole*, per se have an anti-inflammatory component. Alternatively, a combination of an antimycotic and a corticosteroid may be successfully used in the topical treatment of inflammatory forms of tinea pedis. Fixed combinations of miconazole and fluprednidene-21-acetate, clotrimazole and betamethasone dipropionate, clotrimazole and hydrocortisone or clotrimazole plus prednisolone acetate plus an antiseptic (hexamidine diisethionate) are commercially available. Clinical studies on the combined use of an antimycotic agent plus a corticosteroid in inflammatory mycoses did *not* reveal any inferior results compared to monotherapy with the respective antimycotic. Though it has been shown that the use of combination products in the initial phase of inflammatory and eczematous mycoses was found to be advantageous, the treatment duration with the combined preparation should not exceed *two weeks* because of the corticosteroid component. In addition, imidazoles also exhibit good antimicrobial effects against Gram-positive bacteria (staphylococci and streptococci). This proves favorable, for instance, in tinea pedis complicated by secondary bacterial infections.

TINEA UNGUIUM (ONYCHOMYCOSIS)

Onychomycosis is a term used to encompass all fungal infections of the nail and includes those due to dermatophytes as well as non-dermatophytes. It is divided into seven patterns based upon the point of fungal entry into the nail unit (Fig. 5.21).

Patterns of Onychomycosis	Fungi
1. Distal and lateral subungual onychomycosis (DLSO)	Dermatophytes (*Trichophyton rubrum, T. mentagrophytes*), *Candida albicans, Fusarium* spp., *Neoscytalidium* spp., *Scopulariopsis brevicaulis*
2. Superficial onychomycosis (SO) (white or black):	Patchy *T. mentagrophytes, T. rubrum, Fusarium* spp., *Acremonium* spp., *Neoscytalidium* spp. Transverse *T. rubrum, Fusarium* spp.
3. Proximal subungual onychomycosis (PSO) (patchy, striate (transverse) and longitudinal)	*T. rubrum, Fusarium* spp.
4. Endonyx onychomycosis	*T. soudanense, T. violaceum*
5. Totally dystrophic onychomycosis	Dermatophytes, *C. albicans, Neoscytalidium* spp.
6. Mixed onychomycosis; examples include the following on the same nail: DLSO plus SO SO plus DLSO SO plus PSO DLSO plus PSO	*T. rubrum* *T. rubrum, Fusarium* spp. *T. rubrum* *T. rubrum, Fusarium* spp. *T. rubrum, T. rubrum*
7. Paronychia With onychomycosis (usually or PSO) Without onychomycosis	*Candida* spp., *Fusarium* spp., *Neoscytalidium* spp.

Organism

Tinea unguium refers specifically to dermatophyte infection of the nail unit. It occurs worldwide, affects men more often than women, and is frequently associated with chronic tinea pedis. Trauma and other

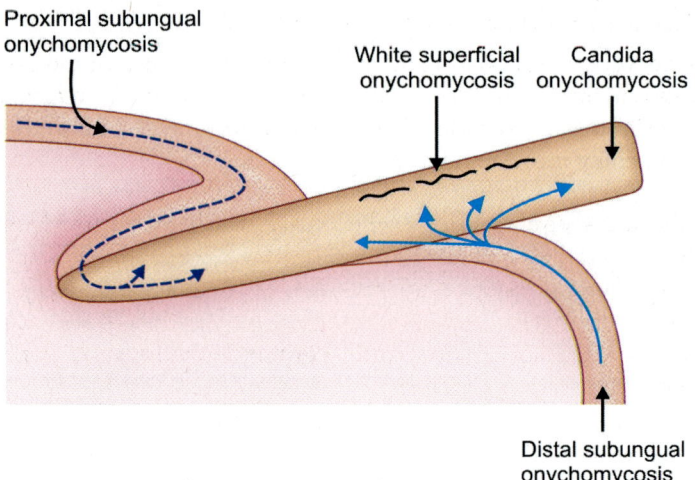

Fig. 5.21: A diagram depicting the patterns of onychomycosis based upon the point of fungal entry into nail unit

nail disorders represent predisposing factors. All dermatophytes can cause tinea unguium, but the most common causative pathogens are *T. rubrum*, *T. mentagrophytes* and *E. floccosum* (and, rarely, Microsporum spp.). Though dermatophytes account for ~90% of cases of onychomycosis, remainder are due to yeasts or non-dermatophyte molds (Table 5.4). *Candida* spp. are often found in association with chronic paronychia, and infection of the nail may occur in this setting. The fingernails are usually affected, with ridging, yellow discoloration and onycholysis. *Candida* spp. are a relatively common cause of onychomycosis in children less than 3 years of age, and nail involvement also represents a manifestation of chronic mucocutaneous candidiasis.

Table 5.4: Non-dermatophyte molds that can cause onychomycosis

Fungus	Key features
Fusarium spp.	Superficial white pattern
Aspergillus spp.	Superficial white pattern
Acremonium	Superficial white pattern
Scopulariopsis brevicaulis	Lateral yellow-brown discoloration KOH of nail reveals lemon-shaped conidia and atypical hyphae
Scytalidium hyalinum	Whitish discoloration of the nail
Scytalidium dimidiatum	Black discoloration of the nail

Predisposing Factors for Onychomycosis

1. **Genetic predisposition.** There is an autosomal dominant susceptibility to infection with *Trichophyton rubrum* onychomycosis. *Trichophyton rubrum* onychomycosis frequently occurs in several members of the same family in different generations. The infection is rare in persons marrying into infected families. Predisposed individuals may acquire *T. rubrum* infection in childhood from their infected parents. The infection remains asymptomatic and localized to the plantar region. Nail invasion begins in adult life, possibly from nail trauma.

2. Circulatory disorders (chronic venous insufficiency, peripheral arterial circulatory disorder)

3. *Local defects:* Malalignment of the feet including hallux valgus or hammer toe, toenail deformities/onychodystrophy, strong perspiration/hyperhidrosis pedum, lymphedema in the lower extremities

4. *Cutaneous disorders:* Psoriasis vulgaris and psoriasis unguium, ichthyosis vulgaris
   - Diabetes mellitus, immunosuppression (HIV/AIDS), patients with trisomy 21
   - Nail and nailbed microtrauma due to sporting activities.

Clinical Features

Distal Subungual Onychomycosis

Distal subungual onychomycosis is the most common pattern of nail invasion. Fungi invade the hyponychium, the distal area of the nail bed. The distal nail plate turns yellow or white as an accumulation of hyperkeratotic debris causes the nail to rise and separate from the underlying bed. Fungus grows in the substance of the plate, causing it to crumble and fragment (Fig. 5.22a). A large mass composed of thick nail plate and underlying debris may cause discomfort with footwear.

White Superficial Onychomycosis

This is caused by surface invasion of the nail plate, most often by *T. mentagrophytes*. The surface of the nail is soft, dry, and powdery and can easily be scraped away. (Fig. 22b) The nail plate is not thickened and remains adherent to the nail bed. There is a deep variant of white superficial onychomycosis (WSO). This occurs in the following three situations:

1. Mould infections (particularly *Fusarium* species and *Aspergillus* species infections),

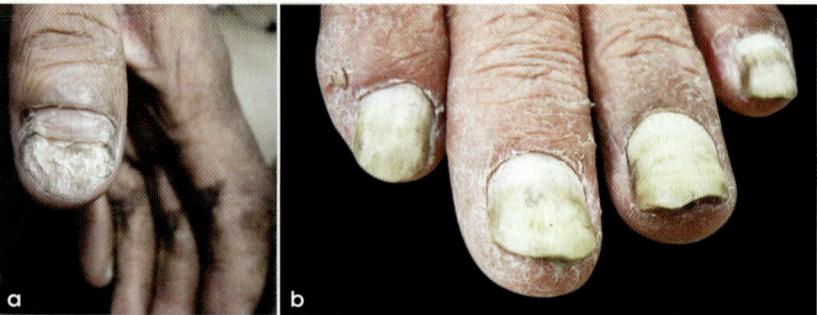

Fig. 5.22a and b: (a) A case of distal onychomycosis with loss of the distal nail plate and visible debris. (b) White superficial with proximal subungual onychomycosis

2. Children with Candida or *Trichophyton rubrum* infection, and
3. Immunocompromised patients with *T. rubrum* infection.

Deep WSO is characterized by diffuse involvement of the nail plate and the presence of fungi in both the superficial and the intermediate layers. WSO is a progressive disease that may infect the entire nail plate. Deep WSO infections require systemic therapy and may be less likely to respond to antifungal drugs.

Proximal Subungual Onychomycosis

Microorganisms enter the posterior nailfold-cuticle area, migrate to the underlying matrix, and finally invade the nail plate from below. Infection occurs within the substance of the nail plate, but the surface remains intact (Fig. 5.22c). Hyperkeratotic debris accumulates and causes the nail to separate. Transverse white bands begin at the proximal nail plate and are carried distally with outward growth of the nail plate. *T. rubrum* is the most common cause. This is the most common pattern seen in patients with AIDS.

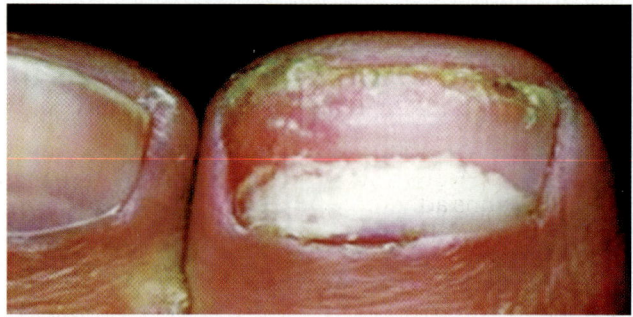

Fig. 5.22c: A case of proximal subungual onychomycosis

Candidal Onychomycosis

It is the nail plate infection caused by *C. albicans* (Fig. 5.21d and e) and the most florid manifestation is seen in chronic mucocutaneous candidiasis. It generally involves all the fingernails. The nail plate thickens and turns yellow-brown.

There are many other patterns of infection. Linear, yellow or dark brown streaks appear at the distal end and grow proximally in some patterns. In others, some or all of the nail plate may appear yellow; in these areas, the nail can be separated from the underlying bed.

Treatment

Oral Agents

Terbinafine, itraconazole, fluconazole.

Oral therapy is recommended when

- Involvement of > 50% of distal nail plate/multiple nail involvement
- Involvement of nail matrix
- Topical drug penetration is expected to be suboptimal.

These drugs penetrate keratinizing tissue. The levels reached in the nail plate exceed those in plasma. Therapeutic levels persist in the nails for at least 1 month after discontinuation of therapy. Terbinafine has higher cure rates and a slower relapse rate. Also itraconazole can influence the level of many drugs, whereas terbinafine is relatively free of interactions.

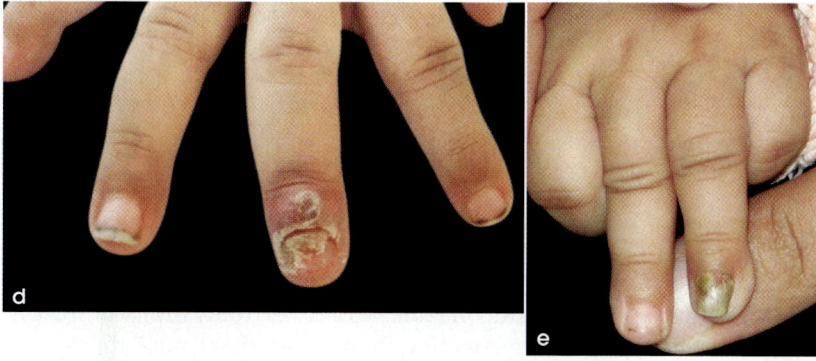

Fig. 5.22d and e: (d) Erythema and swelling of the nailfolds with onychomycosis, a case of candidal onychomycosis; (e) A case of congenital candidal onychomycoses treated with ciclopirox olamine 8% nail lacquer. (Sardana K *et al.* Br J Dermatol. March 2006; 154(3): 573–5.)

First line

1. Continuous terbinafine: It is the optimal therapy for onychomycosis. Continuous terbinafine 250 mg/day (for 6 weeks in fingernails and 3 months in toenails) is significantly more effective.
2. Intermittent itraconazole (400 mg/day for 1 week every 4 weeks for 2–3 months in fingernails and 3–4 months in toenails).

Second line

1. Griseofulvin 1 gm for 4–8 months.

It is less effective than the newer antifungal agents. Periodic debridement of infected nail during the course of treatment may increase the cure rate.

Some other regimens have been suggested for onychomycosis and are listed below:

Terbinafine	1. *Conventional regimen* 250 mg 12 weeks for toenail; 6 weeks for fingernail 2. *Intermittent regimen* 250 mg × 5–14 days, f/b 250 mg (1 tablet) weekly until clinical cure is achieved (recommendation level = "expert opinion") 3. *Pulse dose regimen* Terbinafine 250 mg daily for four weeks followed by a four-week interval, again followed by another four-week course
Itraconazole	1. *Interval therapy* (pulse therapy) 200 mg twice daily for one week, followed by an interval of 3 weeks 3 cycles (= 3 months), up to 4 intervals possible, shorter treatment possible for fingernails 2. *Continuous dose* 100 mg BD × 3 months

A recent comparative review of different treatment regimens in onychomycosis revealed that *terbinafine* 250 mg daily for 12 to 16 weeks resulted in *higher* clinical cure rates than *itraconazole* pulse therapy or weekly administration of fluconazole. Moreover, daily oral administration of terbinafine is more effective than terbinafine pulse therapy.

Topical Therapy

Indications for topical monotherapy include:

- Involvement limited to distal 50% of nail plate in 3 or 4 nails.
- No matrix area involvement.

- Superficial white onychomycosis (SWO).
- In children with thin, fast growing nails.
- As prophylaxis in patients at risk of recurrence.
- Patients where oral therapy is inappropriate.

Topical medications for onychomycosis are often unable to fully penetrate the nailplate and therefore, complete fungal eradication with these medications alone is difficult. For example, ciclopirox solution 8%, in a nail lacquer formulation applied daily to the entire nail and surrounding skin has a clinical cure rate of only 5. 5% after 48 weeks of therapy.

Amorolfine has been shown to persist in the nail plate significantly longer than ciclopirox, allowing a durable "reservoir effect" making once weekly application feasible. The clinical efficacy of amorolfine has been reported to be 75–80%.

Naftifine (Naftin), terbinafine (Lamisil), and ciclopirox (Loprox) creams similarly have low efficacy. Two recent studies of efinaconazole 10% solution, a triazole antifungal developed for distal lateral subungual onychomycosis (DLSO), showed complete cure rates of 17.8% and 15.2% after 48 weeks of use in patients with DLSO, suggesting that this medication may be more efficacious than other topical treatments.

Various other modified regimens have been suggested and are listed in Table 5.5.

Adjuvant Measures

a. *Mechanical reduction of infected nail plate.* A nail clipper with plier handles may be used to remove substantial amounts of hard, thick debris. One should insert the pointed tip of the instrument as far down as possible between the diseased nail and the nail bed. Adherent thick nail plate can be reduced by sanding or cutting the surface layers with the clippers. Removal of the infected nail may accelerate resolution of the infection.

b. *Surgical removal.* Painful or extremely infected nails (usually the nail of the first toe) can be removed by a simple surgical procedure.

c. *Nonsurgical avulsion of nail dystrophies.* If nails are very thick at baseline, consider occlusion with 40% urea cream under tape in addition to oral therapy. Symptomatic dystrophic nails may be painlessly removed with a urea compound. The technique has its greatest application in removing hypertrophic mycotic nails and can be used to treat other hypertrophic nail conditions, such as psoriatic nails. The procedure also facilitates subsequent treatment with topical antifungal agents. The technique removes only grossly

Table 5.5: Modified regimens for onychomycoses

Combination therapy	Sequential therapy	Supplementary	BOAT/BATT
The combination of oral and topical drugs may allow reduction in oral dosing resulting in increased patient tolerance and compliance while improving efficacy and reducing relapse.	Sequential therapy combines use of two oral antifungals acting on two different pathways in ergosterol metabolism	Supplementary therapy involves microscopic examination and culture at 24 weeks or 6 months following initiation of therapy and extended administration of oral antifungal (4 weeks of daily terbinafine or another pulse of itraconazole) in patients who are found positive.	The boosted oral antifungal treatment (**BOAT**) is designed to target dormant chlamydospores and arthroconidia within the nail plate in order to produce sensitive hyphae which are less refractory to antifungal treatment by securing a piece of SDA onto the affected nail plate for 48 hr following weekly pulse of itraconazole. Boosted antifungal topical treatment (**BATT**) is designed to improve the therapeutic efficacy of amorolfine nail lacquer in a similar way

diseased or dystrophic nails, not normal nails. Forty percent urea gel or cream is commercially available or by prescription.

d. *Lasers* are one of the devices that have gained FDA approval for the treatment of onychomycosis. Although the exact mechanism by which lasers treat onychomycosis is unknown, they are thought to have a fungicidal effect by exploiting the sensitivity of fungi to temperatures over 55°C. Both the neodymium-doped yttrium-aluminum-garnet (Nd: YAG) laser and diode laser are approved by the FDA for onychomycosis treatment; however, evidence-based data on the efficacy of these lasers are poor.

e. *Photodynamic therapy (PDT)* is also being investigated for the treatment of onychomycosis. PDT uses a spectrum of visible light to activate a topically applied photosensitizing agent, generating reactive oxygen species and inducing apoptosis. Several clinical trials have tested the efficacy of the heme biosynthesis inter-mediates 5-aminolevulinic acid and methyl aminolevulinate as photosensitizers for treating onychomycosis. Further studies are necessary to determine the exact clinical efficacy of this treatment method.

f. *Iontophoresis* uses a low-level electrical current to increase drug transport across a semipermeable barrier. Combining this technique with terbinafine therapy may optimize terbinafine's penetration of the nail bed and matrix, leading to higher cure rates of onychomycosis. Clinical trials on such devices are currently underway.

Response to Treatment

Cure of all 10 toenails may be unattainable even after all the measures are taken (Box 5.1). A nail plate with a normal appearance is not always attainable after a successful therapeutic onychomycosis regimen. Some residual change is likely after chronic infection. Successful eradication of the fungus may leave the nail abnormal and the residual changes may be unrelated to infection or be a result of damage to the nail unit from long-standing disease (e.g., onycholysis). Clinical and mycologic criteria are important to ascertain both the diagnosis and the resolution of onychomycosis. In severe cases of onychomycosis, up to 10% of the nail surface is likely to remain abnormal in appearance even when mycologic studies indicate a cure of fungal infection.

It takes 12 to 18 months for a newly formed toenail plate and 4 to 6 months for a fingernail to replace a diseased nail. Immediately after completion of therapy the nail usually does not appear to be clear

Box 5.1: Summary of measures to treat onychomycosis

1. Confirm the diagnosis (e.g. culture, nail biopsy) before systemic treatment.
2. Identify poor prognostic signs: thick nails, total onychodystrophy; poor perfusion, immunocompromised status, diabetes.
3. Debride and trim thick nails.
4. Treat tinea pedis, it is the likely reservoir for relapse.
5. Use antifungal spray or powders in shoes daily.
6. Treat close family contacts.
7. Keep feet cool and dry, wear "flip flops" at pools, in locker rooms.
8. Consider occasional pulse or "booster" therapy with a systemic agent to decrease the chance of relapse or re-infection. For example, treat at months 6 and 9 after a traditional 3 month systemic course for recalcitrant toenail disease.
9. Use poroper footwear: wide toe box; limit high heels or narrow-toed shoes, which cause micro- or macro-trauma to the normal nail barrier, breaking the seal between the nail plate and nailbed.
10. Trim toenails regularly, cutting straight across and not rounded or in a V-shape at the free margin.
11. Avoid sharing nail clippers and files.

of infection. A proximal area of normal-appearing nail, representing newly formed nail plate that is devoid of infection, may be present. Visible clearance of the infection will occur after the process of nail plate turnover is complete. If onychomycosis is suggested on the basis of clinical observation, diagnostic laboratory tests should be performed. If these produce negative findings, they should be repeated. Clinical manifestations of other nail disorders—such as psoriasis, neoplasms, and lichen planus-may mimic those of onychomycosis but can be diagnosed by nail-unit biopsy.

The factors that can determine a poor overall prognosis for ultimate cure of onychomycosis are given in Box 5.2 and Fig. 5.22f.

Recurrence Rates

The administration of systemic terbinafine to treat the first episode of onychomycosis may provide better long-term success than itraconazole.

Studies of terbinafine and itraconazole demonstrated that at 5 years, 23% of terbinafine-treated patients and 53% of itraconazole-treated patients experienced a relapse or reinfection, after achieving mycologic cure at 1 year. At 5-year follow-up, 13% of the itraconazole group and

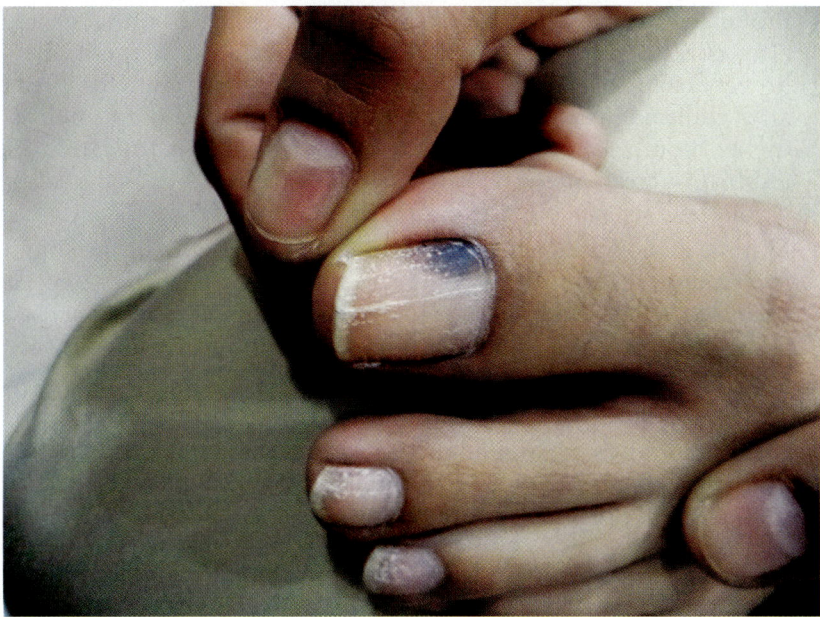

Fig. 5.22f: Longitudinal white streaks, a poor prognostic sign for onychomycosis

Box 5.2: Poor prognostic factors in the treatment success of onychomycosis
1. Area of nail involvement >50%
2. Significant lateral disease
3. Subungual hyperkeratosis >2 mm
4. White-yellow or orange-brown streaks in the nail
5. Total dystrophic onychomycosis (with matrix involvement)
6. Nonresponsive organisms (e.g. Scytalidium mould)
7. Patients with immunosuppression
8. Diminished peripheral circulation

46% of the terbinafine group remained disease-free. Another study showed that 11% of terbinafine responders showed evidence of relapse 18 to 21 months after cessation of treatment.

Patients treated with itraconazole or terbinafine who experience recurrence of onychomycosis can be retreated with response rates similar to those of the initial course.

Preventing Recurrence

- Preventing recurrence of tinea pedis may prevent recurrence of onychomycosis.

- Prolonged use of a topical antifungal agent applied around the toes, after clinical response of onychomycosis to an oral agent, may prevent nail reinfection. Use of a topical antifungal cream for 1 year after clinical cure of onychomycosis has prevented reinfection in the 12-month follow-up period. A twice weekly application of terbinafine cream in the nail area, between the toes and on the soles, would be a reasonable prevention program.
- Trauma to the tips of nails from tight-fitting shoes may be the single most important event for encouraging hyphae invasion in the region of the hyponychium that leads to distal subungual onychomycosis. Shoes or boots that create a confined, damp, and warm atmosphere facilitate the development of fungal infection.
- Protect feet in communal showers.
- Medicated powders applied directly to the toe webs and soles (not poured into shoes) will help maintain a dry environment but will probably not prevent recurrence.

CAUSES OF POOR CLINICAL RESPONSE TO ANTIFUNGAL DRUGS

A resistant infection is not the same as *in vitro* resistance and as actual *in vitro* resistance is uncommon most cases are best described as recalcitrant infections. The various drug related causes include:

1. Non-compliance failure to take the drug or taking reduced doses.
2. Drug lost/not absorbed from gut (vomiting or diarrhea)
3. Drug degraded by microsomal enzymes in liver
4. Drug-drug interactions:
   a. Taking itraconazole with antacid
   b. Displacement of protein bound drugs by other substance in circulation
   c. Enzyme inducers like phenobarbital, warfarin, cimetidine, rifampicin, etc. decreases the concentration of drug
5. Drug failing to reach the stratum corneum.
6. Drug reabsorbed or washed out of stratum corneum.
7. Relative or absolute microbial resistance
8. Associated co-morbidity like obesity, diabetes mellitus, HIV/AIDS, etc.

Drug Resistance

It is the ability of a microorganism to grow both *in vitro* and *in vivo* in the presence of an antibiotic that would be expected to kill or at least inhibit the organism. This phenomenon is sufficiently uncommon among dermatophytes to make routine testing necessary, but where treatment failure occurs without any other explanation, it is possible to estimate the sensitivity of the causal organism. This should be performed by a specialized laboratory. This can be classified as follows:

Clinical resistance: It is the failure to eliminate fungal infection, despite giving a drug with *in vitro* activity against the organism.

Microbiological resistance

1. *Primary (intrinsic):* It is present before exposure to antifungals, arising through the process of evolution.
2. *Secondary (acquired):* Develops after exposure to antifungals owing to stable or transient genotypic alterations.

Absolute resistance: No inhibition of fungal growth observed at highest concentration of drug.

Relative resistance: Organisms grow in low concentration of drug. This is important for griseofulvin, particularly with *T. rubrum* because griseofulvin is static fungi and not cidal fungi.

Molecular aspects in resistance development:

1. *Structural alterations or modifications in target enzymes.*
2. *Increased drug efflux:* Overexpression of genes encoding ATP-binding cassette (ABC) transporters leads to multi-drug resistance like phenomena in *T. rubrum*. The genes involved are: TruMDR1 gene-1511 aa protein and TruMDR2 gene-1331 aa protein.
3. *Stress response related proteins:* HSP (heat shock proteins) responds to a specific stress condition and that cohort of HSP facilitates fungal survival under various environmental challenges. Chemical inhibition of HSP 90 resulted in increased susceptibility of the fungus to itraconazole and micafungin, and decreased growth in human nails *in vitro*.
4. *Modification and degradation of drug*
5. *Biofilms:* These are differentiated masses of microbes that adhere to surfaces and are surrounded by a matrix of extracellular polymers, increasing resistance to standard drugs.
6. *Dermatophytoma:* It is a fungal ball formed by collection of fungal spores and filaments with sometimes biofilm formation within. They are refractory to standard antifungal drugs and thus need surgical removal of diseased nail.

(A detailed focus on recalcitrant dermatophyte infection follows in Chapter 5D).

Bibliography

1. Ardeshna KP, Rohatgi S, Jerajani HR. Successful treatment of recurrent dermatophytosis with isotretinoin and itraconazole. Indian J Dermatol Venereol Leprol 2016;82:579–582.

2. Arrese JE, Piérard GE. Treatment failures and relapses in onychomycosis: A stubborn clinical problem. Dermatology 2003;207:255–260.

3. Baran R, Hay R, Haneke E, Tosti A, editors. Onychomycosis: The current approach to diagnosis and therapy. London: Informa Healthcare; 2006.

4. Christopher E. M. Griffiths, Jonathan Barker, Tanya Bleiker, Rook's textbook of dermatology. 9th ed: 32. 49 Aptara Inc: New Delhi, India.

5. Cole GW, Stricklin G. A comparison of a new oral antifungal, terbinafine, with griseofulvin as therapy for tinea corporis. Arch Dermatol 1989;125:1537–1539.

6. Elewsld BE, Hazen PG. The superficial mycoses and the dermatophytes. J Am Acad Dermatol 1989;21:655–673.

7. Havlickova B, Czaika VA, Friedrich M. Epidemiological trends in skin mycoses worldwide. Mycoses 2008;51 Suppl 4:2;15.

8. Holmes JG, Gentles JC. Diagnosis of foot ringworm. Lancet 1956;271:62–63.

9. Kanafani, Zeina A Perfect, John R. Resistance to antifungal agents: mechanisms and clinical impact. 2008/01/01, clinical infectious diseases.

10. Kurade SM, Amladi SA, Miskeen AK. Skin scraping and a potassium hydroxide mount. Indian J Dermatol Venereol Leprol 2006;72:238–241.

11. Leyden JJ, Kligman AM. Interdigital athlete's foot. The interaction of dermatophytes and resident bacteria. Arch Dermatol 1978;114:1466–471.

12. Lowell A, Stephen IK. Fitzpatrick's dermatology in general medicine. 8th edn. New York: McGraw-Hill; 2012.

13. Nenoff P, Constanze K, Schaller J, et al. Mycology—an update Part 2: Dermatomycoses: Clinical picture and diagnostics. J Dtsch Dermatol Ges. 2014:12(9);749–777.

14. Nenoff P, Kruger C, Ginter-Hanselmayer G, et al. Mycology—an update Part 1: Dermatomycoses: causative agents, epidemiology and pathogenesis. J Dtsch Dermatol Ges 2014:12(3);188–209.

15. Odom R. Dermatologic manifestations of AIDS. J Am Podiatr Med Assoc 1988;78:127–129.

16. Rippon JW. Cutaneous infections: dermatophytosis and dermatomycosis. In: Medical mycology. The pathogenic fungi and the pathogenic actinomycetes. 3rd edn. Philadelphia: WB Saunders 1988;169–275.

17. Roberts SOB, Hay RJ, Mackenzie DWR. The superficial mycoses. In: A clinician's guide to fungal disease. New York: Marcel Dekker 1984;37–102.

18. Roderick J Hay, H Ruth Ashbee. Fungal Infections. Christopher EM Griffiths, Jonathan Barker, Tanya Bleiker. Rook's textbook of dermatology. 9th edn: 32. 49 Aptara Inc: New Delhi, India.

19. Sahai S, Mishra D. Change in spectrum of dermatophytes isolated from superficial mycoses cases: First report from Central India. Indian J Dermatol Venereol Leprol 2011;77:335–336.

20. Sahoo AK, Mahajan R. Management of tinea corporis, tinea cruris, and tinea pedis: A comprehensive review. Indian Dermatol Online J 2016;7:77–86.

21. Singal A, Khanna D. Onychomycosis: Diagnosis and management. Indian J Dermatol Venereol Leprol 2011;77:659–672.

22. Sinski JT, Kelley LM. A survey of dermatophytes from human patients in the United States from 1985 to 1987. Mycopathologia 1991;114:117–126.

23. Tainwala R, Sharma Y. Pathogenesis of dermatophytoses. Indian J Dermatol 2011;56:259–261.

24. Taplin D, Meinldng TL. Scabies, lice, and fungal infections. Prim Care 1989;16:551–568.

25. Walsh TJ, Viviani MA, Arathoon E, Chiou C, Ghannoum M. New targets and delivery systems for antifungal therapy. Med Mycol 2000;38 Suppl 1:335–347.

B. MALASSEZIA INFECTIONS: SKIN MANIFESTATIONS

TINEA VERSICOLOR/PITYRIASIS VERSICOLOR

Definition

Tinea versicolor is a chronic superficial fungal infection characterized by discrete or confluent scaly discoloured or hypopigmented areas on upper trunk, caused by members of the fungal genus Malassezia (Pityrosporum), which are considered normal skin flora (Fig. 5.22). Environmental and immunologic changes may cause conversion of the yeast form to the hyphal form leading to pigmentary changes in the skin.

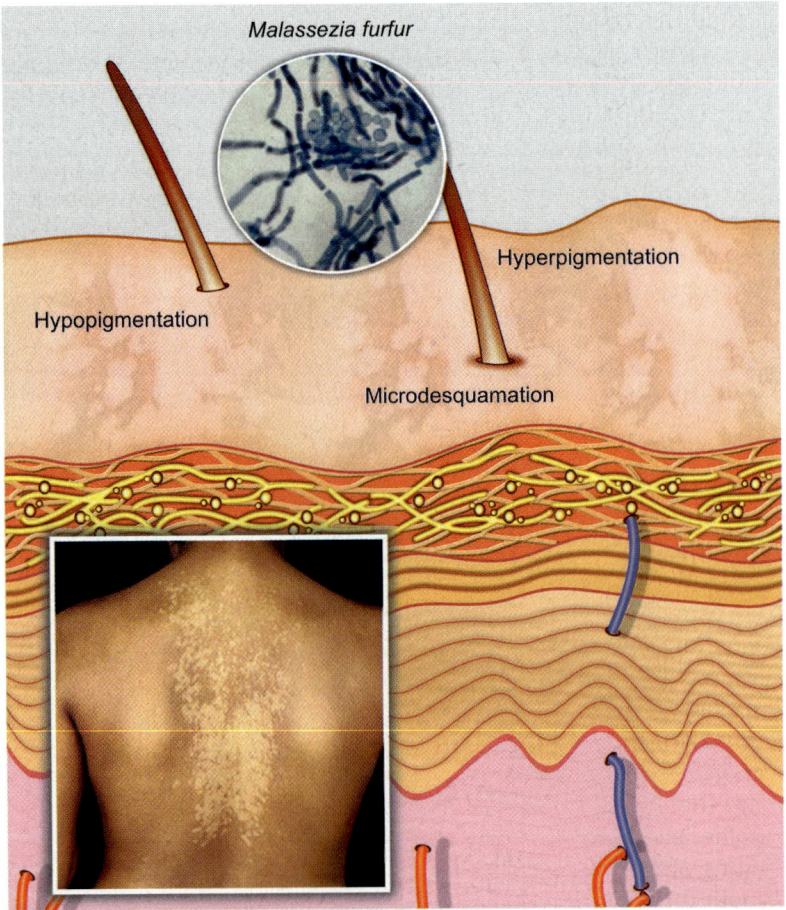

Fig. 5.23: A figurative depiction of the infections caused by Malassezia (pityriasis versicolor)

Causative Organism

It is caused by a group of lipophilic yeasts classified in the genus *Malassezia* which include various species like *M. sympodialis, M. globosa, M. restricta, M. slooffiae, M. furfur, M. obtuse, M. dermatis, M. japonica, M. yamotoensis, M. nana, M. caprae, M. equina* and *M. cuniculi.* The most common of these are *M. globosa* followed by *M. furfur* and *M. sympodialis.*

Epidemiology

The disease may occur at any age, but it is much more common during the years of higher sebaceous activity (i.e. adolescence and young adulthood). Some individuals, especially those with oily skin, may be more susceptible. Whether the disease is contagious is unknown but familial clustering is seen at times.

Certain predisposing endogenous factors (adrenalectomy, Cushing's disease, pregnancy, malnutrition, burns, corticosteroid therapy, depressed cellular immunity, oral contraceptives) or exogenous factors (excess heat, humidity) cause the yeast to convert from its budding yeast form to its mycelial form, leading to the appearance of tinea versicolor. Pityriasis versicolor does not appear to be more common in AIDS patients.

Clinical Features

The eruption is usually asymptomatic, although rarely mild pruritus may be noted. The primary lesion is a sharply demarcated macule, sometimes slightly erythematous, characterized by fine minimal scaling (Fig. 5.24a) which might be accentuated by firm scraping or stretching of the skin, or with a sticky tape strip. The eruption may form large confluent areas or scattered oval patches (Fig. 5.24b). Under the Wood's lamp, the scaly lesions may show pale yellow fluorescence. The cosmetic concern is on account of the lesions that vary in color from white and pink to light-brown (Fig. 5.24c) or fawn-colored lesions (term versicolor refers to varying color of the scales) on the upper trunk and neck, though rarely the face is also involved (forehead) (Fig. 5.25a). Facial lesions occur more commonly in children, and when seen in adults (Fig. 5.25b), women are affected more than men. Sometimes the limbs can also be affected. Patients usually present during summer months when the hypopigmented lesions are accentuated by tanning of surrounding normal skin. The residual depigmentation may remain for many months without any scaling. Malassezia species do not attack the hair shaft, nails or mucous membranes. Occasionally tinea corporis can be seen with pityriasis versicolor (Fig. 5.25c).

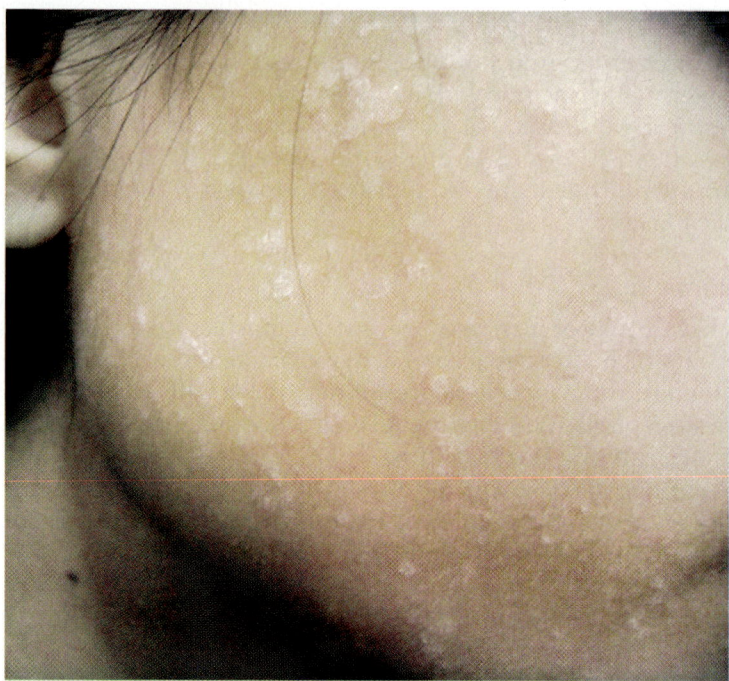

Fig. 5.24a: Pityriasis versicolor: Multiple scaly macules on the face of a adult female

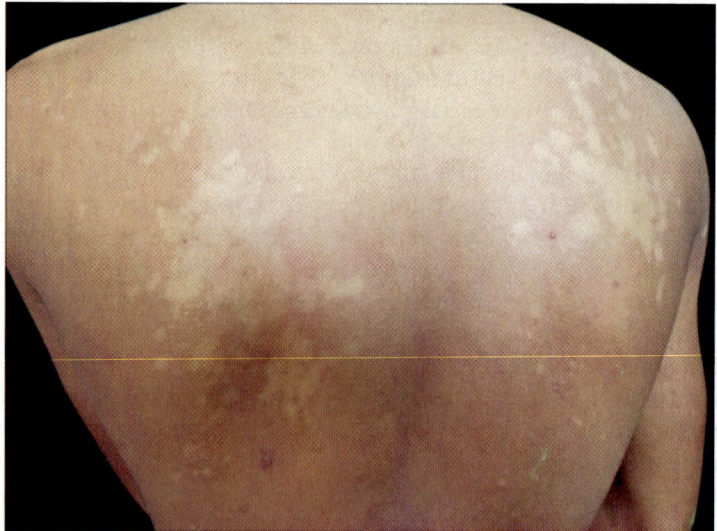

Fig. 5.24b: Depigmented well-circumscribed macules coalescing at places over back of a 25-year-old male

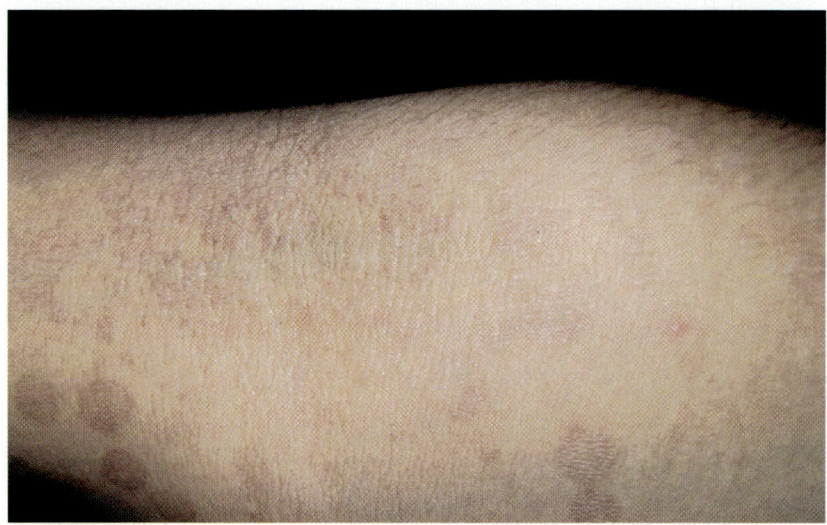

Fig. 5.24c: Hyperpigmented scaly macules on the arms in a patient

There have been several mechanisms postulated for the alterations in pigmentation, including the production of dicarboxylic acids produced by *Malassezia* species (e.g. azaleic acid) which cause competitive inhibition of tyrosinase and perhaps a direct cytotoxic effect on hyperactive melanocytes. The explanation for the hyperpigmentation seen in fair-skinned subjects remains obscure, although electron microscopy reveals abnormally large melanosomes in hyperpigmented lesions, and smaller than normal melanosomes in hypopigmented ones.

Investigations

Microscopy of the scales reveals coarse mycelium, fragmented to short filaments 2–5 μm wide and up to 25 μm long, together with spherical, thick-walled yeasts 2–8 μm in diameter. However, it is the mycelium that is the diagnostic feature, and predominates in a few cases. The characteristic appearance is commonly called 'spaghetti and meatballs' or 'bananas and grapes'.

Histopathology shows hyperkeratosis, parakeratosis and slight acanthosis, with a mild inflammatory infiltrate including mast cells in the upper dermis. The infecting organism is usually present in the upper layers of the stratum corneum.

Immunophenotyping of the infiltrates has revealed a dominance of memory T cells, an accumulation of macrophages and a lack of B cells.

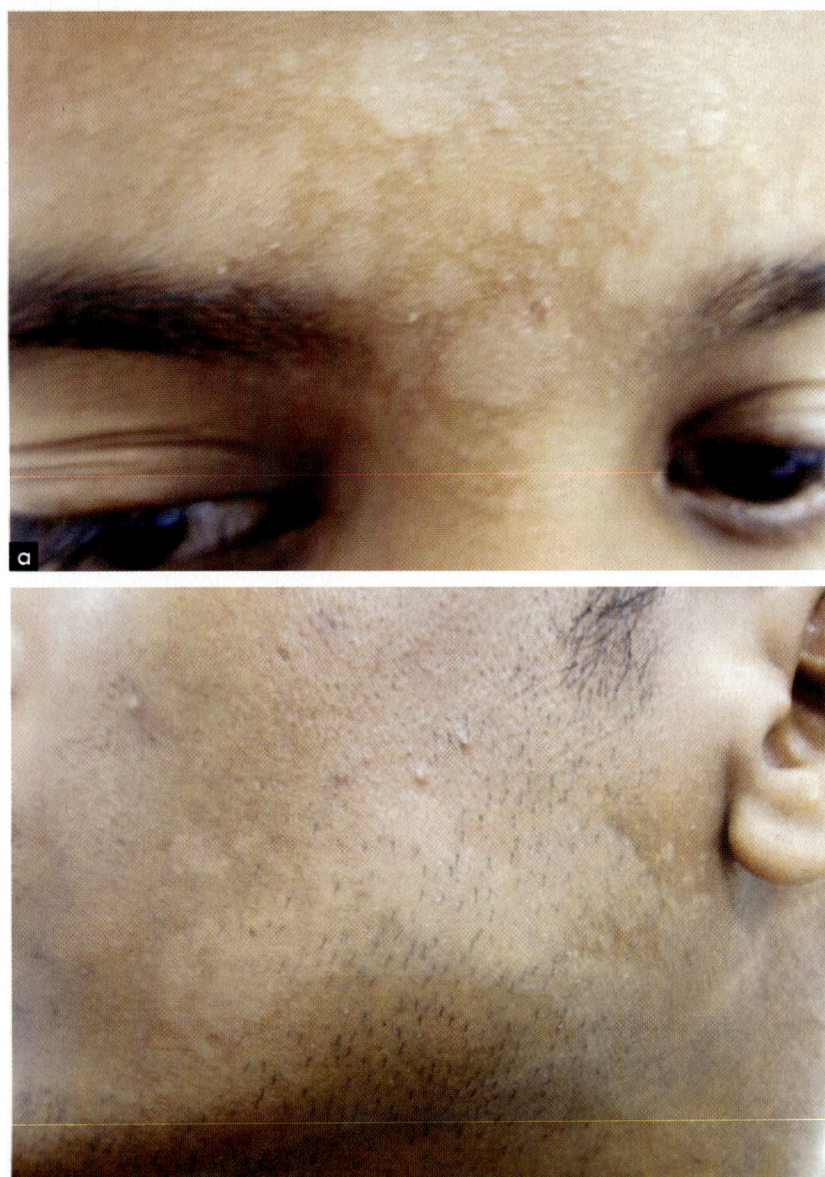

Fig. 5.25a and b: Facial involvement which is seen commonly in children but sometimes also in adults

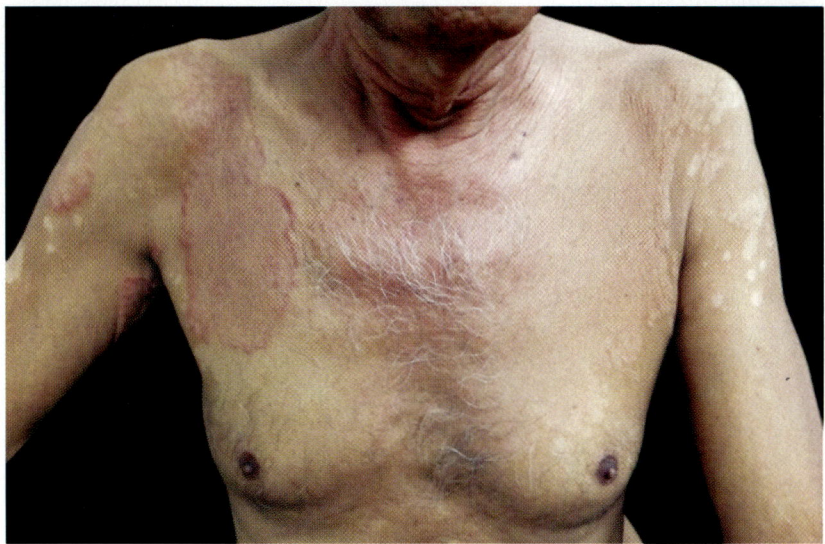

Fig. 5.25c: Concomitant tinea corporis and pityriasis versicolor present in a single patient. Treat patient with the azoles instead of terbinafine

Treatment

A variety of medicines may eliminate the fungus, but relief is usually temporary and recurrences are common (40 to 60%). Patients must understand that the hypopigmented areas will not disappear immediately after treatment. Sunlight accelerates repigmentation. The inability to produce powdery scale by scraping with a #15 surgical blade indicates the fungus has been eradicated. Fungal elements may be retained in frequently worn garments that are in contact with the skin; discarding or boiling such clothing might decrease the chance of recurrence. Patients without obvious involvement who have a history of multiple recurrences might consider repeating a treatment program just before the summer months to avoid uneven tanning.

Treatment options for tinea versicolor are abundant (Table 5.6). Topical antifungal therapy is usually sufficient, but in more widespread disease, systemic therapy may be preferred. Topical treatments should be applied to the entire torso from the neck to the waist, because lesions may be widespread as well as clinically unapparent. Although the appearance of the rash will improve within days, patients should be counseled that it may take months for pigmentary changes to resolve. Of the non-imidazole topical agents, zinc pyrithione shampoo appears most effective. Sulfur salicylic acid shampoo is also effective. Longer durations of treatment and higher concentrations of active agents produce greater cure rates.

Table 5.6: Overview of therapy of pityriasis versicolor

Mode of therapy	Agents	Dose
Topical agents	Ketoconazole 2%* Selenium Sulphide‡ Ciclopirox olamine ZPTO	Apply for 14 days for **10 min and then wash it off**
	Imidazole creams Allylamines	Twice a day for 1–4 weeks
Systemic	Ketoconazole Itraconazole Fluconazole	200 mg/day × 5 days 200 mg/day × 5 or 7 days 150 mg once a week for 4 weeks 300 mg once a week for 2 doses 300 mg single dose repeated 2 weeks later

*Another regimen is for 3 days, ‡Apply the lotion and wash it off in 24 hours. This is repeated once each week for a total of 4 weeks.

Systemic therapy with ketoconazole, fluconazole or itraconazole is often used but it must be remembered that all these drugs are cytochrome P450 inhibitors and thus have numerous interactions. In randomized controlled trials of oral ketoconazole, cure rates varied from 84% (200 mg × 5 days) to 100% (200 mg × 5 weeks), while a cure rate of 100% was observed in several randomized controlled trials following a 5-day course of oral itraconazole (200 mg daily). One open-label trial of oral fluconazole (300 mg once weekly for 2 weeks) reported a 98% cure rate; there are a few comparative studies of oral antifungal medications.

The rate of **recurrence** of pityriasis versicolor is very high, especially in hot humid climates. Patients at high risk for recurrence may be helped by using once-weekly application of ketoconazole 2% shampoo (Nizoral), applied as a lotion to the neck, trunk, and proximal extremities 5 to 10 minutes before showering. Another preventative measure is once-monthly dosing of oral ketoconazole (400 mg), fluconazole (400 mg) or itraconazole (400 mg).

Treatment Ladder

First line

- Topical azoles twice daily for 2–3 weeks
- Terbinafine 1% cream twice daily for 2–3 weeks
- Ketoconazole shampoo twice weekly for 2–3 weeks
- 2.5% selenium shampoo alternative days for 2–3 weeks

Second line

Itraconazole 200 mg daily for 5 days.

PITYROSPORUM/MALASSEZIA FOLLICULITIS

Definition

Pityrosporum folliculitis is an infection of the hair follicle caused by the yeast *Pityrosporum orbiculare*, the same organism that causes tinea versicolor, usually affecting back and upper trunk.

The presence of diabetes mellitus and the administration of broad-spectrum antibiotics or corticosteroids are predisposing factors. It is also seen following holiday in the sun. Follicular occlusion may be the primary event, with yeast overgrowth as a secondary occurrence. Hodgkin's disease may predispose to Pityrosporum folliculitis.

Clinical Features

Most often seen in teenagers or young adult males, it presents as asymptomatic or slightly *itchy* follicular papules and pustules localized to the upper back and chest, upper arms, and neck (Fig. 5.26). Occlusion and greasy skin may be important predisposing factors. It is frequently diagnosed as acne.

Pityrosporum folliculitis is very common in the tropics, where it presents as a polymorphous eruption with the following characteristics. The primary lesion is a keratinous plug that underlies four clinical types of lesion: Follicular papules (dome-shaped papules with a central depression), pustules, nodules, and cysts. The lesions evolve from follicular plugs colonized by Pityrosporum. The face is often affected—this is the most common site in female patients and

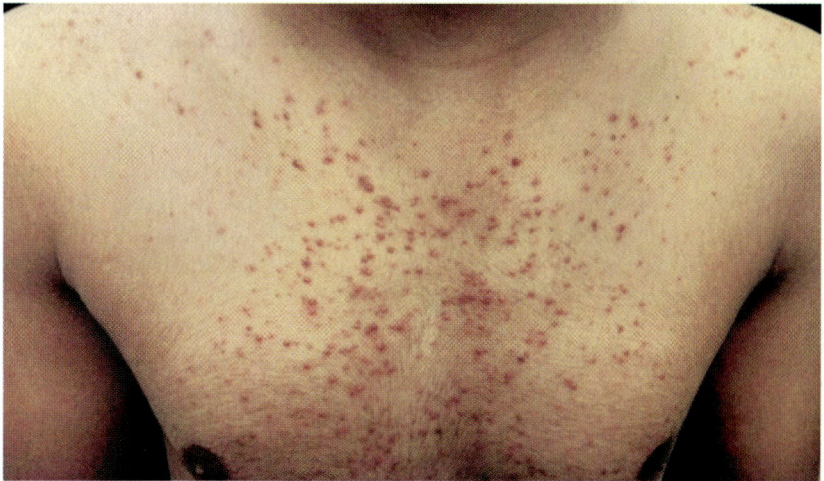

Fig. 5.26a: A case of P. folliculitis with follicular bright red papules on upper chest

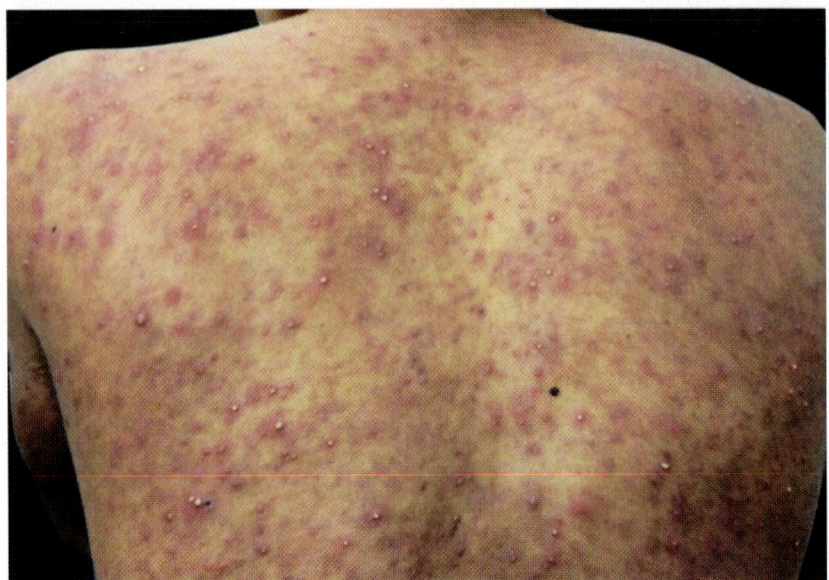

Fig. 5.26b: Follicular papules and pustules on the upper back of a patient with P. folliculitis

the second most common site in male patients. The lesions are localized to the *mandible, chin,* and *sides* and *forehead* (hair line) of the face. This is in contrast to the usually more central facial location of acne vulgaris. They can also be seen on the neck. The lesions are bright red and both itch and hurt. A case of acne not responding to antibiotics can be a case of P. folliculitis. Lesions can also be seen on the nape of the neck, abdomen, buttocks, and thighs.

Treatment

Treatment is the same as that for tinea versicolor. Combined ketoconazole shampoo and systemic ketoconazole (200 mg daily for 4 weeks) produced clearance of the lesions in 100% of patients, whereas systemic therapy alone resulted in only a 75% clearance rate. Salicylic acid wash is keratolytic and an effective therapeutic option.

SEBORRHEIC DERMATITIS
Definition

Seborrheic dermatitis and dandruff are common, chronic, relapsing, scaling disorders which share a similar origin. Seborrheic dermatitis (SD) is thought to affect up to 5% of the general population, and its milder counterpart, dandruff, has been found to affect up to 50% of the population.

Dandruff is a non-inflammatory, mild form of seborrheic dermatitis of the scalp caused by excessive physiologic desquamation. In comparison, seborrheic dermatitis is an inflammatory, erythematous, scaling eruption in areas of the skin with a high number of sebaceous glands.

The exact cause of seborrheic dermatitis is unknown, but its etiology is believed to be multifactorial. **Sebum** production, the presence of and the **immune** response to certain Malassezia (previously Pityrosporum) yeast species (most commonly *Malassezia globosa* and *Malassezia restricta*), atmospheric **humidity**, and **stress** may all be contributing factors. Although seborrheic dermatitis and dandruff occur in areas with a high density of sebaceous glands, there is **no** direct correlation between sebum production and the presence or activity of disease. Furthermore, reducing the amount of sebum production does not eliminate dandruff or seborrheic dermatitis. In contrast, a reduction in the number of Malassezia yeast after treatment with antifungals has been shown to improve seborrhea.

The prevalence of SD is seen to be higher in patients with human immunodeficiency virus (HIV) infection, HTLV infection and chronic neurological disease.

Pathophysiology

Adult-type seborrheic dermatitis appears to be directly related to Malassezia yeasts but not to a single species. The relationship between infant seborrheic dermatitis and these organisms is less well established. *Malassezia* are primarily found in the infundibulum of the sebaceous gland where lipids, their main energy source, are freely available. They usually exist as skin commensals in a state of symbiosis. The mechanisms by which the balance is altered and skin changes are induced and not fully known, although direct lipase activity or inflammatory responses initiated by *Malassezia*-produced aryl hydrocarbon inhibitors such as malassezin and indolocarbazole have been described. Oxidative stress either due to overproduction of oxygen radicals or inadequate antioxidants has also been proposed to contribute to the pathogenesis of SD. Keratinocytes can also produce pro-inflammatory cytokines after stimulation with *Malassezia* cells, and the response is species-specific.

Clinical Features

The lesions tend to be asymptomatic or mildly pruritic (seborrheic dermatitis worse than dandruff), with episodic exacerbations associated with cold weather, stress, and infection. The lesions of dandruff appear as nonerythematous, noninflammatory, white greasy scaling throughout the scalp (Fig. 5.27a). The lesions of seborrheic dermatitis appear as erythematous, inflammatory, greasy, yellow to brown scaly patches or plaques affecting the scalp, face (eyebrows, eyelids, nasal alar crease, mouth, and ears), and body (central chest and genital region in adults, diaper region in infants) (Fig. 5.27b and c). It typically runs a chronic relapsing course.

Scalp: It presents with ill-defined patches on the crown and parietal regions of the scalp and anterior hairline (Fig. 5.27a).

Face: There are dry, mildly erythematous, scaly lesions that can progress to thick, greasy, exudative areas. They may be localised to the area around the nose or eyelids (seborrheic marginal blepharitis) (Fig. 5.27b and c) or may be associated with ocular rosacea or mild conjunctivitis. Hypopigmentation may be a prominent feature in dark-skinned individuals.

Trunk: Several presentations may be seen. In men, involvement of the presternal area is typical with petaloid (petal-shaped) lesions that may be localized. More widespread involvement may extend to the upper back, umbilicus, axillae, groins and submammary area. The 'pityriasis-form' variant of SD comprises a generalized erythematosquamous eruption, similar to but more extensive than pityriasis versicolor, with involvement of the neck up to the hair margin. Ano-genital involvement may occur in both sexes.

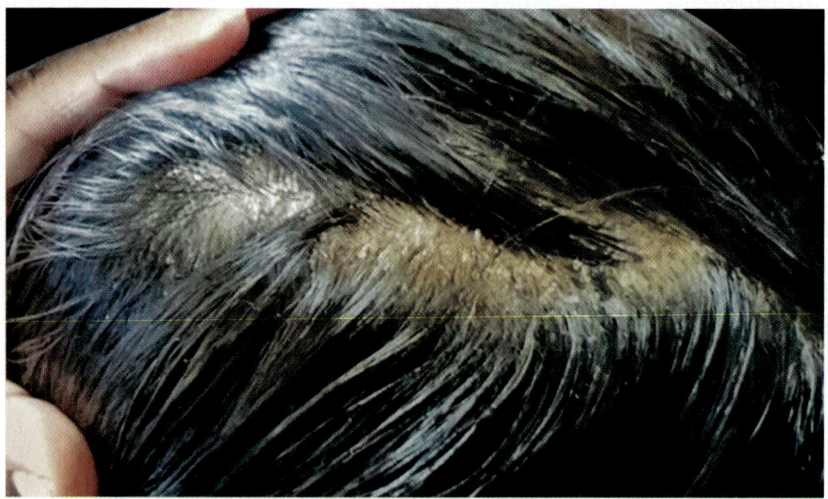

Fig. 5.27a: Scaling on the scalp associated with itching in a case of mild seborrheic dermatitis

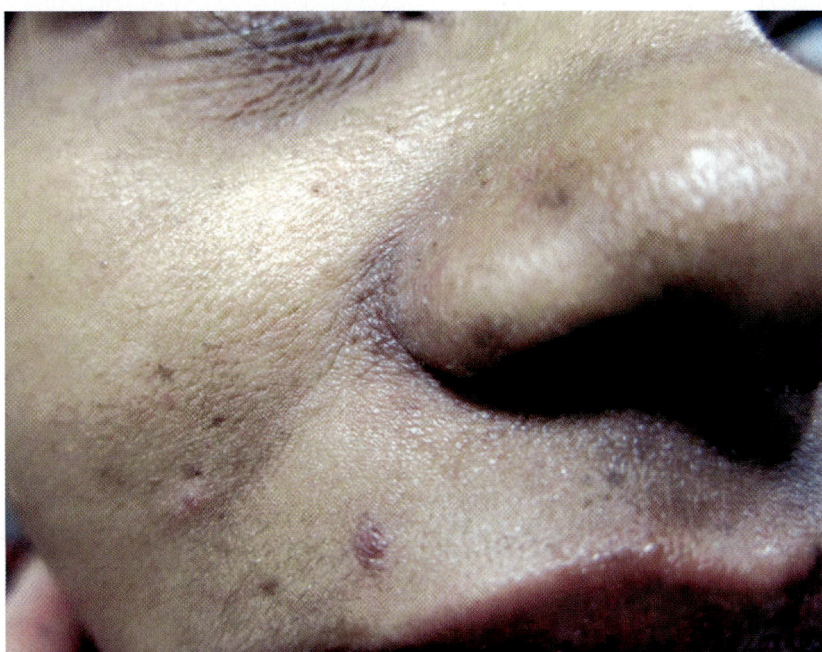

Fig. 5.27b: Greasy scales on the nasolabial fold in a case of seborrheic dermatitis

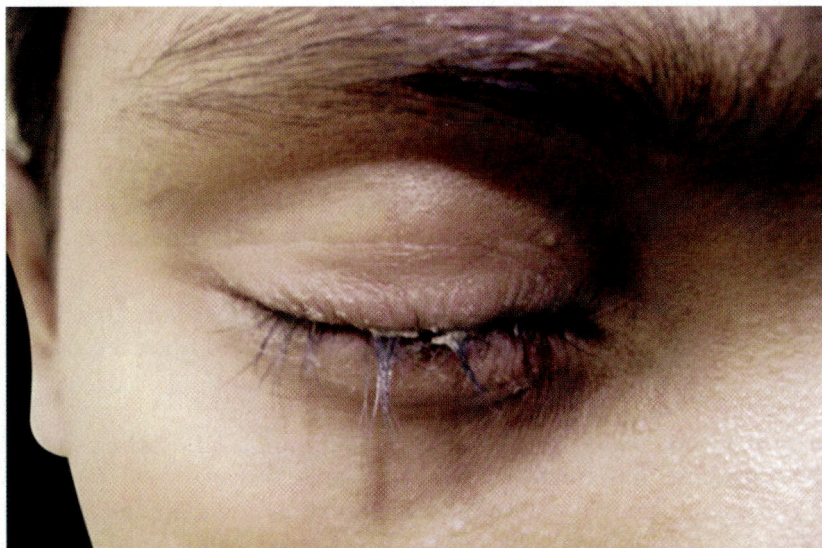

Fig. 5.27c: Greasy scales adherent to the base of eyelashes with erythema of the eyelid seen in a case of SD

Infantile seborrheic dermatitis: This typically involves the vertex of the scalp (cradle cap), flexural surfaces, and diaper region. Pruritus is not as common in infants and the disease is often self-limited, with presentation in the first few months of life and resolution by 1 year. Involvement of eyebrows, paranasal areas and large flexures is often present and helps in distinguishing infantile SD from atopic eczema. However, many authors consider that a distinction between infantile SD and atopic eczema is not clear-cut.

Differential Diagnosis

Psoriasis: Scaling is usually more circumscribed, thicker and silvery, nail changes may be seen and typical psoriatic plaques may be evident elsewhere. Dermoscopy may help with SD showing a characteristic vascular pattern of arborizing vessels, atypical vessels and the absence of red dots and globules (which are features of psoriasis).

Sebopsoriasis: This has been used to describe patients with psoriasiform scaling in a SD distribution, but this entity is not clearly defined.

Allergic contact dermatitis: Patch testing should be considered in atypical cases

Perioral dermatitis: This also affects the nasolabial folds and may be associated with superficial scaling, however, additional involvement of the skin below the lateral lower lips and presence of small papules is characteristic, with a distinctive diamond-shaped distribution.

Others: Darier disease, Hailey-Hailey disease, pemphigus foliaceus and pemphigus erythematosus, pityriasis rosea, early cutaneous T-cell lymphoma, erythrasma.

Drugs: A range of drugs may produce SD-like eruptions, including captopril, d-penicillamine, gold sodium thiomalate, lithium, methyl-dopa, chlorpromazine and cimetidine.

Differential diagnoses in *infants* include histiocytosis, zinc deficiency (acrodermatitis enteropathica), Leiner's disease and tinea capitis.

Investigations

The diagnosis is usually made on clinical grounds. HIV testing should be considered in refractory and severe cases.

Histology is not diagnostic and usually shows overlapping features of psoriasis and chronic dermatitis. The primary histological lesion of SD is the 'squirting papilla' which involves capillary dilatation in the papillae, followed by migration of granulocytes into the epidermis where they incite spongiosis. As the inflammation subsides, there is an increase in epidermal proliferation with focal parakeratosis and increased desquamation.

Treatment

Treatment for seborrheic dermatitis and dandruff is focused on eliminating the visible disease (scale and erythema) and symptomatic relief (especially pruritus) through the use of antifungal, anti-inflammatory, and keratolytic agents.

A. *Antifungals*

Topical antifungals are considered first-line medications for the treatment of seborrheic dermatitis. Topical ketoconazole is a safe, effective, and well-tolerated treatment for seborrheic dermatitis, with minimal to no systemic absorption. Ketoconazole is available as a 2% shampoo and a 2% cream for non-scalp seborrheic dermatitis.

Ketoconazole 2% shampoo is used twice weekly and left on for 5 to 10 minutes prior to rinsing for approximately 4 weeks, followed by a weekly maintenance application. For non-scalp seborrheic dermatitis, ketoconazole 2% cream applied twice daily for 4 weeks is effective.

Ciclopirox is another antifungal agent found to be safe, effective, and well tolerated. Ciclopirox 1% shampoo is used twice weekly for 4 weeks, and ciclopirox 1% cream is applied twice daily for 1 month followed by once daily application for maintenance.

Other antifungals found to be effective against seborrheic dermatitis include miconazole 2% cream, terbinafine 1% solution or 1% cream and fluconazole and newer azoles such as sertaconazole.

Some strains of *Malassezia globosa* and *M. restricta* are resistant to azole antifungals and this may be associated with treatment failure. In such cases allylamines like terbinafine and naftitine has been reported to be effective despite their lack of activity against *Malassezia* species, suggesting other mechanisms.

Oral antifungal therapy is occasionally advocated for recalcitrant or widespread SD, but the evidence for its efficacy is limited. Itraconazole has been the most frequently reported oral treatment for SD and a pulse regimen has generally been associated with good clinical and mycological responses.

B. *Topical Corticosteroids*

Topical corticosteroids are useful in the treatment of severe or very inflammatory cases of seborrheic dermatitis. They are inexpensive and effective at rapidly decreasing the inflammation and pruritus associated with seborrheic dermatitis. Low to midpotency corticosteroids treat most cases of seborrheic dermatitis, but higher potency steroids followed by a taper may be necessary to treat refractory scalp cases. High potency steroids should be avoided on the face. Due to the potential side effects, treatment with topical steroids should be limited to a few weeks.

Non-scalp seborrheic dermatitis can be treated with over-the-counter hydrocortisone 1% cream applied one to three times daily for a few weeks at a time. Refractory or extensive lesions on the scalp may be treated with corticosteroid lotions, solutions, sprays, or foam. Formulations include betamethasone valerate 0.1% lotion and clobetasol propionate 0.05% foam. Fluocinolone acetonide 0.01% scalp oil usually used with occlusion is another effective treatment.

C. Topical Calcineurin Inhibitors

The calcineurin inhibitors, tacrolimus 0.03%, 0.01% ointment and pimecrolimus 1% cream, are immunomodulators that decrease inflammation by inhibiting T-cell function. Twice daily application of pimecrolimus cream may be as effective at treating moderate-to-severe seborrheic dermatitis as antifungals and corticosteroids without the side effect profile of prolonged corticosteroid use. FDA has warned against a potential increased risk of skin cancer and lymphoma after extensive, widespread use of calcineurin inhibitors. Thus antifungals remain the first-line treatment.

D. Other Nonsteroidals

Preparations containing 2.5% selenium sulfide or 1 to 2% zinc pyrithione are also effective at treating seborrheic dermatitis. Selenium sulfide has both antimitotic and antifungal properties.

Zinc pyrithione has cytotoxic, antimicrobial, and antifungal properties. Application of the **selenium sulfide 2% shampoo** three times weekly for a treatment period of 5 to 10 minutes is nearly as effective as ketoconazole in treating seborrheic dermatitis. Unfortunately, it is less effective at preventing relapse of disease. **Tar shampoos**, like selenium sulfide containing shampoos, inhibit mitotic activity, thus decreasing the amount of scale. **Salicylic acid** disrupts the bonds between cells within the stratum corneum. However, this product has not been well studied in adults and salicylic acid/sulfur shampoos are less effective than other keratolytics. Hair discoloration is one of the major side effects of both selenium sulfide and tar shampoos. Overnight application of keratolytic gel or a 30-minute application of warm mineral oil prior to shampooing may help remove thick crusts.

Table 5.7: 'NICE' recommendations for treatment of SD

Type of SD	First line	Second line	Additional therapy
Scalp and beard	2 % ketoconazole shampoo or selenium sulphide shampoo	Zinc pyrithione, coal tar or salicylic acid shampoos	Topical keratolytic or mineral/olive oil for the removal of scale and crust. Potent topical corticosteroid scalp application for 4 weeks if there is severe scalp itch
Face and body in adults	Ketoconazole 2% cream od/bd, clotrimazole 1% cream bd/tds, econazole 1% cream bd, miconazole 2% cream bd, to be applied for 4 weeks	Mild topical corticosteroids for 1–2 weeks	Antifungal shampoo, e.g. 2% ketoconazole, as a body wash Hygiene measures for eyelid involvement using cotton buds moistened with baby shampoo
Severe SD	Review diagnosis, consider specialist referral, HIV testing		
Infants	Removal of scalp crusts with baby shampoo and gentle brushing. Overnight soak of petroleum jelly or warmed vegetable oil if needed. Daily bathing with soap substitute	Topical imidazole cream: clotrimazole 1% cream bd/tds, econazole 1% cream bd, miconazole 2% cream bd	Topical corticosteroids not advised but may be used for nappy rash

In patients suffering from both facial seborrheic dermatitis and rosacea, metronidazole 0.75% or 1% gel, 4% *nicotinamide* cream and *azelaic* acid 15% gel are safe, well tolerated, and effective. **Metronidazole 1% gel** is typically applied once daily at bedtime, and azelaic acid gel is applied once to twice daily. Photodynamic therapy with indole-3-acetic acid have also been useful in such cases.

Topical *lithium gluconate* has anti-inflammatory effects in SD and probably via increased expression and secretion of IL-10 and reduced expression of TLR2 and TLR4.

A nonsteroidal cream with no active ingredients has shown antiinflammatory and antifungal activity **(Promiseb)**, gaining the Food and Drug Administration (FDA) approval for the treatment of seborrheic dermatitis. NICE recommendations for treatment of SD is given in Table 5.7.

Other Cutaneous Disorders Associated with Malassezia Yeasts

Malassezia yeasts have also been associated with other skin conditions such as confluent and reticulate papillomatosis and sebopsoriasis.

Bibliography

1. Back O, Faergemann J, Hornquist R. Pityrosporum folliculitis: a common disease of the young and middle aged. J Am Acad Dermatol1985;12:56–61.

2. Christopher EM Griffiths, Jonathan Barker, Tanya Bleiker. Rook's textbook of dermatology. 9th edn: 32.49 Aptara Inc: New Delhi, India.

3. Crespo Erchiga V, Delgado Florencio V. Malassezia species in skin diseases. Curr Opin Infect Dis 2002;15:133–142.

4. Gupta AK, Kohli Y, Faergemann J, *et al*. Epidemiology of Malassezia yeasts associated with pityriasis versicolor in Ontario, Canada. Med Mycol 2001;39:199–206.

5. Gupta AK, Bluhm R, Summerbell R. Pityriasis versicolor. J Eur Acad Dermatol Venereol 2002;16:19–33.

6. Mathes BM, Douglas MC. Seborrheic dermatitis in patients with acquired immunodeficiency syndrome. J Am Acad Dermatol 1985;13:947–951.

7. Salkin IF, Gordon MA. Polymorphism of *Malassezia furfur*. Can J Microbiol 1977;23:471–475.

8. Sugita T, Tajima M, Takashima M, *et al*. A new yeast, *Malassezia yamotoensis*, isolated from a patient with seborrhoeic dermatitis, and its distribution in patients and healthy subjects. Microbiol Immunol 2004;48:579–583.

C. CANDIDOSIS (Moniliasis)

The yeast-like fungus *Candida albicans* can affect the skin, mucous membrane, and internal organs. It is a normal flora of the mouth, vaginal tract, and gut, and it reproduces through the budding of oval yeast forms. Pregnancy, oral contraception, antibiotic therapy, diabetes, skin maceration, topical steroid therapy, certain endocrinopathies, and factors related to depression of cell-mediated immunity may allow the yeast to become pathogenic and produce budding spores and elongated cells (pseudohyphae) or true hyphae with septate walls.

A depiction of various forms of cutaneous candidosis is made in Fig. 5.28.

Pathophysiology

1. *Agent Factors*

C. albicans is the most common pathogen in skin disease, although other species are isolated increasingly in vaginal infections and from immunocompromised patients.

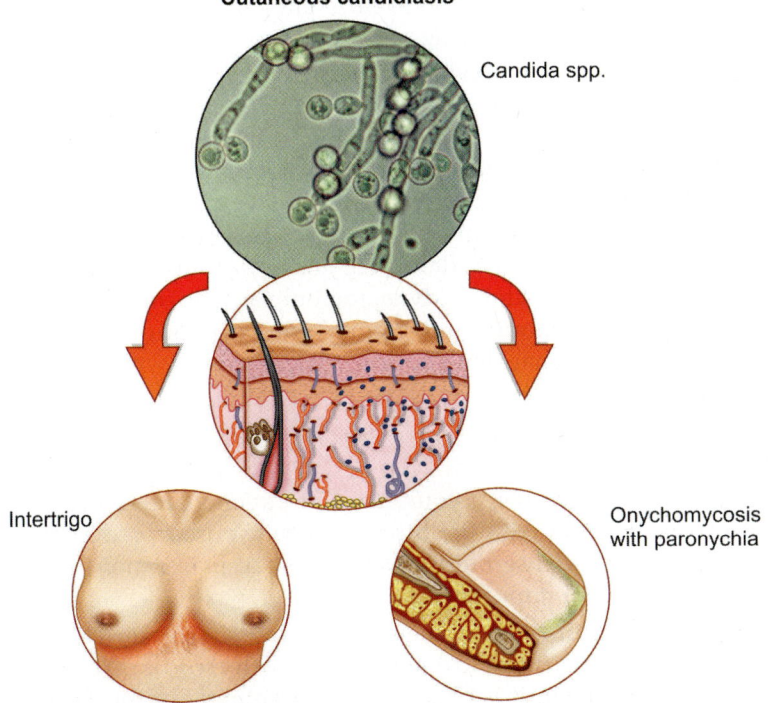

Fig. 5.28: An artistic depiction of the various forms of cutaneous candidiasis

Factors that predispose to infection include: (i) A local environment of moisture, warmth, and occlusion; (ii) systemic antibiotics, corticosteroids and other immunosuppressive agents, or birth control pills; (iii) pregnancy; (iv) diabetes; (v) Cushing disease; and (vi) debilitated states. Immune reactivity to Candida is reduced in infants up to 6 months of age and in patients with lymphoproliferative diseases or acquired immunodeficiency syndrome. However, most women with recurrent vulvovaginal candidiasis have normal cellular immunity.

The production of hyphae may contribute to fungal virulence and *in vitro* multiple factors are known to stimulate mycelium formation, however, their extrapolation to *in vivo* situation is doubtful.

The resident bacteria on skin inhibit the proliferation of *C. albicans*. Cell-mediated immunity plays a major role in the defense against infection. In addition, *C. albicans* can activate complement through the alternative pathway. The innate immune system appears to respond to mannan, a *C. albicans* cell wall polysaccharide, through toll-like receptors 2 and 4. Production of a secreted aspartyl protease and melanin by certain strains of *C. albicans* are known to affect pathogenicity. Candida's ability to form a biofilm on certain surfaces may also lead to the expression of different genes affecting virulence or drug resistance such as drug efflux pumps.

The yeast infects only the outer layers of the epithelium of mucous membranes and skin (the stratum corneum). The adhesion to epithelial cells is an important prequel of tissue invasion and may be mediated through receptor interactions and through proteinase production. The primary lesion is a pustule, the contents of which dissect horizontally under the stratum corneum and result in its separation. Clinically, this process results in a red, denuded, glistening surface with a long, cigarette paper-like, scaling, advancing border. The infected mucous membranes of the mouth and vaginal tract accumulate scale and inflammatory cells that develop into characteristic white or white-yellow curdy material.

2. Host Factors

The elderly, diabetics, very young and ill patients are susceptible to oral thrush. Patients with dentures are predisposed predominantly by formation of a dense biofilm. On the skin, maceration resulting from occlusion is of importance.

Endocrine factors like diabetes, Cushing's disease, Addison's disease, hypoparathyroidism and hypothyroidism may also predispose. However, it is observed that treatment of the endocrine abnormality does not improve the Candida infection.

Immunological factors especially cell-mediated immunity is of paramount importance, however, circulating antibodies or secretory IgA may have some role. The susceptibility of elderly and severely ill people, especially those with leukaemia, lymphomas or carcinomatosis or those with AIDS, probably results from depression of cell-mediated immunity.

Investigations

As *C. albicans* may be a normal commensal, a scanty growth of the same obtained from any site may be meaningless without evidence of infection from a positive direct microscopy.

Direct microscopy: It reveals oval, thin-walled yeasts buds on a narrow base usually accompanied by filaments, either true hyphae or pseudohyphae. Filaments are usually absent when a non-*albicans* yeast is present. The size and shape of the yeasts observed may also suggest the presence of a non-*albicans* yeast.

Culture: Isolation and identification of *C. albicans* is done at 37°C, on media free of cycloheximide. Colonies usually appear within 1–3 days, however, growth from thicker skin and nail material can be slower, so plates should be held for a week before reporting as negative. *Candida albicans* colonies on glucose-peptone agar are white to cream and soft in texture. The production of filaments is best examined on depleted media, such as cornmeal agar, or rice extract agar supplemented with Tween 80. Other Candida species produce colonies that vary slightly in texture, colour and production of obvious pseudohyphae.

Histology: Pathological changes vary with different range of clinical manifestations. However, there are certain common features seen. Fungal elements are almost always restricted to the outer layers of epithelium, including the stratum corneum, however, they may be sparse in acute infections. Acute oral candidosis is further characterized by inflammatory changes with the formation of a pseudomembrane of epithelial and inflammatory cells. The infiltrate in skin and mucosa consists predominantly of polymorphs, which may form micro-abscesses or subcorneal pustules. Splitting of the epidermis often follows. In the dermis, the inflammatory infiltrate is a mixture of lymphocytes, plasma cells (especially in the mouth) and histiocytes. In chronic cases, hyperplasia with parakeratosis and acanthosis of the epithelium is associated with a mixed, chronic, inflammatory infiltrate. In chronic cutaneous lesions, hyperkeratosis with acanthosis may be seen, and in Candida granuloma of the skin, a dense mixed cell infiltrate may include giant cells.

VULVOVAGINITIS

Vulvovaginal candidiasis (VVC) is usually caused by *C. albicans*, but occasionally is caused by other *Candida* spp. or yeasts. This condition affects around 75% of women of child-bearing age.

Clinical Features

Symptoms include pruritus, vaginal soreness, dyspareunia, external dysuria, and abnormal vaginal discharge.

1. Uncomplicated Vulvovaginal Candidiasis

Candida vaginitis presents with external dysuria and vulvar pruritus, pain, swelling, and redness. Signs include vulvar edema, fissures, excoriations, or thick, curdy white vaginal discharge.

The diagnosis can be made when either (1) a wet preparation (saline, 10% KOH) or Gram stain of vaginal discharge which demonstrates yeasts, hyphae, or pseudohyphae or (2) a culture which yields a yeast species. Candida vaginitis may be associated with a normal vaginal pH (4.5) and, therefore, pH testing is not a useful diagnostic tool. Identifying Candida by culture in the absence of symptoms or signs is not an indication for treatment, because approximately 10 to 20% of women harbor *Candida* spp. and other yeasts in the vagina.

Treatment

Short-course topical formulations (i.e. single dose and regimens of 1 to 3 days) are effective. The topically applied azole drugs are more effective than nystatin.

Topical

1. Clotrimazole 1% cream 5 gm intravaginally for 7–14 days OR Clotrimazole 2% cream 5 gm intravaginally for 3 days.
2. Miconazole 2% cream 5 gm intravaginally for 7 days OR miconazole 4% cream 5 gm intravaginally for 3 days OR miconazole 100 mg vaginal suppository, one suppository for 7 days OR miconazole 200 mg vaginal suppository, one suppository for 3 days OR miconazole 1200 mg vaginal suppository, one suppository for 1 day.

   Miconazole is pregnancy category C and clotrimazole is a category B medication.

   Any woman whose symptoms persist after using an over-the-counter (OTC) preparation or who has a recurrence of symptoms within 2 months should be evaluated with office-based testing. Unnecessary or inappropriate use of OTC preparations is common and can lead to a delay in the treatment of other diseases. Patients should be instructed to return for follow-up visits only if symptoms persist or recur within 2 months of onset of the initial symptoms. VVC is not usually acquired through sexual intercourse; no data support the treatment of sexual partners.

VVC frequently occurs during pregnancy. Only topical azole therapies, applied for 7 days, are recommended for use among pregnant women. Therapy for VVC in HIV-infected women does not differ from that for seronegative women.

Systemic

A Single Oral Dose of 150 mg of fluconazole has been US Food and Drug Administration (FDA) approved for the treatment of vaginal candidiasis. Its efficacy is equivalent to topical therapy and to oral itraconazole 200 mg at two doses 12 hours apart.

Slightly greater efficacy may be achieved with fluconazole 100 mg/day for 5 to 7 days or itraconazole 200 mg/day for 3 to 5 days.

2. Complicated Vulvovaginal Candidiasis (Recurrent/Severe/ Non *C. albicans*/Women with Uncontrolled Diabetes, Debilitation, or Immunosuppression)

a. Recurrent Vulvovaginal Candidiasis (RVVC)

RVVC, usually defined as **four or more** episodes of symptomatic VVC in 1 year, affects a small percentage of women (5%). The pathogenesis of RVVC is poorly understood, and most women with RVVC have no apparent predisposing or underlying conditions. Vaginal cultures should be obtained from patients with RVVC to confirm the clinical diagnosis and to identify unusual species (including non-*albicans* species), particularly *Candida glabrata*.

Although *C. glabrata* and other non *Candida albicans* species are observed in 10 to 20% of patients with RVVC, *C. glabrata* does *not* form pseudohyphae or hyphae and is not easily recognized on microscopy. Conventional antimycotic therapies are not as effective against these species as they are against *C. albicans*.

Also it is important to rule out other causes of vaginosis or *Chlamydia* infection as sometimes the clinical picture is confusing. Molecular typing of isolates from women suffering from recurrent episodes has demonstrated that in most cases the same strain is responsible for the recurrences, suggesting that clearance of the organism was not achieved by standard courses of antifungal therapy. Recently, deficiencies in IL-22 and IDO1 gene products have been associated with susceptibility to recurrent VVC.

In cases of recurrent vulvovaginitis, treatment of the patient's sexual partner is controversial; in contrast, for recurrent balanitis, eradication of Candida from the sexual partner's genital tract is generally recommended.

Treatment

Each individual episode of RVVC caused by *C. albicans* responds well to short-duration oral or topical azole therapy. To maintain clinical and mycologic control, a longer duration of initial therapy (e.g. 7 to 14 days of topical therapy) or a 100-, 150-, or 200-mg oral dose of fluconazole every third day for a total of three doses (days 1, 4, and 7) should be attempted to obtain mycologic remission before initiation of a maintenance antifungal regimen.

Maintenance regimens Oral fluconazole (i.e. 100, 150, or 200 mg dose) **weekly** for 6 months is the first line of treatment. If this regimen is not feasible, topical treatments used intermittently as a maintenance regimen can be considered. Suppressive maintenance antifungal therapies are effective in reducing RVVC. However, 30% to 50% of women will have recurrent disease after maintenance therapy is discontinued. Routine treatment of sexual partners is controversial. Azole resistance in *C. albicans* is rare in vaginal isolates and susceptibility testing is usually not warranted for treating patients individually.

b. *Severe Vulvovaginal Candidiasis*

Severe vulvovaginitis (i.e. extensive vulvar erythema, edema, excoriation, and fissure formation) (Fig. 5.29) is associated with lower clinical response rates in patients treated with short courses of topical or oral therapy. Either 7 to 14 days of topical azole or 150 mg of fluconazole in **two sequential doses** (second dose 72 hours after initial dose) is recommended. In severe or very symptomatic *Candida vulvitis*, a topical corticosteroid for the first 3 to 4 days may be used.

c. *Non-albicans VVC*

The optimal treatment of non-albicans VVC remains unknown. Options include longer duration of therapy (7–14 days) with a non-fluconazole azole drug (oral or topical) as first-line therapy. If recurrence occurs, 600 mg of boric acid in a gelatin capsule is recommended, administered vaginally once daily for 2 weeks. This regimen has clinical and mycologic eradication rates of approximately 70%.

d. *Women with Uncontrolled Diabetes, Debilitation, or Immuno-suppression*

They do not respond well to short-term therapies. Efforts to correct modifiable conditions should be made, and more prolonged (i.e. 7–14 days) conventional antimycotic treatment is necessary.

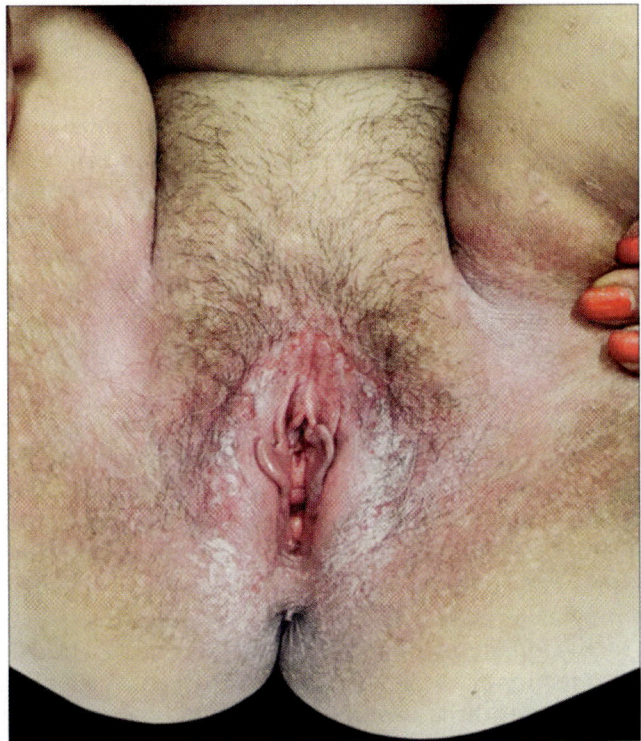

Fig. 5.29: A case of severe vulvovaginal candidiasis characterized by extensive vulvar erythema, edema, excoriation, and whitish deposits

ORAL CANDIDIASIS

Candida is not uncommonly found in the normal mouth but candidosis is more likely to develop when there is local or general immunosuppression resulting from systemic steroid therapy, local application in the form of steroid creams, mouthwashes and lozenges for the treatment of aphthosis or lichen planus or use of steroid aerosols for asthma.

Non-*albicans* Candida species are causing an increasing number of infections. Most of these occur in immunocompromised individuals, especially in those infected with human immunodeficiency virus (HIV). Oral candidiasis is common in advanced cancer. In a study of patients with advanced cancer, the two most prevalent species were *C. albicans* and *C. glabrata*, with fewer numbers of *C. tropicalis*, *C. parapsilosis*, *C. guilliermondii*, and *C. inconspicua*. Non-*albicans* Candida yeasts are common in the mouths of patients with advanced-stage cancer, and these patients may have reduced sensitivity to fluconazole. *Candida dubliniensis* is a recently identified yeast, mostly isolated in HIV-positive individuals with oral candidiasis.

Infants Oral candidiasis in children is called thrush. Healthy, newborn infants, especially if premature, are susceptible. In older infants, thrush usually occurs in the presence of predisposing factors such as antibiotic treatment or debilitation. In the healthy newborn, thrush is a self-limited infection, but it should be treated to avoid interference with feeding. The infection appears as a white, creamy exudate or white, flaky, adherent plaques. The underlying mucosa is red and sore. The mother should be examined for vaginal candidiasis.

Adults In the adult, oral candidiasis occurs for several reasons; clinically, it is found in a variety of acute and chronic forms. Extensive oral infection may occur in patients with diabetes or depressed cell-mediated immunity, the elderly, and patients with cancer, especially leukemia. Prolonged use of corticosteroids, immunosuppressive or broad-spectrum antibiotics, and inhalant steroids may also cause candidiasis. The acute process in adults is similar to the infection in infants. The tongue is almost always involved. Infection may spread into the trachea or esophagus and cause very painful erosions, appearing as dysphagia, or it may spread onto the skin at the angles of the mouth (perlèche). A specimen may be taken by gently scraping with a tongue blade. Pseudohyphae are easily demonstrated. In other cases, the oral cavity may be red, swollen, and sore, with a little or no exudate. In this instance, pseudohyphae are often difficult to find and treatment may have to be started without laboratory verification.

Classification of Mucosal Candidosis

A. Oropharyngeal Candidosis
1. Acute pseudomembranous candidosis or thrush
2. Acute erythematous or atrophic candidosis
3. Chronic pseudomembranous candidosis
4. Chronic erythematous candidosis
5. Chronic plaque-like candidosis
6. Chronic nodular candidosis
7. Angular cheilitis
8. Median rhomboid glossitis

B. Esophageal and Tracheobronchial Candidosis

Clinical Features

Oropharyngeal candidiasis is often asymptomatic but burning or pain on eating spices/acidic foods, with diminished taste sensation is a common complaint.

Acute pseudomembranous candidosis/oral thrush/Candida stomatitis It presents with sharply defined patch of creamy, crumbly, curd-like, white pseudomembrane (which consists of desquamated epithelial cells, fibrin, leukocytes and fungal mycelium that attaches it to the inflamed epithelium), which, when removed, leaves an underlying erythematous base (Fig. 5.30). It occurs most commonly in the first week of life with increased susceptibility in preterm infants. There is generally a local or general predisposing factors. The cheeks, gums or palate may be affected. In immunocompromised patients with neutropenia or HIV/AIDS, the extension of lesions to the buccal mucosa, tongue and esophagus is common.

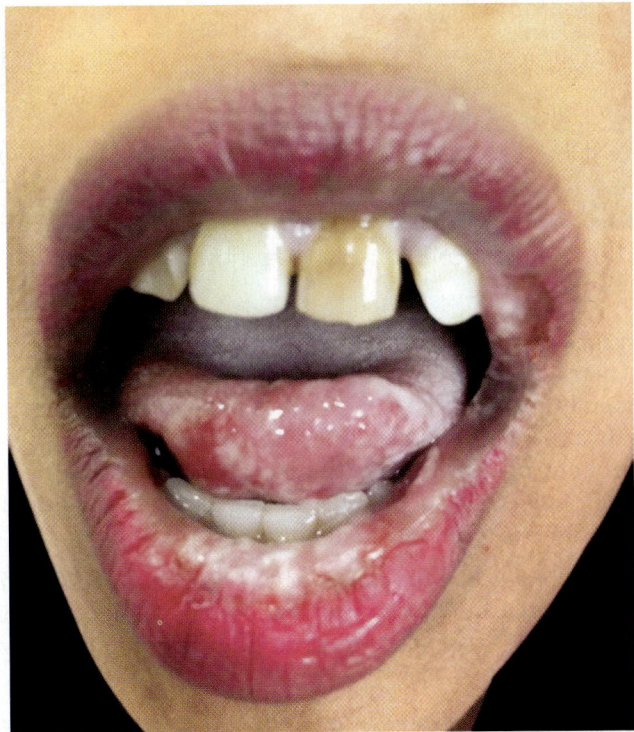

Fig. 5.30: Pseudomembranous candidiasis: White deposits present on the labial mucosa and tongue which on removal leaves an erythematous mucosal surface as seen on the tongue

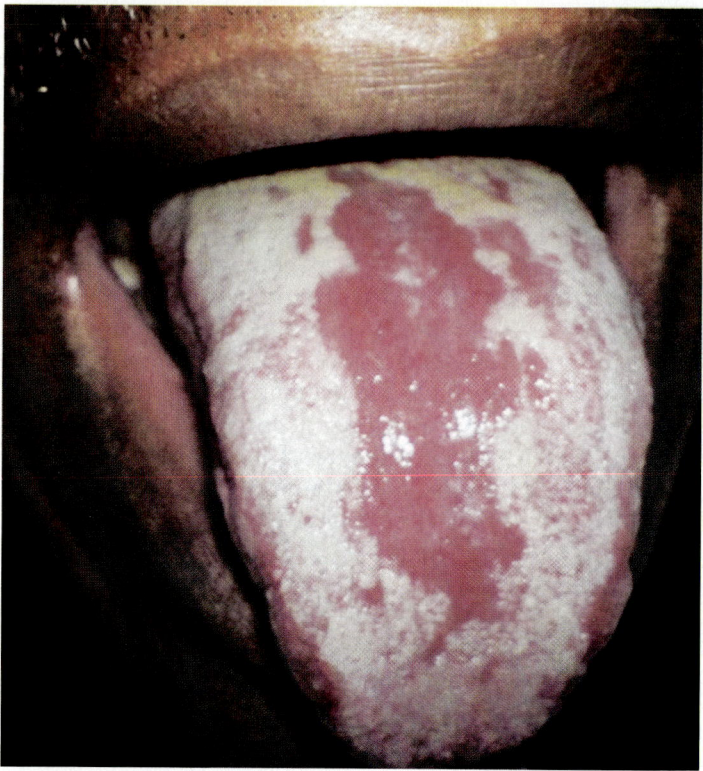

Fig. 5.31: The central part of the tongue shows atrophic erythematous candidiasis

Acute erythematous or atrophic candidosis/antibiotic sore tongue
There is marked soreness with denuded, atrophic, erythematous mucous membranes, particularly on the dorsum of the tongue (Fig. 5.31). Areas of thrush may also be present. This type is specially associated with antibacterial antibiotic therapy, but may also develop in HIV-positive subjects and patients taking inhaled steroids. In these cases, the tongue is often markedly affected.

Chronic pseudomembranous candidosis This does not differ clinically from the acute pseudomembranous variety but as the name suggests, lesions are very persistent. It occurs principally in immunocompromised patients.

Chronic erythematous candidosis/chronic atrophic candidiasis/ denture stomatitis (Fig. 5.32) Seen in denture bearers, the lesions are generally confined to the upper denture-bearing area, i.e. the palate and the gums. The affected mucous membranes show a variable bright

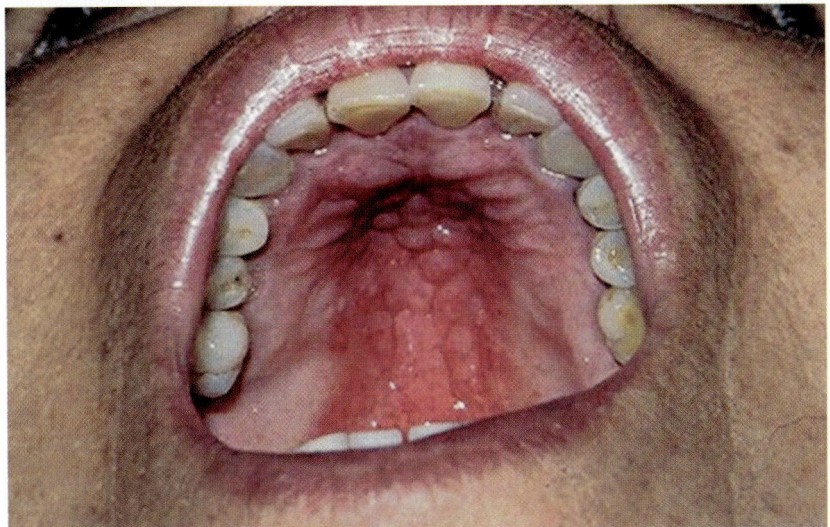

Fig. 5.32: Denture stomatitis also known as chronic erythematous candidosis

red or dusky erythema, fairly sharply defined at the margin of the denture. There is often an associated angular cheilitis. Chronic mechanical irritation and bacterial colonization have an important role in the pathogenesis and elimination of Candida alone does not usually result in complete recovery.

Chronic plaque-like candidosis/Candida leukoplakia Presents with persistent irregular white plaques on the cheeks or tongue that cannot be wiped off but regress with anticandidal therapy (Fig. 5.33). Smokers are particularly prone to develop this form of oral candidosis. The significance of this condition lies in the fact that it must be differentiated from other types of leukoplakia (Fig. 5.34).

Chronic nodular candidosis This is a rare form of oral candidosis, where the tongue is cobbled. It is most often seen in certain patients with chronic mucocutaneous candidosis.

Angular cheilitis **(Fig. 5.35)** Presents as intertrigo at the angles of lips and is usually associated with oropharyngeal colonization with Candida.

Angular cheilitis or perlèche, an inflammation at the angles of the mouth, can occur at any age. Patients may have the misconception that they have a vitamin B deficiency; however, yeast and bacteria may be involved in the process. Lip licking, biting the corners of the mouth, or thumb sucking causes perlèche in the young. Continued irritation may lead to eczematous inflammation.

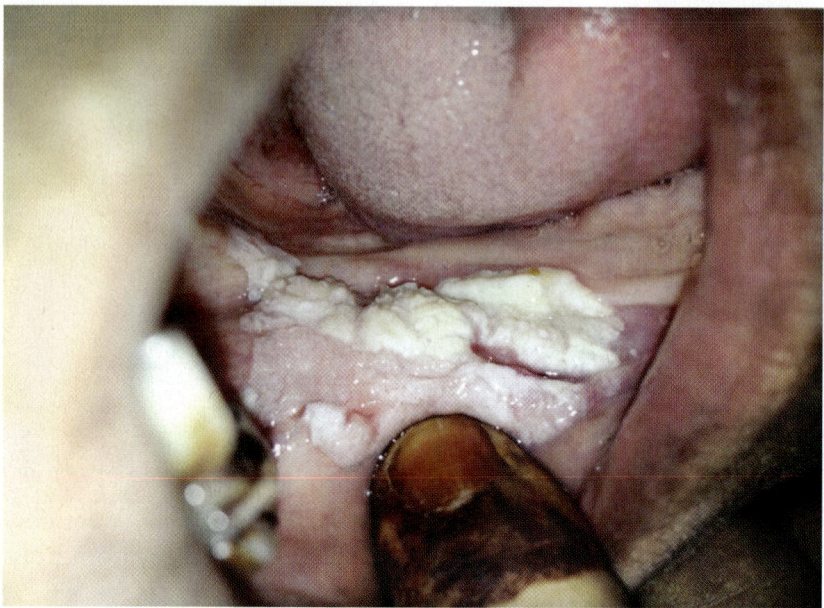

Fig. 5.33: A case of candidal leukoplakia

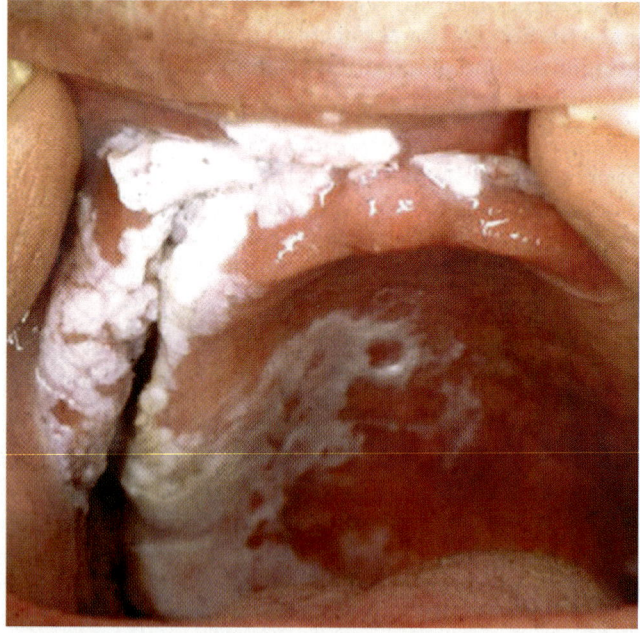

Fig. 5.34: A case of frictional leukoplakia. Candidal leukoplakia should always be differentiated from other types of leukoplakia

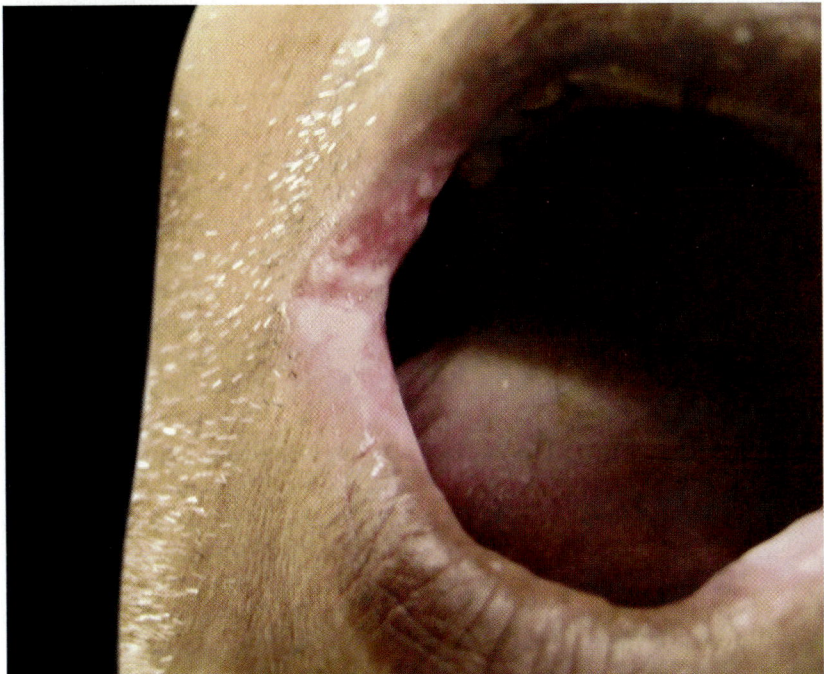

Fig. 5.35: A case of angular cheilitis. Skin folds at the angles of the mouth are red and eroded

The presence of saliva at the angles of the mouth is the most important factor. Excess saliva occurs as a result of mouth breathing secondary to nasal congestion and of malocclusion resulting from poorly fitting dentures and compulsive lip lickng. Aggressive use of dental floss may cause mechanical trauma to mouth angles. A moist, intertriginous space forms in skin folds at the angles of the mouth as a result of advancing age, congenital excessive-angle skin folds, sagging that occurs with weight loss, or abnormal vertical shortening of the lower one-third of the face from loss of teeth and resultant resorption of the alveolar bone. Capillary action draws fluid from the mouth into the fold, creating maceration, chapping, fissures, erythema, exudation, and secondary infection with Candida organisms and/or staphylo-cocci.

Median rhomboid glossitis This is an acquired condition, characterized by a diamond-shaped area on the dorsum of the tongue with loss of papillae. It has been regarded in the past as a developmental abnormality but current opinion suggests that it is simply a variant of chronic plaque-like candidosis.

Treatment

A. Oral Candidiasis

1. **Fluconazole** Fluconazole (200 mg/day × 7 days for adults) is the first-line management option for the treatment and prophylaxis of localized and systemic *C. albicans* infections. It is effective, well tolerated, and suitable for use in most patients with *C. albicans* infections, including children, the elderly, and those with impaired immunity. Second-line therapy with a wider spectrum antifungal, such as itraconazole, should be sought if treatment with fluconazole is not successful. *Candida* spp. other than *C. albicans* may develop resistance to fluconazole in a patient who is repeatedly exposed to the drug.

2. **Itraconazole** Itraconazole is as effective as fluconazole but is less well tolerated as first-line therapy. Itraconazole oral solution is a useful therapy in the treatment of HIV-infected patients with fluconazole refractory oropharyngeal candidiasis. HIV-infected patients with oropharyngeal candidiasis for whom fluconazole therapy (200 mg/day) failed were treated with 100 mg of itraconazole administered twice daily (200 mg/day) for 14 days. Patients who demonstrated an incomplete response to treatment were treated for an additional 14 days (28 days total).

3. **Clotrimazole** Children and adults are effectively treated by slowly dissolving a clotrimazole troche in the mouth five times a day for 14 days.

4. **Amphotericin B** (80 mg/ml) may be used as a rinse.

5. **Gentian violet solution** 1 to 2% may be tried in difficult or recurrent cases.

B. Oropharyngeal Candidiasis

Fluconazole 200 mg po on day 1, then 100–200 mg po daily, continue treatment for 7–14 days after clinical resolution.

[Recommended as first-line treatment for HIV-infected patients (or other immunosuppressed individuals) with moderate to severe disease, recurrent infection or a CD4+ count of <200 cells/mcl.]

C. Esophageal Candidiasis

- Fluconazole 200–400 mg po on day 1, then 100–400 mg daily
- Itraconazole 200 mg po daily
- Voriconazole 200 mg po or iv bid

- Posaconazole 400 mg po bid
- Caspofungin 50 mg po iv daily

Continue treatment for 7–14 days following resolution of symptoms, for a minimum of 21 days total.

CANDIDA BALANITIS

The uncircumcised penis provides the warm, moist environment ideally suited for yeast infection, but the circumcised male is also at risk. Candida balanitis sometimes occurs after intercourse with an infected female and is more common in those who had vaginal intercourse than in those who had anal intercourse within the previous 3 months.

Clinical Features

Tender, pinpoint, red papules and pustules appear on the glans and shaft of the penis. The pustules rupture quickly under the foreskin and may not be noticed (Fig. 5.36). Typically, 1–2 mm, white, possibly confluent rings are seen after the pustules break. In some cases pustules never evolve, and the multiple red papules may be transient, resolving without treatment. The presence of pustules is highly suggestive of candidiasis.

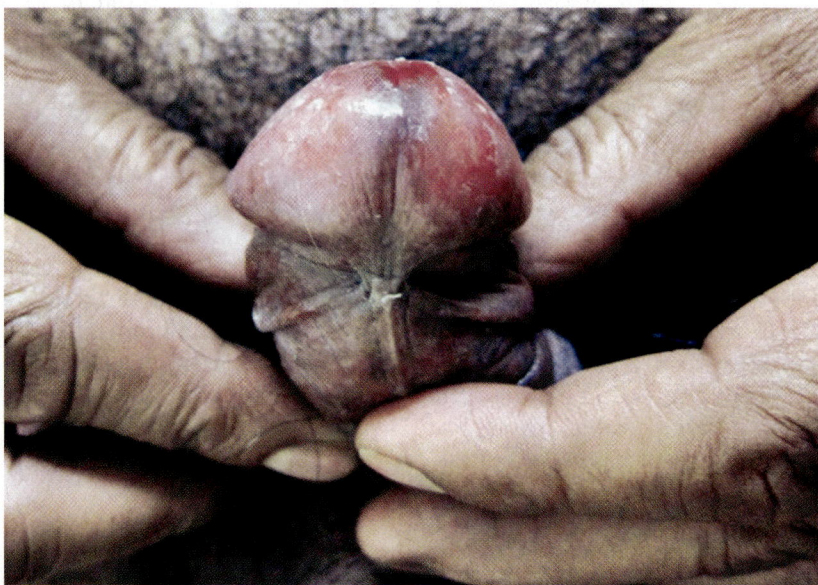

Fig. 5.36: A case of candidal balanitis, with multiple pustules on a erythematous base

Another presentation is edema, ulcerations, and fissuring of prepuce. White exudate similar to that seen in Candida vaginal infections may be present. The infection may occur and persist without sexual exposure.

Diabetes should always be considered in cases of genital yeast infections, as florid persistent lesions spreading beyond the genitalia are seem most likely to be associated with it.

Treatment

The eruption responds quickly with twice-a-day application for 7 days of miconazole or clotrimazole. Relief is almost immediate, but treatment should be continued for 7 days. Preparations containing topical steroids give temporary relief by suppressing inflammation, but the eruption rebounds and worsens, sometimes even before the cortisone cream is discontinued.

A single 150-mg dose of fluconazole was comparable in efficacy and safety to clotrimazole cream applied topically for 7 days when administered to patients with balanitis.

CUTANEOUS CANDIDIASIS

In the skin the most common site of infection is in the skin folds, also called candidal intertrigo. This is seen under pendulous breasts, between overhanging abdominal folds, in the groin and rectal area, and in the axillae.

Skin folds (intertriginous areas where skin touches skin) contain heat and moisture, providing the environment suited for yeast infection. Hot, humid weather, tight or abrasive underclothing, poor hygiene, and inflammatory diseases occurring in the skin folds such as psoriasis, make a yeast infection more likely. The various presentations of cutaneous candidiasis are described below.

1. Intertrigo

Obese people are at greatest risk. Itching, burning, and stinging are the most common symptoms. Apposing skin folds retain moisture and become warm, macerated, and inflamed. Candida is the most common secondary infection but bacteria, fungi, or viruses may be a factor. Erosions are possible. Sweat, feces, urine, and vaginal discharge may aggravate intertrigo. The course can be recurrent and chronic.

Clinical Features

There are two presentations. In the first type, pustules form but become macerated under apposing skin surfaces and develop into red papules with a fringe of moist scale at the border. Intact pustules may be found outside the apposing skin surfaces.

The second type consists of a red, moist, glistening plaque that extends to or just beyond the limits of the apposing skin folds. The advancing border is long and sharply defined and has an ocean wave-shaped fringe of macerated scale. The characteristic pustule of candidiasis is not observed in intertriginous areas because it is macerated as soon as it forms. Pinpoint pustules do appear outside the advancing border and are an important diagnostic feature. There is a tendency for painful fissuring in the skin creases (Figs 5.37 and 5.38).

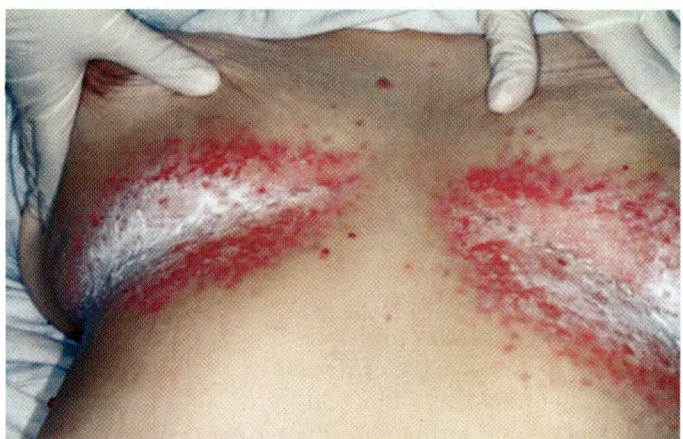

Fig. 5.37: Intertrigo with central maceration and peripheral pustules (candidiasis)

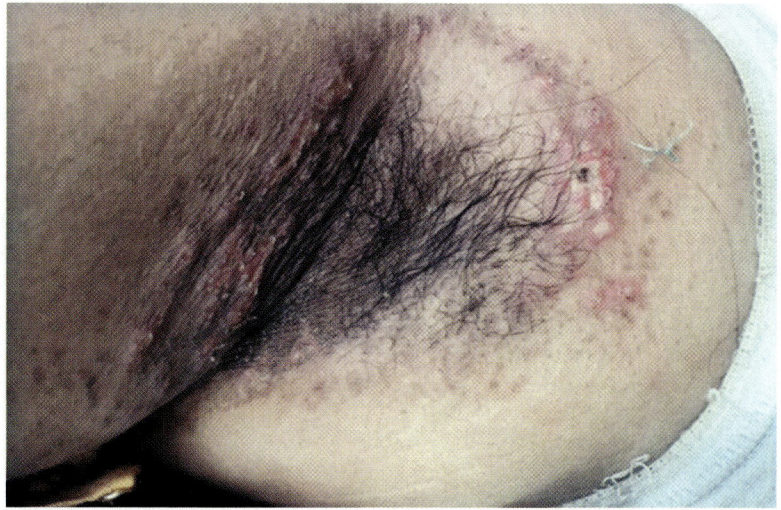

Fig. 5.38: Pinpoint pustules seen at the advancing border are an important clue for diagnosing candidal intertrigo

Treatment

a. *General Measures*

Education about the role of moisture and maceration is important. The following techniques may be recommended: (i) Drying affected areas after bathing using a handheld hair dryer on low heat, at least once a day; (ii) supportive clothing and weight reduction; (iii) air conditioning in warm environments; and (iv) regular application of a plain or medicated powder (nystatin or miconazole) to the areas.

For very inflammatory lesions, open compresses three to four times a day with water or normal saline will expedite relief of symptoms. Cool water compresses applied for 1/2 hour two or three times a day for just a few days are rapidly effective in controlling moisture and suppressing inflammation.

b. *Topical Agents*

A 1- or 2-week course of group VI to VII topical **steroids** (desonide, hydrocortisone) may be all that is necessary. Long-term continuous use of topical steroids in skin fold areas may result in the formation of atrophy and striae; 0.1% **tacrolimus** may be used as an anti-inflammatory agent instead of topical steroids for initial treatment or for cases requiring long-term intermittent treatment. **Ciclopirox** cream or lotion twice daily for 1–2 weeks or until resolved is another option. It is a good practice to add a topical anti-yeast medications such as **miconazole** cream if Candida infection is suspected. Alternate these creams with topical steroids. It is wise to separate and expose skin effectively in order to promote dryness, administer while the patient is in the supine position. After clinical resolution, topical treatments may be continued **twice weekly** to prevent recurrence.

Gentian violet 0.25 to 2.0% and **Castellani paint** (fuchsin, phenol, and resorcinol) are older remedies, which are effective but may sting and will stain clothing, bed linen, and skin.

c. *Systemic Agents*

Outside the setting of chronic mucocutaneous candidiasis, chronic systemic suppressive therapy in immunosuppressed individuals is discouraged due to the risk of colonization with resistant organisms.

Fluconazole
- 50 to 100 mg daily for 14 days
- 150 mg weekly for 2–4 weeks

Itraconazole: 200 mg twice daily for 14 days

2. Diaper Candidiasis

This condition is largely seen in urban population where there is prevalent use of diapers which create an artificial intertriginous area under the wet diaper, predisposing the area to a yeast infection with the characteristic red base and satellite pustules.

Diaper dermatitis is often treated with steroid combination creams and lotions that contain antibiotics. Although these medications may contain the anti-yeast agent clotrimazole, its concentration may not be sufficient to control the yeast infection. The cortisone component may alter the clinical presentation and prolong the disease.

A nodular, granulomatous form of candidiasis in the diaper area also called **granuloma gluteale infantum**, appears as dull, red, irregularly shaped nodules, sometimes on a red base, and may represent an unusual reaction to Candida organisms or to a Candida organism infection modified by steroids. Although dermatophyte infections are unusual in the diaper area, they do occur. Every effort should be made to identify the organism and treat the infection appropriately.

Treatment

a. Dryness should be maintained by changing the diaper frequently or by using a diaper for short periods.
b. Antifungal creams should be applied twice a day until the eruption is clear, in approximately 10 days.
c. Some erythema from irritation may be present after 10 days; this can be treated by alternately applying 1% hydrocortisone cream followed in a few hours by creams active against yeasts. Apply each agent twice a day.
d. Baby powders may help prevent recurrence by absorbing moisture.
e. Mupirocin ointment 2% (Bactroban) applied three or four times daily is effective for severe Candida and bacterial diaper dermatitis.

3. Interdigital Candidiasis

Web spaces are like small intertriginous areas. Cooks, bartenders, dishwashers, dentists, and others who work in a moist environment are at risk.

Clinical Features

White, tender, macerated skin erodes, revealing a pink, moist base. Candidiasis of the toe webs occurs most commonly in the narrow interspace between the fourth and fifth toes, where it may coexist with dermatophytes and Gram-negative bacteria (Fig. 5.39). In the case of

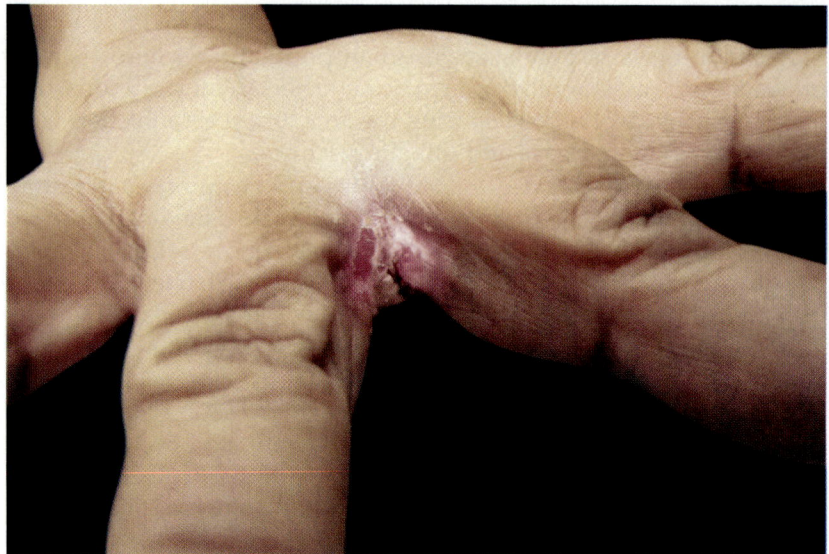

Fig. 5.39: Erosio-interdigitalis blastomycetica is a skin condition where oval-shaped areas of macerated white skin is seen in the web space

hands, some abnormality, including wide, fat fingers, appears to predispose to infection. In this particular syndrome, often known as erosio-interdigitalis blastomycetica or interdigital candidosis, Candida and Gram-negative bacteria are often co-pathogens.

Treatment

Both areas are treated with any of the antifungal creams or lotions listed previously.

As there is a chance of bacterial superinfection oral antibiotics are a useful adjunct to antifungal therapy.

4. Paronychia

This is associated with rounding and lifting of the proximal nail fold, disruption of the cuticle, and erythema and swelling of the fingertip. The nail plate may display transverse ridging or greenish-brown discoloration. In chronic paronychia, the area surrounding the nail is tender, and there is often a history of frequent wetting of the hands. Apart from Candida, bacteria and irritant or allergic contact dermatitis also play a part in its pathogenesis, although the contribution of each varies from patient to patient and with the chronicity of the disease. This condition is chiefly found among those whose hands are frequently immersed in water. Toenail folds are not usually affected.

Treatment

Successful treatment of a chronic paronychia often requires weeks to months, and nails will grow out normally within 3 to 6 months of the paronychia healing.

1. An imidazole, such as ketoconazole , sertaconazole, clotrimazole, miconazole, or ciclopiroxolamine, should be applied several times a day. If there is associated pain or edema, use a combined steroid-antifungal ointment. Overnight application under occlusion may increase effectiveness. In addition, the area should be protected during wet work by wearing waterproof gloves and cotton liners.

2. Amphotericin B (Fungizone) lotion or cream or 1% alcoholic solution of gentian violet may also be used. Because amphotericin B and imidazole agents counteract one another, they should not be used simultaneously.

3. Topical steroid creams (group V) or tacrolimus ointment 0.1% applied twice daily for up to 3 weeks is more effective than systemic antifungal agents.

4. Fluconazole (200 mg/day) for 1 to 4 weeks may sometimes control chronic inflammation. Short courses of fluconazole may have to be repeated as the infection recurs.

Treatment Ladder

First line	Second line
• Azole solution twice daily for 2–4 months depending on clinical response (plus in chronic cases a medium strength topical steroid applied to the nail fold skin once daily) • Itraconazole 100 mg daily for 1–2 months • Fluconazole 100 mg daily for 1–2 months	• 4% thymol solution

5. Candida Onychomycosis

It is an infection of the nail plate caused by Candida species.

Two important predisposing conditions are Raynaud phenomenon or disease and Cushing syndrome. The main clues that the yeast is a significant pathogen are erosion of the distal nail plate, the presence of yeasts and hyphae in the nail on direct microscopy and the isolation of *C. albicans*.

The various presentations are:

• The most common is distal and lateral subungual onychomycosis (DLSO) associated with paronychia.

- Complete destruction of the nail plate is seen in some patients with chronic mucocutaneous candidosis.
- Erosion of the distal and lateral nail plate of the fingernails, not usually progressing to total nail dystrophy. This is most often seen in women.
- Very rarely, Candida may invade the nail plate in the neonatal period, sometimes causing an isolated nail dystrophy with evidence of penetration of the superior aspect of the nail plate.
- Candida may also be isolated from the undersurface of the nail plate in patients with onycholysis resulting from other causes. Antifungal therapy in these circumstances does not produce any improvement.

In proven Candida onychomycosis, fluconazole or itraconazole produce the best responses.

6. Perianal and Scrotal Candidosis

Perianal and scrotal candidosis may occur with, or independently of, genital involvement. Lesions start around the anal margin with non-specific erythema, soreness and irritation, subsequently spreading along the natal cleft with classic features developing as it extends. Involvement of the scrotum is usually in the form of a non-specific erythema and rarely subcorneal pustules. Candidosis must be included in the differential diagnosis of unexplained erythema of scrotal skin. The dense growth of organisms on a swab culture or the presence of diagnostic clinical features such as satellite pustules are usually taken as indications for treatment.

7. Congenital/Neonatal Candidosis

This represents established candidosis, usually of the skin and birth membranes present at the time of birth, and following intrauterine infection.

It is usually associated with prematurity, presence of an intrauterine foreign body like IUCD or following contamination of the skin surface during birth. Such cases are distinct from the more common neonatal systemic candidosis, a septicaemic illness associated with extreme prematurity, where skin involvement is not common.

Clinical features: The amniotic fluid may be turbid at delivery. The skin lesions are present at birth and are typically discrete vesicles or pustules on an erythematous base. The face and chest are first affected by the rash, which generally spreads over the next few days after delivery. In over 10% there is evidence of spread to deep sites such as the lungs.

Although there has been a high level of mortality reported with such cases, the cause of death is usually related to other complications of prematurity rather than candidosis per se.

Management: Topical therapy alone suffices, but where there is systemic involvement, amphotericin B or fluconazole should be considered.

8. Candida Allergy

A variety of clinical features attributed to Candida allergy have been described and include urticaria, ordinary annular erythema, bullous annular erythema, generalized pruritus and palmoplantar pustulosis.

The term Candida allergy or Candida syndrome is also used to describe a constellation of symptoms ranging from headache to malaise and depression, allegedly secondary to colonization of the gastro-intestinal tract with yeasts. However, there is no objective scientific evidence to connect these symptoms with the presence or absence of Candida.

9. Chronic Mucocutaneous Candidosis (CMC)

It is a distinct entity with persistent Candida infection of the mouth, the skin and the nails, refractory to conventional topical therapy and may be associated with a variety of other cutaneous and systemic infections. Many cases form part of the autoimmune polyendocrino-pathy Candida ectodermal dystrophy syndrome (APECED) or CMC associated with hypothyroidism.

Immunological factors point towards defects of delayed hypersensitivity, defects of phagocytosis or killing in both macrophages and polymorphs and raised levels of neutralizing autoantibodies to IFN-α subtypes in patients with Candida endocrinopathy. In addition, it is known that certain antigenic compo-nents of *C. albicans*, such as glycopeptides, are immunomodulatory.

It is a heterogenous group classified by Higgs and Wells into several distinct categories using genetic and clinical criteria. However, patients with an obvious underlying immune defect should be excluded from this syndrome as in them candidosis may be a secondary manifestation rather than a prominent clinical pattern as seen in this condition. Most CMC patients develop signs in early childhood, and usually Candida infection is the presenting feature. It should also be remembered that clinical manifestations may overlap between various categories. The different categories are described below:

1. *Autosomal recessive CMC:* Presenting in first decade with persistent oral and nail plate infections in otherwise healthy individuals with no underlying defects, improve with age.

2. *Autosomal dominant CMC:* Generally, they are more severely affected than those with the recessive variety, and other infections, such as dermatophytosis, may be particularly troublesome.

3. *Idiopathic CMC:* This subgroup is used for individuals where the inheritance is not defined yet, and includes most severely affected patients, who may have other infections and often develop bronchiectasis and pulmonary bullae. Their candidosis is also very severe, with esophageal involvement and the appearance of 'granulomas'. Rarely, the patients develop other systemic diseases, such as cryptococcosis or miliary tuberculosis. Survival into adult life is still not universal in these children.

4. *CMC associated with endocrinopathy*
   a. These patients appear to have the familial polyendocrinopathy syndrome but candida infection may precede endocrine disease by 10 years. It is usually seen in early childhood and inherited in an autosomal recessive pattern. The endocrine abnormalities commonly seen is hypoparathyroidism with hypoadrenocorticalism. In addition, other autoimmune abnormalities can occur such as pernicious anaemia, vitiligo and ovarian failure. The severity of the patient's candidosis is variable even among siblings. This variety is associated with mutations in the autoimmune regulator gene pathway.
   b. This group has CMC with associated hypothyroidism. The inheritance is autosomal dominant and clinical features are similar to those of other patients with endocrinopathy but associated skin infections, including severe dermatophytosis, are more common. This form is associated with mutations in the STAT1 gene.

5. *Late-onset CMC:* Occasionally, adult patients are found to have the syndrome of CMC. Though sporadic cases are known, cases have been associated with thymoma and systemic lupus erythematosus. The sudden onset of chronic oral candidosis in an adult should be investigated as it may be the initial presentation of another condition such as HIV infection.

Clinical Features

1. Persistent oral thrush, which is poorly responding or relapsing in nature. Chronic hypertrophic changes may follow.
2. Cutaneous candidosis. Often intertriginous skin is involved, but also the face, hands, trunk, limbs and rarely scalp may be involved.

In long-standing lesions, the cutaneous changes are often atypical, suggesting ringworm. In some patients, markedly thickened areas with gross hyperkeratosis may form or deep dermal nodules may be seen.

3. Paronychia is commonly a feature, often with extensive nail plate invasion and total dystrophic onychomycosis.
4. Seborrheic dermatitis can be very persistent in some patients. Alopecia areata, vitiligo and other organ-specific inflammation such as keratitis are seen in patients with endocrinopathy.

Management

Treatment of this condition depends on antifungal chemotherapy. Systemic therapy with fluconazole, itraconazole or voriconazole is usually necessary, and treatment may have to be prolonged and repeated.

Attempts have been made to restore T-cell function by the use of: (i) transfer factor (ii) thymosin; (iii) grafting compatible lymphocytes from blood or marrow; (iv) grafting fetal thymic tissue, and (v) non-specific measures such as the restoration of normal iron stores when these are defective.

Maintenance therapy should be avoided where possible to avoid the risk of antifungal resistance. Underlying endocrinopathies should be investigated and treated, although such treatment does not lead to improvement in the candidosis. Where appropriate, parents should be given genetic counselling. The possibility of coexisting dermatophytosis should not be forgotten, but it usually responds satisfactorily to oral treatment with itraconazole or terbinafine.

Bibliography

1. Chandler FW, Watts JC. *Pathologic Diagnosis of Fungal Infections*. Chicago: ASCP, 1987.
2. Christopher EM Griffiths, Jonathan Barker, Tanya Bleiker, Rook's textbook of dermatology. 9th edn: 32.49 Aptara Inc: New Delhi, India.
3. Cooke BED. Median rhomboid glossitis: candidiasis and not a developmental anomaly. *Br J Dermatol* 1975;93:399–405.
4. Hay RJ, Baran R, Moore MK, *et al*. Candida onychomycosis: an evaluation of the role of Candida species in nail disease. Br J Dermatol 1988;118:47–58.
5. Lowell A, Stephen IK Fitzpatrick's dermatology in general medicine. 8th edn.NewYork: McGraw-Hill; 2012.
6. MacCourtis J, Douglas LJ. Relationship between cell surface composition, adherence and virulence of *Candida albicans*. *Infect Immun* 1984;45:6–12.
7. Odds FC. *Candida and Candidosis*. London: Baillie-reTindall, 1988.

8. Odds FC. Genital candidosis. *Clin Exp Dermatol* 1982;7:343–254.

9. Ohman SC, Dahlen G, Moller A, *et al*. Angular cheilitis: a clinical and microbial study. *J Oral Pathol* 1985;15:213–217.

10. Rasmussen SA, *et al*. Vulvovaginal Candidiasis. MMWR Recomm Rep 2015;64:75–78.

11. Rosen T. Cutaneous candidiasis. In: Bodey GP, Fainstein V, eds. *Candidiasis*. New York: Raven 1985;227–240.

12. Samaranayake LP, Yaacob HB. Classification of oral candidosis. In: Samaranayake LP, MacFarlane TW, eds. *Oral Candidosis*. London: Wright 1990;15–21.

13. Sobel JD. Recurrent vulvovaginal candidiasis. *N Engl J Med* 1986;315:1455–1458.

14. Tappeiner J, Pfleger L. Granuloma gluteale infantum. *Hautarzt* 1971;22:383–388.

15. Wells RS. Chronic mucocutaneous candidiasis: a clinical classification. Proc R Soc Med 1973;66:801–802.

D. RECALCITRANT DERMATOMYCOSIS: FOCUS ON TINEA CORPORIS/CRURIS/PEDIS

INTRODUCTION

Before we discuss this topic a summary of the common terms and connotations in recalcitrant dermatomycosis are discussed below and depicted in Fig. 5.40.

Recalcitrant Infection

This is a generic term that may refer to relapse, recurrences, reinfection, persistence and possibly microbiological resistance. In India, this is largely restricted to truncal and crural tinea infections.

Resistance

This is a microbiological term and is ideally to be used when the MIC of the organism isolated is > 0.5 µg/ml for terbinafine. There are reports of resistance of *Trichophyton rubrum* to terbinafine where the *T. rubrum* isolates resistant were due to alterations in the squalene epoxidase gene or a factor essential for its activity. Usual MICs are 0.03 mg/ml in susceptible strains of *T. rubrum*; in these resistant strains, MICs were >1.0 mg/ml.

This term has been loosely used for recalcitrant infection leading to multiple esoteric and largely illogical dose regimens that satisfy primarily the pharmaceutical concerns! Clinically a patient that has a persistent infection or relapses within 4 weeks of an adequate dose regimen and duration of an approved drug can possibly have

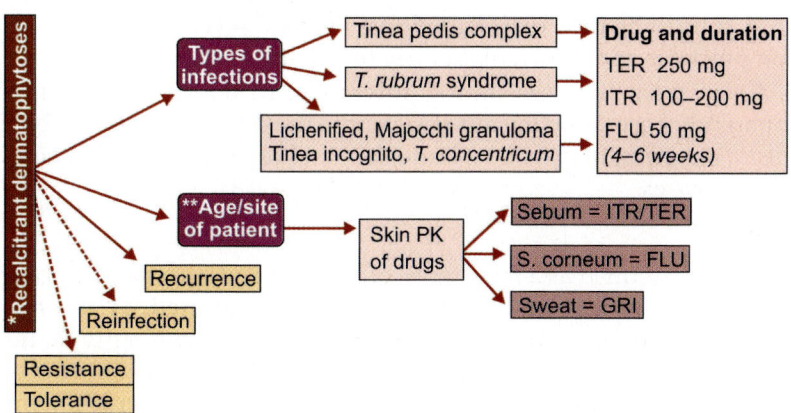

Fig. 5.40: Overview of various scenarios causing recalcitrant dermatophytosis (ITR: Itraconazole, TER: Terbinafine, GRI: Griseofulvin, FLU: Fluconazole) (*Rule out: Compliance, Misdiagnosis, Quality of drug) (**Age: Elderly, children FLU is an ideal drug)

resistance, if the immunological and extraneous factors (steroid suppression) have been excluded.

Clinical resistance: This is defined as failure of therapy due to subtherapeutic drug levels at the site of the infection caused by the *pharmacokinetics* of the drug, drug *interactions* or poor patient *compliance*. Other reasons for clinical failure include overwhelming infection, site of infection, and immune status of the host.

In vitro **resistance:** This is defined as a failure of drug to suppress growth of the test organism under certain specific growth conditions may be a predictor of poor clinical outcome. Two forms of antifungal drug resistance are recognized: Innate and emergent.

a. *Innate/intrinsic/primary:* The isolate was resistant to the drug before treatment started. This is predictable if one knows what the organism is and highlights the need for species identification.

b. *Emergent/acquired/induced/secondary:* The strain became resistant during treatment with the drug. This is the most difficult form of resistance because it is unpredictable.

Importantly a documented *in vitro* resistance does *not* translate always into clinical failure. This is because the levels achieved by the antifungal drug in the skin as opposed to the plasma, are much higher than the levels *in vitro*. Hence the drug may exceed the MIC many times over and the AUC/MIC ratio may exceed the *in vitro* MIC. This said, it is also known that in India the MIC to terbinafine is higher than itraconazole, but clinically ITR does not consistently show superior results. Griseofulvin has low MIC but by itself is a clinically ineffectual drug. It must be thus understood that the MIC levels reflect prescription practices and with a higher use of ITR the MIC to it will also rise.

Apart from true resistance, **tolerance**, in which the organism apparently becomes clinically resistant to the drug in the tissues but is *sensitive in vitro*, may also be important and may explain the scenario in some cases.

Relapse

This can be defined as a recurrence of the infection usually *after 4 weeks* of approved systemic therapy has been completed. It can have numerous causes including, humidity, sweating, clothing type, host immune response, barrier dysfunction and of course reinfection. A lack of adequate dose, compliance or an inimical drug interaction may also play a role.

It is a common occurrence in fungal infection and simple advise can help in preventing this, including, wearing cotton clothes, use of absorbent powders, treating hidden sites and barrier repair.

Persistence

This is a scenario where the patient does not respond in spite of correct appropriate fungicidal therapy for the appropriate duration. If all the above described scenarios are satisfied, such cases might be due to resistance. But in most cases these are merely the well established *difficult clinical types* where the correct duration of therapy is not administered, namely:

Tinea incognito, tinea imbricata, tinea pedis (non-dermatophye etiology), *T. rubrum* syndrome and of course Majocchi granuloma/ tinea profunda.

In India, use of steroids is the most important cause of persistence, amply certified by the fact that one does not see recalcitrant tinea capitis, tinea unguim, tinea pedis sites where steroids are rarely misused!

Chronic Dermatopytoses

Chronic dermatophytosis is defined as an infection that persists for 6 months to one year.

PATHOGENESIS

To understand the "epidemic" of recalcitrant and relapsing tinea infections it is important to understand the intricate relationship and interaction of the host defense mechanisms and the organisms as most of the cases of so-called "resistance" are actually cases where there is a local immune imbalance between the host and organism and *no in vitro* resistance.

Dermatophytoses, or tinea infections, are the most common superficial fungal infections in humans. They are caused by dermatophytes which may be classified as anthropophilic (*T. rubrum*, *Trichophyton tonsurans*), zoophilic (*Trichophyton mentagrophytes*, *Arthroderma benhamiae*) or geophilic (*Microsporum gypseum*). The steps of pathogenesis involve fours steps are depicted in Fig. 5.41.

1. Adhesion and Invasion of Tissue

In contrast to Candida and Malassezia, dermatophytes are not opportunists but are obligate pathogens that require keratin found in the skin stratum corneum, hair and nails for their survival. Thus, the ability to degrade *keratin* is a dermatophyte virulence factor. Dermatophytes produce several *proteases* such as subtilins and fungalysins and *A. benhamiae* has been shown to exhibit different protease gene expression profiles *in vitro* and *in vivo*, which suggests that these enzymes may perform roles other than keratin degradation. Furthermore, the gene encoding the serine protease subtilisin 6, a major allergen in *T. rubrum* (also called Tri r2) and putatively linked to host inflammation, are found to be strongly upregulated during *A. benhamiae* infection.

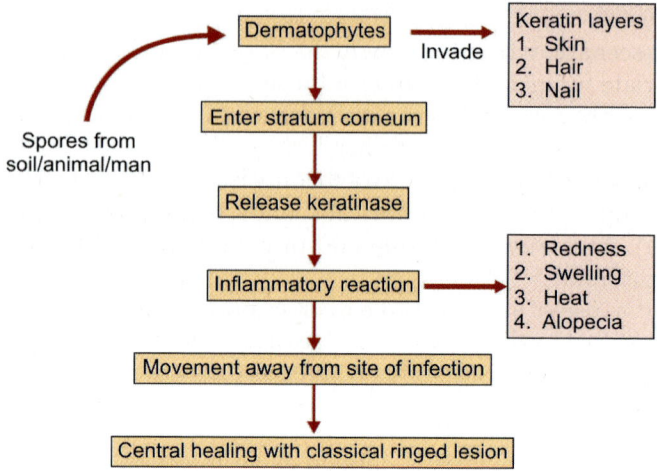

Fig. 5.41: A depiction of the salient steps of dermatophyte infection

Barrier defects: The cutaneous barrier helps to keep the dermatophyte out of the skin and any impairment like in ichthyosis and atopic skin precludes to invasion. The concomitant itching is another cause for impairment of this barrier. Importantly *T. rubrum* activates the Th2 response that stimulates B cells and leads to increase IgE levels that in turn causes itching and can explain the chronic dermatophyte infection due to *T. rubrum*. It has been also shown that dermatophytes alter the barrier function of the epidermis.

2. Host Factors

Genetic

HLA 26/DR 2, blood group A, atopy and raised IgE levels have been linked to chronicity. An AD predisposition to chronicity has been described.

Immune Response

Probably the most important aspect of pathogenesis and persistence of infection lies in understanding the host immune response (Fig. 5.42).

a. Pathogen-associated molecular patterns (PAMPs) and damage-associated molecular patterns (DAMPs) that are present during fungal infections are recognized by pattern recognition receptors (PRRs). The major **PRRs** are toll-like receptors **(TLRs)**; C-type lectin receptors **(CLRs**; such as dectin 1 (also known as CLEC7A), **dectin 2** (also known as CLEC6A), DC-specific ICAM3-grabbing non-integrin **(DC-SIGN)**, mincle and the mannose receptor); galectin family proteins (such as **galectin 3**) and receptor for advanced glycation end-products **(RAGE)** (Fig. 5.43).

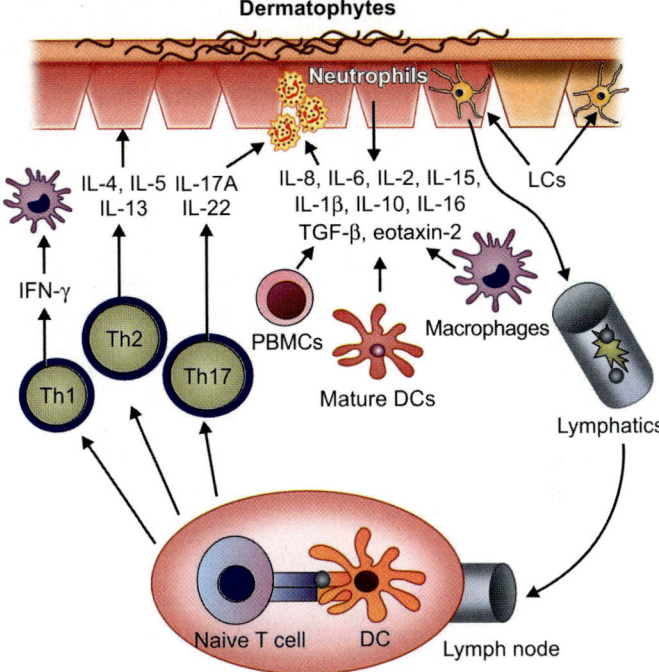

Fig. 5.42: Immune responses to dermatophytes. Anthropophilic dermatophytes such as *Trichophyton rubrum, Trichophyton schoenleinii* and *Trichophyton tonsurans* induce the production of interleukin (IL)-8, IL-6, IL-1β and eotaxin-2 in keratinocytes, peripheral blood mononuclear cells (PBMCs) and THP-1 cells, macrophages and dendritic cells (DC), while zoophilic dermatophytes such as *Arthroderma benhamiae* induce a wide range of cytokines including IL-1B, IL-6, IL-8, IL-10, IL-2, IL-15, IL-16, transforming growth factor (TGF)-β, interferon (IFN)-γ T helper (Th1), IL-17 (Th17), IL-4, IL-5 and IL-13 (Th2), leading to various pro-inflammatory processes such as neutrophil chemoattraction as well as macrophage and DC activation resulting in fungal killing and clearance

b. *TLRs* and *CLRs* activate multiple intracellular pathways upon binding to specific fungal PAMPs, including *β-glucans, chitin, mannans* and fungal *nucleic acids*. These signals activate canonical or non-canonical nuclear factor-κB (NF-κB) and the NOD-, LRR- and pyrin domain-containing 3 (NLRP3) inflammasome, and this culminates in the production of defensins, chemokines, cytokines, reactive oxygen species (ROS) and indoleamine 2, 3-dioxygenase (IDO) (Fig. 5.43).

c. The PRR like **TLR2** and **TLR4** as well as **dectin-1**, which are reported to mediate responses to *T. rubrum* conidia in HaCat KC by

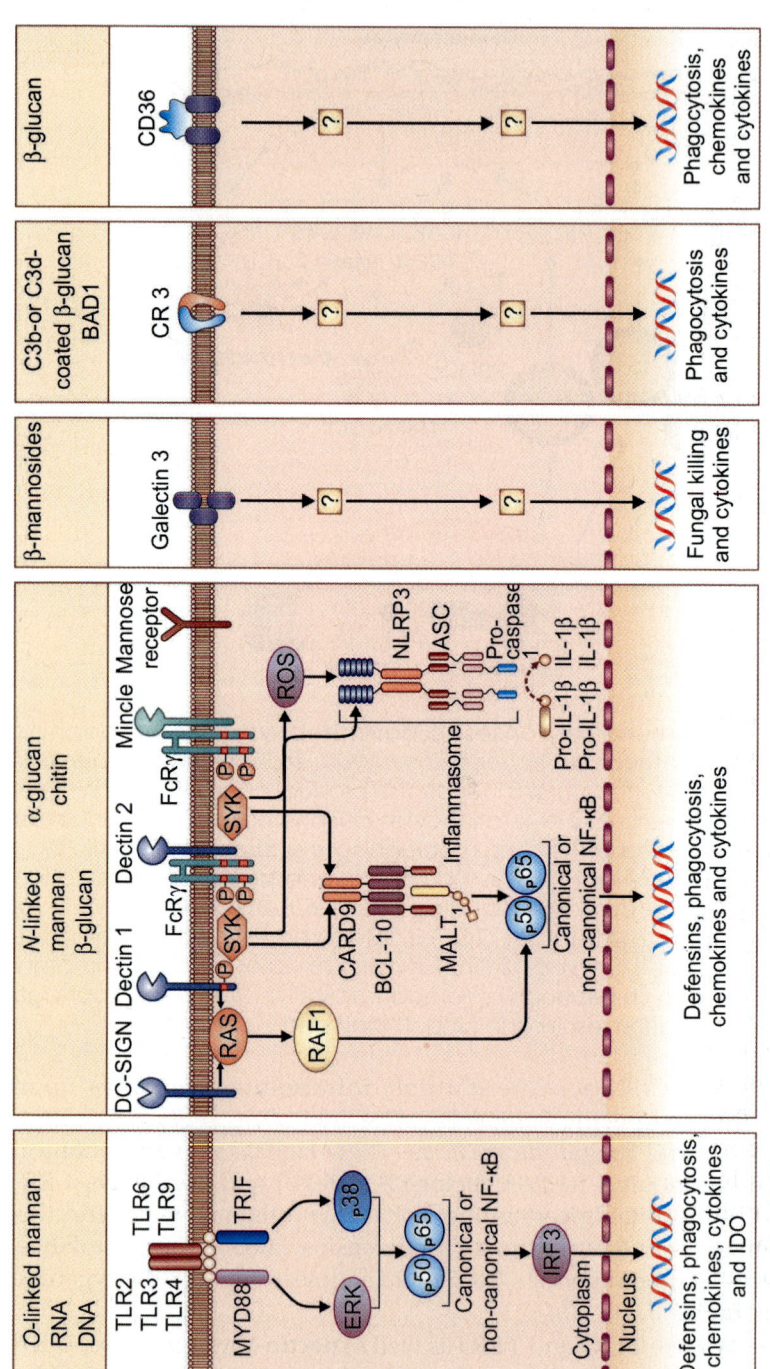

Fig. 5.43: Signaling pathways involved in the recognition of fungi by the host immune response

upregulation of IL-8, IFN-γ, IL-6 and IL-13. **DC-HIL**, a highly glycosylated type I transmembrane protein that is constitutively expressed at high levels in DC and macrophages, serves as a PRR for dermatophytic fungi by binding to *T. rubrum* and *M. audouinii* but not *C. albicans*. On the other hand, *Trichophyton schoenleinii*, the causative agent of trichophytosis and tinea favosa of the scalp, is shown to induce the production of IL-1β in THP-1 cells, a human monocytic cell line, through activation of the inflammasome via NLRP3.

The interactions between the PRR and the host receptors trigger phagocytosis, respiratory burst (via the NADPH oxidase) and the killing of fungi, and also trigger intracellular signalling pathways that lead to the activation of transcription factors, such as nuclear factor-κB (NF-κB). These transcription factors induce the production of many pro-inflammatory cytokines and chemokines that are important for host defence against fungi.

c. Infections caused by anthropophilic dermatophytes are generally *chronic* and accompanied by minimal to varying inflammation. On the other hand, infections with zoophilic fungal species such as *A. benhamiae*, a teleomorph of *T. mentagrophytes*, can induce more severe inflammation in the human host. In a study comparing the cytokine secretion profiles of *T. tonsurans* and *A. benhamiae*, Shiraki et al. reported that *T. tonsurans*-infected KC secreted only eotaxin-2, IL-8 and IL-16, whereas *A. benhamiae* induced the production of a broad variety of pro-inflammatory and immunomodulatory cytokines/chemokines. It has been reported that Trichophyton-induced inflammation involves the proliferation of PBMC and IFN-γ production. IFN-γ gene expression is seen in *T. rubrum* infections indicating that Trichophyton-induced dermatophytosis is a Th1-type contact hypersensitivity.

These findings indicate that the cutaneous acquired immune responses to dermatophyte infections involve **Th1**, **Th2** and **Th17** components, and this is in line with other studies involving *Trichophyton* spp. (Fig. 5.42).

Importantly a **Th2** response leads to **persistence** of infection. The multiple, functionally distinct signalling pathways in antigen-presenting cells ultimately affect the local Th cell/Treg cell balance, and are likely to be exploited by fungi to allow commensalism or opportunism.

Other factors: It is plausible that reinfection from family members may play a role as is infection from nails, and vellus hair. The other factors include DM, HIV and systemic immunosuppression.

The Ph, CO_2 levels, sebum levels and transferrin levels are other factors that have been shown to play a role in persistent infections. There are a plethora of factors that have been used to explain the host predisposition and the list is ever growing, some bordering on fanciful thinking.

These include hygiene, migration of infection, pollution and clothing, which are hard to substantiate as in other countries which are worse off in all these parameters do not have the same extent of affliction as in India.

3. Fungal Specific Factors

It is well accepted that there is an intricate mechanism of interaction of the fungal receptors and the host receptors that determine the pathogenicity (Fig. 5.43). This include the type of species, *virulence* factors, *toxins*, *keratinases* and *mannans*. These preclude to the invasion into the stratum corneum. Though the commonest species is still *T. rubrum* which is usually non-inflammatory (anthropophilic), a larger proportion is now *T. mentagrophytes* that has two variants, the *granulosa* and var. *intertidigitale*, which are variably zoophilic and anthrophilic.

Dermatophytes, like *T. rubrum* and *T. tonsurans*, are highly adapted to humans and can evade or silence the immune response, causing chronic dermatophytosis. *Trichophyton rubrum* cell wall mannans (TRM) seem to be involved in apart from immunosuppression.

a. In a dose-dependent manner, TRM are able to inhibit *in vitro* lymphoproliferative response of mononuclear leukocytes in response to several antigens (dermatophytic or not) and mitogens; paradoxically, they are a major T-cell antigen. Although specific suppressor T-cells are eventually activated during persistent infections, target cells for TRM action appear to be monocytes rather than lymphocytes.

b. TRM may also inhibit stratum corneum turnover, directly or via lymphocyte function alteration.

c. The level of interleukin (IL)-1α produced by *T. rubrum*-treated keratinocytes is significantly lower than that induced by *T. mentagrophytes*, which could be related to the different clinical expression of the two types of infection.

    Trichophyton rubrum could thus evade the immune response by killing macrophages or modulating their activation program.

d. The complex relationship existing between dermatophytosis and allergic diseases has to be discussed here. The predisposing role of atopy in chronic dermatophytosis is not clearly established; on the other hand, it is now accepted that chronic dermatophytosis, associated with immediate hypersensitivity skin test reactions and Th2 cytokines, can contribute to the pathogenesis of allergic diseases, especially asthma.

e. The fact is that most tinea infections seen by dermatologists are caused by *T. rubrum* which induce immune-suppression through toll-like receptor 2 (TLR2) mediated IL-10 release, and this leads to generation of CD4+, CD25+ T-regulatory cells with immunosuppressive potential. Thus there is a lack of a Th1-type cell response. Consequently, there would be increased Th2-type responses that are inadequate to fight fungal infections. This would allow a chronic and extensive infection to set in.

These findings indicate that inflammatory mediators differentially regulate Trichophyton-induced contact hypersensitivity depending on the status of host immunity, signifying that varying acquired immune responses may be noted in patients with different immunological statuses.

In conclusion, the interaction between pathogenic fungi and the immune system is highly complex and involves an entire range of responses. Furthermore, certain fungi have adaptive mechanisms and have immunomodulatory capabilities that enable them to survive on the skin. Lessons drawn from understanding the mechanisms that underlie the cutaneous immune responses to superficial skin fungal infections may shed light on future strategies in antifungal treatment.

FACTORS DETERMINING RECALCITRANT INFECTION

The practical relevance of host immune response is that it can explain the recalcitrant infection, the various factors which are listed in Box 5.3 and will help the clinician to look beyond just the antifungal drug, which is a small part of the complex interaction that determines the ultimate clinical picture of recalcitrant infection.

1. **Clinical type:** There are certain types of tinea which are inherently recalcitrant and this is important as often standard dose regimens

---

Box 5.3: Determinants of recalcitrant mycoses

- Clinical type of tinea corporis
- Fungal species (*T. rubrum*) and type (zoophilic/anthropophilic)
- Barrier integrity
- Host immunity
- Local host factors
- Drug: PK/PD and quality
- Reinfection and persistence
- *In vitro* resistance
- Antifungal use in agriculture

are given which do *not* treat them adequately. This include the lichenified tinea corporis, tinea incognito, tinea profunda, Majocchi granuloma and tinea concentericum. These warrant a longer dose regimen up to *6 weeks*.

Tinea pedis is caused also by *non-dermatophytes* and the ideal therapy is *itraconazole*. When secondary bacterial infection is involved, the condition may be referred to as *dermatophytosis complex* and is recalcitrant to therapy. *T. mentagrophytes*, a fungus of animal origin, can be responsible for an especially fulminating form of the disease, including ulceration of the epidermis, purulent vesicle fluid, and rapid spread.

2. **Species:** The type of organism is important with *T. rubrum* being more *chronic* than other infections. Recalcitrant dermatophyte infections are often caused by *T. rubrum*. *T. rubrum* may invade beyond the stratum corneum to involve the follicles, progressing to form chronic inflammatory lesions. Re-infection with a new genetically unrelated strain can also be a cause. It has been proposed that the virulence of species has increased and is related to a change from zoophilic to anthropophilic but this is as yet conjectural.

   Is a co-pathogen or secondary infection present? This should be considered in the feet, kerion, and perhaps in groin infections. In nails, the coexistence of non-dermatophyte fungus should be considered. *Scopulariopsis brevicaulis*, apart from causing infections of the toenails in its own right, may coexist with *Trichophyton rubrum* or *T. interdigitale* and seems, at least on occasions, to cause failure of treatment. Nail removal may be indicated in this instance.

3. The **host immune response**, Th1/17 being protective and Th2 helping in chronicity of infection (Fig. 5.42).

4. **The barrier defect:** The skin barrier is important and thus it is crucial to administer a good antihistamine to reduce itching and take care of barrier repair as the lack of this simple measure may cause recurrences.

5. **Local factors:** Heat, humidity, sweating and type of cloth are also proposed to play a role.

6. **Pharmacological factors:** Has the patient been taking the tablets *regularly*? Is the patient taking any potentially *competitive* drugs? In spite of taking them correctly, is the patient failing to *absorb* the antibiotic? An estimation of itraconazole levels, which is sometimes poorly absorbed, may be helpful. Also the *cutaneous PK* of the antifungal drugs with the variable concentration in the skin of drugs (Fig. 5.40) depending on the route of secretion is also crucial and is detailed in the chapter on drugs. In India there is a definite issue of quality and is seen with various brands of itraconazole.

7. **Reinfection:** As ringworm fungi can frequently be isolated from the environment, when there are cases of ringworm of the scalp, and from clothing after laundering, it is highly likely that patients whose infection has been eradicated may be reinfected from these sources. Unfortunately, there is no proven way to avoid this.

8. **Recurrence:** Although a response may be obtained with topical or systemic therapy, there is recurrence in 60 to 70% of patients. These infections require prolonged therapy with systemic and topical agents for 2 to 3 months or longer. Even after such infections appear to be cleared, it may be difficult to prevent recurrences.

   Recurrence may sometimes be caused by failure to eradicate the original infection rather than by reinfection. In India one of the most important causes for this is *undertreatment*. Patients frequently stop applying topical therapy when their symptoms improve. Also the systemic therapy is costly and the patients stop the same once the initial improvement occurs. For that reason, when a patient has a recurrence of tinea pedis or tinea cruris, culture frequently reveals the same organism that was found in the initial infection.

9. **Antifungal resistance:** This phenomenon is sufficiently *uncommon* among dermatophytes to make routine testing unnecessary, but where treatment failure occurs without any other explanation, it is possible to estimate the sensitivity of the causal organism. This should be performed by a specialist laboratory. Apart from true resistance, tolerance, in which the organism apparently becomes clinically resistant to the drug in the tissues but is sensitive *in vitro*, may also be important.

Of all the factors listed above, the *cardinal factors* that determine chronicity are:

a. The *clinical type* of tinea infection
b. The *host's defense* against receptors of the fungi
c. The *virulence* potential of the infecting strain or species.

MANAGEMENT OF RECALCITRANT DERMATOPHYTES: PRINCIPLES AND PRACTICES

Though most clinicians are obsessed with the issue of failure of antifungal drugs, we have in this section looked at the other relevant factors and we give a summary of the common clinical practices adopted, the rationale therein and then discuss a treatment approach, using a step by step algorithm.

Failure of Topical Therapy

Most failures of topical therapy are caused by inaccurate diagnosis or by inappropriate use of topical therapy (e.g. in hairy areas) or because the treatment is not used. Once or twice daily application for several weeks is usually required for success, and many patients, particularly if their symptoms are minor, will not achieve this unless they are carefully supervised and enthusiastically encouraged. Paradoxically, some non-fungal conditions may be improved considerably by one of the antidermatophyte preparations, although these remedies should not be used empirically to establish the diagnosis of ringworm infection. Many dermatoses respond, at least temporarily, to any bland application, and imidazole compounds in particular have considerable antibacterial properties.

Failure of Oral Therapy

When a patient fails to respond to terbinafine, fluconazole or itraconazole, the following points should be checked:

1. Is the **diagnosis** correct? If necessary, repeat scrapings.
2. **Compliance:** Has the patient been taking the tablets regularly? With the more expensive brands, patients rarely take the therapy and a good practice is to write for 10 days and then call the patients for reveiw.
3. **Interactions:** Is the patient taking any potentially competitive drugs?
4. **Absorption:** In spite of taking them correctly, is the patient failing to absorb the antibiotic? An estimation of itraconazole levels, which is sometimes poorly absorbed, may be helpful. This is a good argument of giving terbinafine. A problem of *quality* is a valid concern and this makes a difference to the therapeutic results.
5. In some patients with onychomycosis, poor **penetration** of drugs into defined linear streaks or nail edge areas of nail plate infection may account for treatment failure. Surgical removal of these abnormal nail areas, often after softening with urea ointment, may be useful.
6. Is there coexisting pathology such as HIV/AIDS or arterial disease? Another common cause of chronicity is DM.
7. Antifungal resistance. This phenomenon is sufficiently uncommon among dermatophytes to make routine testing unnecessary, but where treatment failure occurs without any other explanation, it is possible to estimate the sensitivity of the causal organism. Apart from true resistance, *tolerance*, in which the organism apparently becomes clinically resistant to the drug in the tissues but is sensitive *in vitro*, may also be important.

Common Antifungal Prescription Practices and Strategies to Overcome Recalcitrant Infection

As actual *in vitro* resistance is uncommon most cases are best described as recalcitrant infections. Most of the listed points are based on common practice and are largely restricted to tinea corporis/cruris and pedis/mannum, these being the prevalent concern in India.

1. **Increased antifungal dose and duration:** Many practitioners are using *higher doses* of terbinafine and itraconazole, up to 500 mg (*terbinafine*) once daily and for longer durations, up to 4–6 weeks.

   This has been detailed in the chapter of drugs and as shown in Fig. 5.40, the PK of the drugs vary and the ideal scenario would be to know the AUC and MIC in the skin. In most cases the skin AUC is **10–40 times** the plasma and exceeds the MIC and thus there is a little logic in high dose regimens. A high dose of **itraconazole** beyond 200 mg a day has again a little rationale as the drug has non-linear PK. A 100 mg BD dose is better than giving a 200 mg OD dose if required. This is why DCGI has not approved the 200 mg capsule in India as yet though numerous companies have launched 200 mg, with local FDA approval.

2. **New drug delivery system:** It includes bioadhesive films, solid lipid nanoparticles, microparticles, nanosomes, miroemulsion transdermal delivery, buccal adhesive *in situ* gel, microcapsule, liposomal, niosomes, ethosomes, transdermal spray, biodegradable implants, hydrogels, transferosome, etc. but none of these are yet available in India.

3. **Combination of antifungal drugs:** This will broaden antifungal coverage, have synergistic effect, decrease chances of development of resistance and decrease the toxicity. Thus, combining drugs of two different classes, one in topical form and other as systemic, for example topical allylamine + oral azole is believed to be a preferred combination.

   This approach is again strictly *off label* and unless *in vitro* 'checkerboard' study can show its synergism it may be counter-productive. A classic example is amphotericin B and azoles which are *antagonistic* and thus should *not* be combined. Ciclopirox olamine and terbinafine are *synergistic* but the former is not available in a cream form.

4. **Topical salicylic acid 6%:** It is a useful co-prescription and can help achieve the dual effect of increasing the levels of the topical antifungal drug and remove the stratum corneum wherein the fungus lies. Salicylic acid is a keratolytic and at concentrations between 3% and 6% causes softening of the horny layers and shedding of scales. It produces this desquamation by solubilizing

the intercellular cement and enhances the shedding of corneocytes by decreasing cell-to-cell cohesion. In concentrations >6%, it can be destructive to tissue. Application of large amounts of the higher concentration of salicylic acid can also result in systemic toxicity.

5. **Systemic ketoconazole and griseofulvin:** Their use is contrary to skin PK studies as the highest sebum concentration is of terbinafine and itraconazole and that in the stratum corneum is of fluconazole (daily dose). Ketoconazole is not superior, at least, as far as skin infections are concerned. The low MIC of griseofulvin reported by mycologists is of no clinical importance as the drug rarely achieves high levels in the skin and does not persist apart from its fungistatic effect, except in patient who sweat profusively, where it may be a preferred drug.

6. **Oral isotretinoin combined with other antifungals:** The major drawback often is that this drug can negate the action of lipophilic drugs which happen to be terbinafine and itraconazole, the most commonly prescribed medications. Some use oral vitamin A which may offer similar effects as isotretinoin without effecting sebum.

APPROACH TO TREATMENT OF RECALCITRANT DERMATOPHYTOSIS

Our approach is given in Fig. 5.44 and is based on scientific data and is based on two prerequistes, the first is **compliance** and the second is use of a good **quality** brand, both of which most clinicians are adept at handling in clinical practice. The approach is based on the pathogenesis, but we are at the moment unable to propose a method of overcoming the immune suppression, except for proposing a longer duration of therapy. It is more relevant to understand that some tinea infections, like incognito, Majocchi granuloma, tinea profunda and

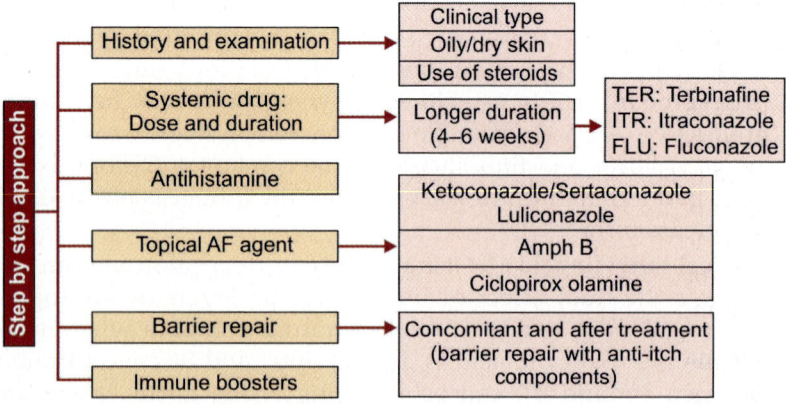

Fig. 5.44: An approach to treatment of recalcitrant dermatophytoses

concentericum, need a prolonged duration of therapy and thus the so-called clinical failure is because we are given a short duration of therapy. Such cases require 6 weeks of therapy for an adequate response. This is also due to a local immunosupprression consequent to the use of steroids which take about 3 weeks to recover.

We are detailing an approach to this problem and the attached clinical cases (Figs 5.45–5.49) detail the various scenarios depicted in Fig. 5.44.

Step 1: History and examination

Assess **steroid** use, if steroids have been used, a 3 weeks lack of response is expected. Also a **Majocchi granuloma** is bound to take more time to respond as the infection is within and around the hair follicle. A **lichenified** look suggests a *T. rubrum* infection and again a prolonged course may be needed. Also it is a good idea to assess whether the patient has a **dry or oily** skin as TER and ITR both are lipophilic and may not work in a patient with dry skin, here fluconazole is a better option.

Step 2: Drug: Dose and duration

There is a form of persistent tinea infection usually caused by *T. rubrum* at sites in the groin or the trunk which, while responding initially to treatment with either terbinafine or itraconazole, relapses quickly. Different treatment regimens have been tried including combinations of azole or allylamine oral medications plus topical azoles or allylamines. In contrast tinea infections of the skin in immunosuppressed patient including those with HIV/AIDS usually respond to treatment although it is often necessary to double the normal dose. A summary of the dose and duration is given below.

1. Terbinafine

The usual adult dose is **250** mg once daily. The duration of treatment depends on the site and severity of the infection. It is usually **2–6** weeks in tinea pedis, **2–4** weeks in tinea cruris and **4** weeks in tinea corporis.

a. Tinea corporis and tinea cruris: 250 mg daily for **4 weeks**
b. Tinea pedis and mannum: 250 mg daily for **2–6 weeks**
c. Tinea imbricata: 250 mg PO qd for **4 weeks**
d. **Off label** double dose (250 mg BD). This has been recommended only in immunosuppressed patients including those with HIV/AIDS.

2. Itraconazole

It is active against a wide range of dermatophytes and is effective in regimens of 100 mg for 15 days in tinea cruris and corporis or 30 days in dry-type tinea pedis. The currently preferred regimen by clinicians uses 400 mg a day, given as two daily doses of 200 mg. In tinea corporis, 1 week of therapy at this dosage is sufficient and in dry-type tinea pedis 2 weeks. Occasionally, longer periods of treatment are needed.

a. **Tinea corporis, tinea cruris**

  Itraconazole : 100 mg 7 to 14 days

  : 200 mg 7 days

b. **Tinea pedis and mannum**

  100 mg/day for 30 days

  200 mg daily for 2–4 weeks

  200 mg bid for 7 days

c. **Majocchi granuloma**

  Majocchi's granuloma: 200 mg PO bid for 7 days, then off for 14 days (repeat 3 times total)

d. **Tinea imbricata:** 100 mg PO qd for 4 weeks

3. Fluconazole

Fluconazole 50–100 mg for 20 days.

Step 3: Antihistamines

This is important to prevent skin damage which is one of the causes for penetration of the fungi. Most clincians give hydroxyzine, some administer Doxepin but being a H_2 blocker it reduces the absorption of Itraconazole, hence an alternative drug should be used in case doxepin is prescribed.

Step 4: Topical ketoconazole, setraconazole, terbinafine, ciclopirox olamine, amphotericin B.

Topical agents are useful as it enhances skin PK levels which exceed serum levels by 100X. It should be continued for 2 weeks after resolution. A good adjuvant is topical salicylic acid 6%, which helps to increase the penetration and desquamates the stratum corneum, the site of infection by dermatophytes.

Step 5: Barrier repair

This is a crucial step and should be added to the therapy with and after resolution. A good non-keratolytic moisturiser with barrier repair will prevent recurrence. The cheaper option is Secalia™ and Emoderm™ while an expensive option is Atopiclair Lotion™, the latter being particularly useful as it has an antifungal component.

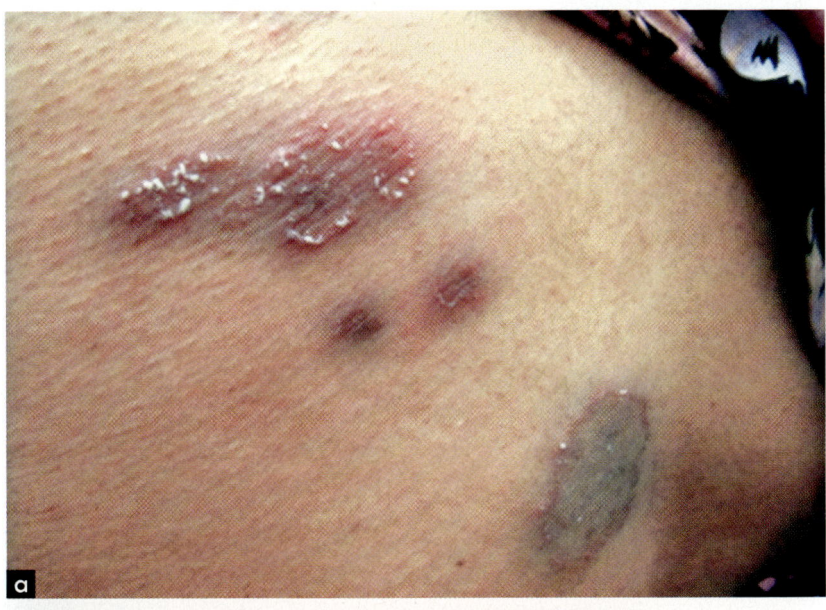

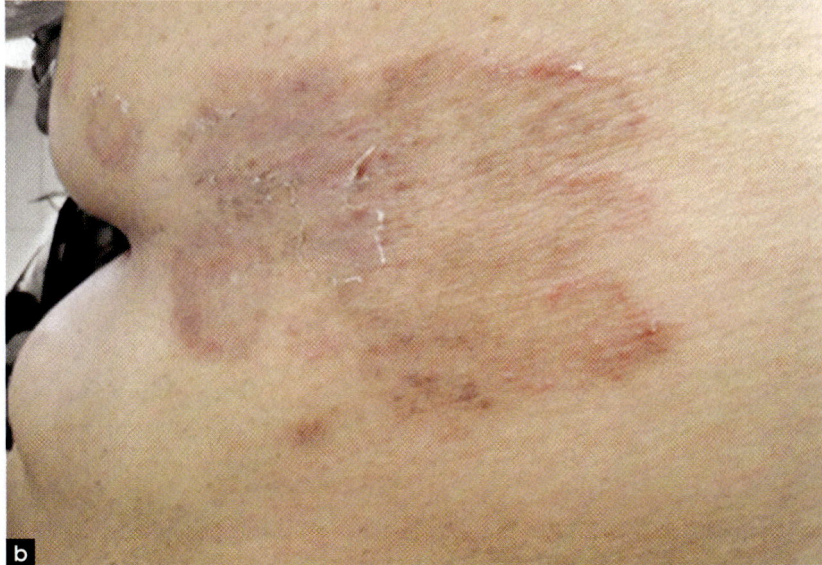

Fig. 5.45a and b: A 50-year-old diabetic female with dry skin who had failed therapy with terbinafine and itraconazole. Note the pustules which are indicative of Majocchi granuloma. The dry skin and failure of conventional systemic AF led to the use of fluconazole 50 mg bd for 20 days with marked improvement. Topical ketoconazole and barrier creams are to be continued for a further 2 weeks

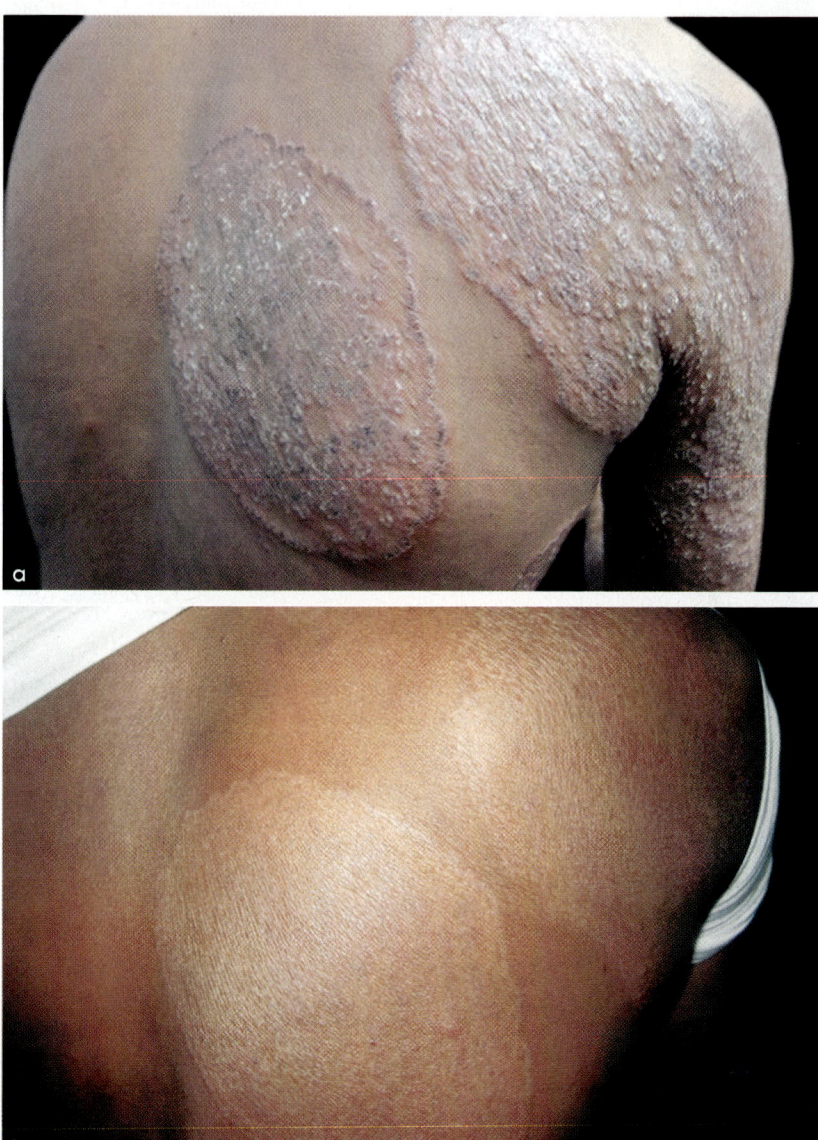

Fig. 5.46a and b: This patient had extensive tinea corporis with papules s/o Majocchi granuloma. He had applied every conceivable steroid combination and used oral AF. As this was a case of localised immunosuppression we administerd double dose terbinafine (250 mg bd) with topical ketaconazole and salicylic acid 6%, the response after 4 weeks is a happy outcome. A barrier cream was advised subsequently to be used for 4 weeks

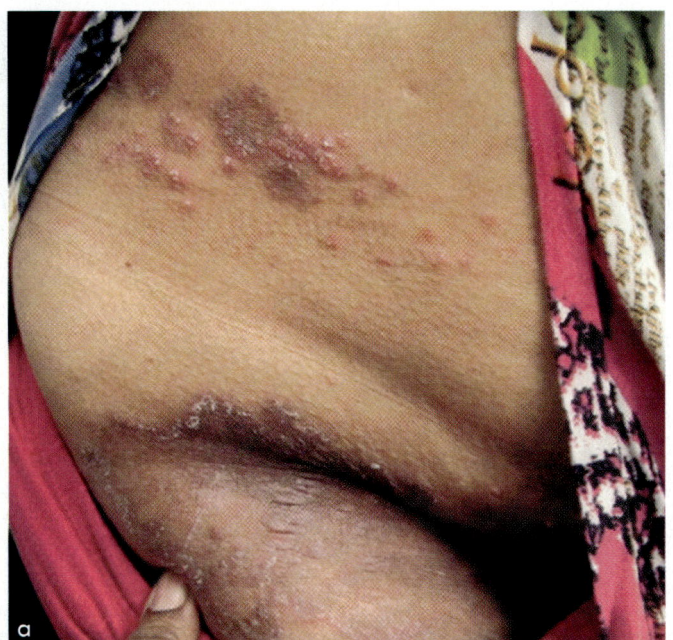

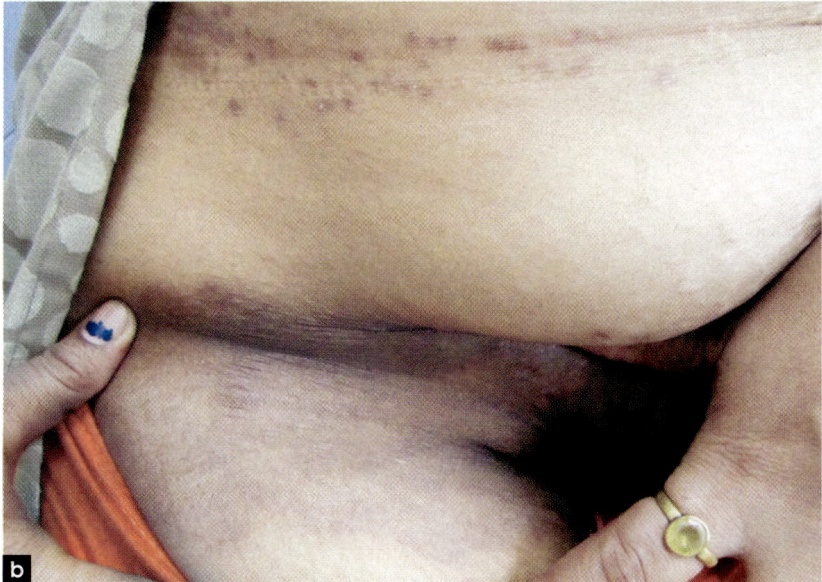

Fig. 5.47a and b: This patient had failed terbinafine 500 mg and was also applying a steroid combination. The patient was administered 100 mg bd itraconazole with topical salicylic acid 6% and ketoconazole. Being a lipid-rich site itraconazole is a useful option in this patient

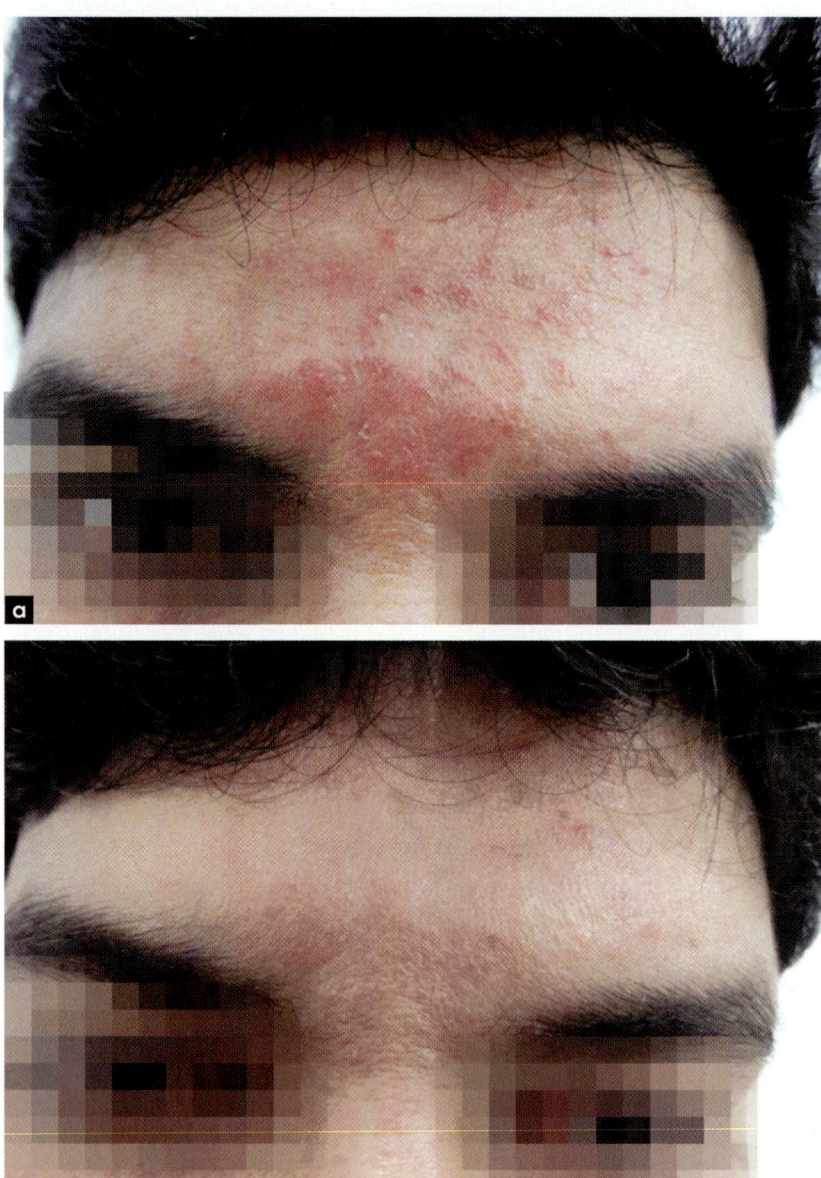

Fig. 5.48a and b: This patient was being treated as a case of acne with oral doxycycline 100 mg, in today's times dermatophytosis is the "great mimicker" possibly replacing syphilis. He responded to oral terbinafine 250 mg for 3 weeks. Being on the face a oil-rich site either terbinafine or itraconazole are equally good options

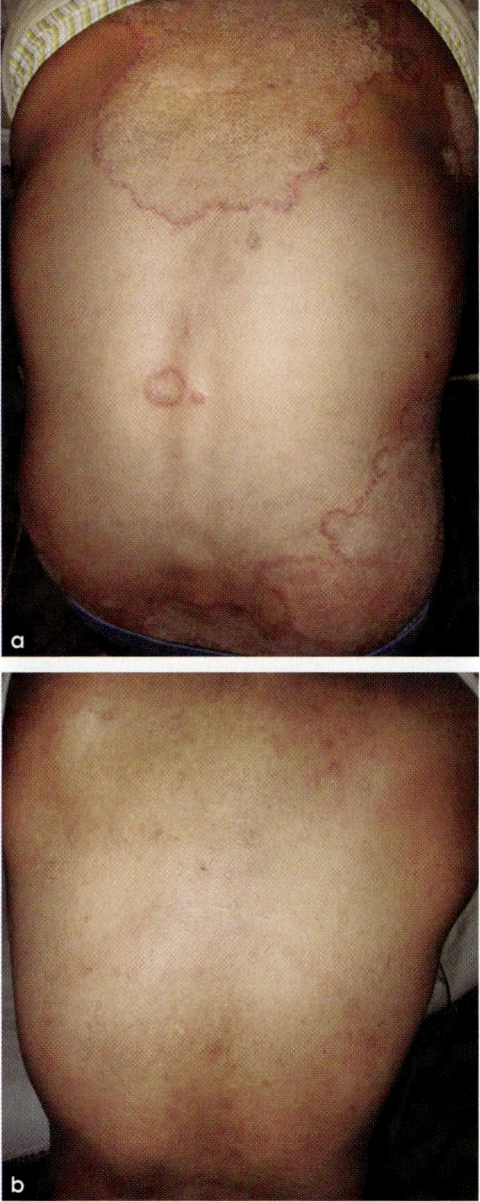

Fig. 5.49a and b: Extensive tinea corporis patient with a history application of numerous triple combination steroids who was given terbinafine 250 mg bd (as it is a case of localised immunosuppression and the trunk is a lipid-rich site) with marked improvement after 5 weeks. Note the dose and duration, a lesser duration would have labelled this as a "resistant case"

CONCLUSIONS

Despite running through the various factors and following the steps listed above dermatologists may not come up with an adequate explanation for treatment failure in all cases (Fig. 5.50). Resistance is more "on the lips than in the lab" and very few genuine cases exist, and if one appreciates the PK and MIC levels in the skin of the oral AF, they would exceed the MIC many times over. Most importantly, it is the host immunity that is crucial and this is the only reason why India is the hot bed of chronicity. All the other host factors are discounted for as they are common worldwide, but those countries do not report chronicity. It is hard to logically believe that all the various factors listed in the text above have all combined to cause chronicity in India. But if one appreciates the elaborate immunological pathways (Figs 5.42 and 5.43) it will be obvious that, herein lies the answer, as its only in India that has the "perfect storm" of OTC steroids and a plethora of prescription based AF-steroids, with a little prescription control that leads to an immunological compromise.

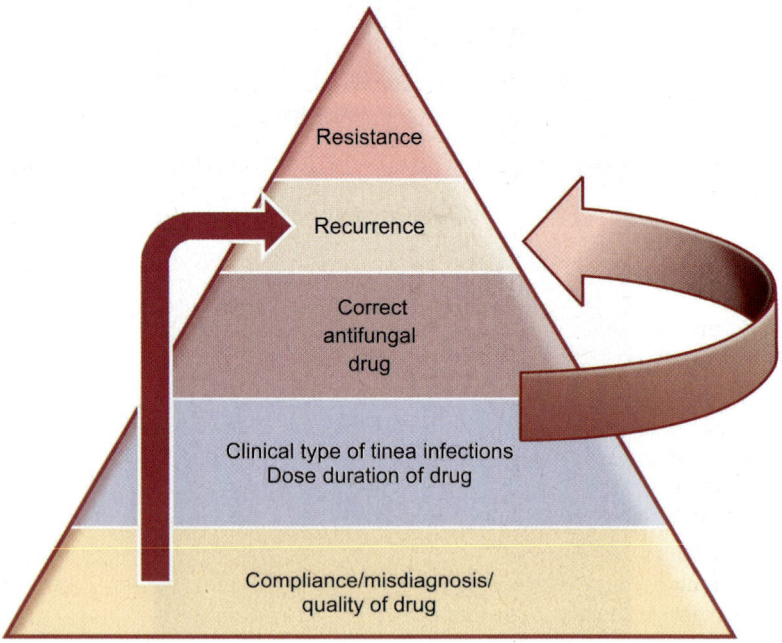

Fig. 5.50: A depiction of the relative contribution of factors that cause recalcitrant dermatophytoses, note that a combination of compliance and improper dose and duration of drug may cause most of the recurrence, which is not the same as resistance, which is decidedly uncommon

In essence the problem is localised immunosuppression due to topical steroids and without that being addressed most aggressive, antifungal measures are likely to fail.

Though it is our belief that the type of species and the subverted immune response predicts most recalcitrant infections, possibly quality of the drugs and compliance may also be important. The final answer may be an amalgamation of the varied factors described in the chapter, but this may well be re-written in the future!

Bibliography

1. Blake JS, Dahl MV, Herron MJ, Nelson RD. An immunoinhibitory cell wall glycoprotein (mannan) from *Trichophyton rubrum*. J Invest Dermatol 1991; 96:657–661.

2. Bressani VO, Santi TN, Domingues-Ferreira M et al. Characterization of the cellular immunity in patients presenting extensive dermatophytoses due to *Trichophyton rubrum*. Mycoses 2013; 56: 281–288.

3. Cambier L, Weatherspoon A, Defaweux V et al. Assessment of the cutaneous immune response during *Arthroderma benhamiae* and *A. vanbreuseghemii* infection using an experimental mouse model. Br J Dermatol 2014; 170: 625–633.

4. Favre B, Ghannoum MA, Ryder NS. Biochemical characterization of terbinafine-resistant Trichophytonrubrum isolates. Med Mycol 2004;42:525–529.

5. Gazit R, Hershko K, Ingbar A et al. Immunological assessment of familial tinea corporis. J Eur Acad Dermatol Venereol 2008; 22: 871–874.

6. Grando SA, Hostager BS, Herron MJ, Dahl MV, Nelson RD. Binding of *Trichophyton rubrum* mannan to human monocytes in vitro. J Invest Dermatol 1992;98:876–880.

7. Grando SA, Hostager BS, Herron MJ, Dahl MV, Nelson RD. Binding of *Trichophyton rubrum* mannan to human monocytes in vitro. J Invest Dermatol 1992;98:876–880.

8. Koga T, Ishizaki H, Matsumoto T, Hori Y. In vitro release of interferon-gamma by peripheral blood mononuclear cells of patients with dermatophytosis in response to stimulation with trichophytin. Br J Dermatol 1993; 128: 703–704.

9. MacCarthy KG, Blake JS, Johnson KL, Dahl MV, Kalish RS. Human dermatophyte-responsive T-cell lines recognize cross-reactive antigens associated with mannose-rich glycoproteins. Exp Dermatol 1994;3:66–71.

10. Shiraki Y, Ishibashi Y, Hiruma M, Nishikawa A, Ikeda S. Cytokine secretion profiles of human keratinocytes during *Trichophyton tonsurans* and *Arthroderma benhamiae* infections. J Med Microbiol 2006; 55: 1175–1185.

11. Slunt JB, Taketomi EA, Woodfolk JA, Hayden ML, Platts-Mills TA. The immune response to *Trichophyton tonsurans*: distinct T cell cytokine profiles

to a single protein among subjects with immediate and delayed hypersensitivity. J Immunol 1996; 157: 5192–5197.

12. Staib P, Zaugg C, Mignon B et al. Differential gene expression in the pathogenic dermatophyte Arthroderma benhamiae in vitro versus during infection. Microbiology 2010; 156: 884–895.

13. Verma S, Hefferman MP. Superficial fungal infection: dermatophytosis, onychomycosis, tinea nigra, piedra. In: Wolff K, Goldsmith L, Katz S, Gilchrest B, Paller A, Lefell D, eds. Fitzpatricks Dermatology In General Medicine, 7th edn. New York: McGraw-Hill Professional 2007; 1807–1821.

14. Weitzman I, Summerbell RC. The dermatophytes. ClinMicrobiol Rev 1995; 8: 240–259.

15. Woodfolk JA, Wheatley LM, Piyasena RV, Benjamin DC, Platts-Mills TA. Trichophyton antigens associated with IgE antibodies and delayed type hypersensitivity. Sequence homology to two families of serine proteinases. J Biol Chem 1998; 273: 29489–29496.

16. Zaugg C, Monod M, Weber J et al. Gene expression profiling in the human pathogenic dermatophyte *Trichophyton rubrum* during growth on proteins. Eukaryot Cell 2009; 8: 241–250.

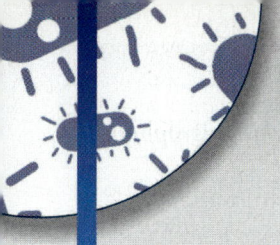

CHAPTER 6

Subcutaneous Mycoses

The classification of subcutaneous mycoses is detailed in Chapter 1, we will be covering the commonly seen disorders in clinical practice and the rare disorders can be referenced from specialized textbooks.

1. MYCETOMA (Madura Foot/Madura Mycosis)

Pooja Arora Mrig, Kabir Sardana

DEFINITION

Mycetoma is derived from the Greek word meaning "fungal tumor". It is a granulomatous infection of skin and subcutaneous tissue that is caused by fungi (eumycetoma) or actinomycetes (actinomycetoma). It is characterised by local edema, formation of abscess and draining sinuses that discharge grains.

Epidemiology

Mycetoma is endemic in tropical and subtropical countries. Eumycotic mycetoma is more prevalent in Africa whereas Actinomycotic mycetoma is endemic in Central and South America. It usually affects adult males in the age group 20–50 years. Agricultural workers are more susceptible due to their nature of occupation. Mycetoma is rare in children.

Etiology

At least 30 species of fungi are associated with human eumycetoma. The etiologic agents of eumycetoma, depending upon the type of grain, are classified into those that produce **black grains** and those that produce **white or grayish grains**. The most important are:

- *Eumycetoma* caused by *black* fungi or phaeohyphomycetes: *Madurella mycetomatis, M. grisea, Leptosphaeria senegalensis, Leptosphaeria tompkinsii, Pyrenochaeta romeroi, Pyrenochaeta mackinnonii, Cladophialophora bantiana, Cladophialophora mycetomatis* (spp. *nova*), *Curvularia lunata*, *Curvularia geniculata*, *Exophiala jeanselmei*, *Phialophora verrucosa*.

- *Eumycetomas* caused by *whitish* fungi (hyalohyphomycetes):
  Pseudallescheria boydii (*Scedosporium apiospermum*), *Acremonium falciform kiliense*, *Acremonium recifei*, *Neotestudina rosati*, *Fusarium moniliforme*, *Fusarium solani*, *Aspergillus nidulans*, *Aspergillus flavus*, *Cylindrocarpon cyanescens*, and *Dermatophytes* (*Trichophyton rubrum*, *Microsporum audouini*, *Microsporum canis*).

More than 90% of eumycetomas reported worldwide are caused by only four agents: *M. mycetomatis*, *M. grisea*, *P. boydii*, and *L. senegalensis*. Depending on their geographic location, some of these fungi are reported with greater frequency in certain regions; for example, *Acremonium* spp. and *M. grisea* are common in South America, and *M. mycetomatis* has the most extensive distribution worldwide, predominantly in India and Africa, and in regions like Sudan, it is responsible for up to 70% of the diagnosed cases of mycetoma.

Pathogenesis

Various species of fungi and actinomycetes causing mycetoma occur as saprophytes in soil or on plants and are implanted into the skin usually after a penetrating injury. Risk factors for infection include lack of protective footwear, trauma and malnutrition. The organism invades deeper into the muscle and bone over a period of time. The causative organisms form clusters of cells (grains), called sclerotia or sulphur granules that are discharged through the sinuses. These can evade the host defence due to the following protective mechanisms:

  i. *Morphology* of the *grains* helps in survival. A protective matrix is formed by the actinomycetes whereas in case of eumycetoma there is intrahyphal growth of fungus that leads to cell wall thickening.
  ii. *M. mycetomatis* produces *melanin* that gets deposited in the cell wall and surrounding matrix and also binds to antifungal agents.

Clinical Features

The most common site of infection is the foot (Fig. 6.1) followed by the hand, trunk and scalp. The disease starts as firm painless papules that progress to nodules and soft tissue swelling and abscess formation. These breakdown to form draining sinuses that contain characteristic grains or sclerotia (Fig. 6.2). These are fungal colonies and vary in size and color depending on the causative organism (Table 6.1). Involvement of deeper tissues, bones and joints can occur leading to osteomyelitis, periostitis and arthritis. Destruction of bone and serious

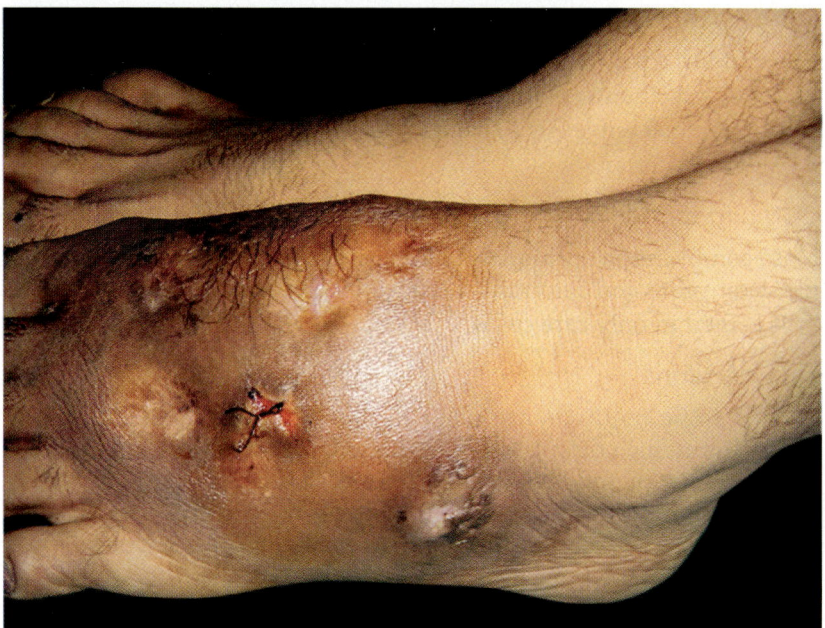

Fig. 6.1: A case of eumycetoma with chronic swelling of the dorsum of foot, tumefaction and sinuses

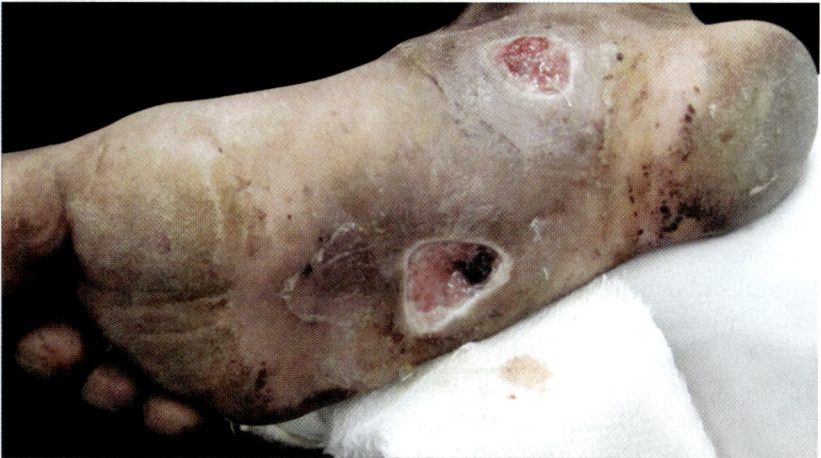

Fig. 6.2: A case of eumycetoma with visible black grains (Courtesy: Dr Ramya RML Hospital)

deformity may result. Inspite of the deeper invasion, the condition is asymptomatic. Local lymph nodes are rarely enlarged.

Differential Diagnosis

- Actinomycosis
- Other subcutaneous fungal infections
- Chronic osteomyelitis (bacterial, tuberculous)
- Actinomycetoma

Complications

Main complication occurs due to invasion of underlying bones leading to osteomyelitis and deformity. Lesion on the chest may invade the lungs.

It is fatal in only rare cases.

Investigations

Morphologic methods are used to identify genus and species of eumycetoma, including direct examination, culture, and histopathology. Immunologic methods have also been described, including enzyme-linked immunosorbent assay to determine specific antibodies. Transmission or scanning electron microscopy has also contributed data to determine the ultrastructure of the grains in the tissues. It is not always possible to diagnose the genus and species by studying pathologic specimens because (1) cultures are often contaminated with bacteria and are negative, and (2)when the culture is positive, the morphologic structures are often difficult to identify.

For this reason, molecular diagnostic techniques, such as polymerase chain reaction (PCR) in its various forms have been introduced, including PCR restriction fragment length polymorphism [RFLP], real-time PCR, and DNA sequencing. These techniques have been used to identify the species of eumycetoma from biopsies of lesions and isolation from the environment (soil and plants), for example, *Phaeoacremonium* spp., as well as black grain-producing species, such as *M. mycetomatis, M. grisea, E. jeanselmei, P. romeroi, P. makinnonii, L. senegalensis, L. tompkinsii,* and *C. lunata.*

Molecular techniques have identified some species of fungi that cause phaeohyphomycosis and hyalohyphomycosis, such as *C. bantiana* and *P. krajdenii,* which also cause eumycetoma. Etiologic agents of this disease are numerous (Table 6.1).

Here we will focus on investigations that can be done in conventional institutional settings:

    i. **Microscopic examination of grains (direct or in KOH):** Pus exuding from the lesion should be examined under the microscope to look for grains. The *fungal* mycelia are *broader* (2–6 µm) whereas actinomycotic grains comprise much narrower filaments (0.5–1.0 µm).

Table 6.1: Main eumycetoma agents*

Agent	Frequency	Grain color
Acremonium falciforme	Rare	White
Acremonium kiliense	Occasional	White
Acremonium recifeid	Occasional	White
Aspergillus flavus	Rare	White
Aspergillus nidulans	Rare	White
Cladophialophora bantiana	Rare	Black
Cochliobolus spicifer	Rare	—
Corynespora cassicola	Rare	Black
Curvularia geniculata	Rare	Black
Curvularia lunata	Rare	Black
Cylindrocarpon cyanescens	—	—
Cylindrocarpon destructans	—	—
Drechslera rostrata	Rare	Black
Exophiala jeanselmei	Rare	Black
Exserohilum rostratum	—	Black
Fusarium spp.	—	White
Fusarium moniliforme	Rare	White
Fusarium oxysporum	Rare	White
Fusarium solani	Rare	White
Leptosphaeria senegalensis	Occasional	Black
Leptosphaeria tompkinsii	Rare	Black
Madurella grisea	Occasional	Black
Madurella mycetomatis	Frequent	Black
Neotestudina rosati	Rare	White
Phaeoacremonium krajdenii	—	White
Phialophora cyanescens	—	Black
Plenodomus avramii	Rare	Black
Polycytella hominis	—	—
Pseudallescheria boydii	Frequent	White
Pseudochaetosphaeronema larense	Rare	Black
Pyrenochaeta mackinnonii	Rare	Black
Pyrenochaeta romeroi	Occasional	Black
Scedosporium apiospermum	—	White

*Estrada R, et al.

The *colour* of the grains helps in identifying the causative agent. Black grains are caused by fungi and red grains by actinomycetes. Eumycetoma can be dark-grain (hard or brittle grains with brown-cement like substance) or pale-grain (white or yellow grains) eumycetomas.

ii. **Biopsy:** Suppurative and granulomatous inflammation is seen in the dermis and subcutis. Fibrosis may be seen. Grains will be seen as tightly packed colonies of fungal organisms. Special stains may be used to identify the fungus. The grains can be seen in the center of the abscesses. Special stains-Grocott, periodic acid–Schiff (PAS), and hematoxylin and eosin help to distinguish the different varieties of grain.

Cytology (FNAC): An alternative that facilitates obtaining samples is fine-needle aspiration for cytologic diagnosis (Gabhane SK). It has a sensitivity of 87.5% and 85.7% for eumycetoma and actinomycetoma, respectively. This procedure is quick and easy to perform, readily providing material for culture and direct mycologic study, histopathology, and molecular techniques for the specific identification of the causative agent.

iii. **Culture:** Identification of the fungus requires culture. Prior to inoculation the grains should be washed with saline containing antibacterials to remove the contaminating bacteria. Half strength cornmeal agar may be used for subculture.

Madurella mycetomatis: Colonies are initially pale and leathery but later become brown or grey in color with a diffusible brown pigment.

iv. **Imaging:** The various imaging methods help to determine the extent of disease and bone involvement. An increase in volume of the soft tissues (93%), bone sclerosis (56%), bone cavities—geodes (32%), periosteal reaction (27%), and osteoporosis (19%) are frequently observed.

a. *Ultrasound imaging:* It is a useful and specific imaging technique for detecting mycetoma. Mycetoma grains, capsules and granuloma have a characteristic ultrasonic appearance. It can be used to differentiate between mycetoma and non-mycetoma lesions. Also eumycetoma grains produce bright sharp hyper-reflective echoes (due to the grain cement material) where as actinomycetoma produces less distinct echoes (due to smaller grains).

b. *Magnetic resonance imaging (MRI):* It is helpful in visualizing the soft tissue involvement and bone destructions. Grains appear as small round hyperintense lesions (2–5 mm) representing granulation tissue surrounded by low-signal-intensity rim. This is known as the "**dot in circle**" appearance that is seem in 80% of patients and is considered diagnostic of eumycetoma.

c. *Computed tomography (CT)*: Has proved to be more sensitive for detecting early bone changes compared with MRI.

Treatment

Contrary to the therapeutic results observed in actinomycetomas, where medical treatment cures most infections without surgery, combined medical and surgical treatment is the standard to follow in eumycetoma. The antifungals used in the treatment of mycetoma since the 1960s have included amphotericin B, clotrimazole, and griseofulvin. The latter two are no longer used. Amphotericin B has been indicated sporadically, with limited success due to its adverse effects,and its use in this disease is now infrequent.

Azoles

The advent of ketoconazole, in the late 1970s, permitted the use of this imidazole in the medical treatment of eumycetoma caused by *M. mycetomatis*, achieving a 40% cure. The treatment frequently used in endemic sites is *ketoconazole* (400 mg/d), given for 9 to 12 months and sometimes longer.

The most notable adverse effects reported with ketoconazole include hepatotoxicity, gynecomastia, dryness and ulceration of the lips, hyperpigmentation of the skin, and decreased libido.

With the emergence of *itraconazole*, a triazole antifungal,the treatment of eumycetoma had a new, effective therapy with fewer side effects and drug interactions. There are isolated reports of cures of eumycetoma achieved with other newer imidazoles such as posaconazole and voriconazole.

Posaconazole: This antifungal is available as a suspension of 40 mg/ mL. The dose of posaconazole is 200 mg orally four times daily for fungal infections refractory to other antifungals. Its effectiveness in eumycetoma was evaluated in six patients with treatment-resistant eumycetoma, five caused by *Madurella* spp and one by *S. apiospermum*. The daily dose was 800 mg orally in two divided doses of 400 mg or 200 mg, four times daily. Four responded with a complete clinical response and one partial response. Two patients, classified as a complete response, relapsed at 10 and 12 months and were retreated with posaconazole, with disappearance of the lesions in one patient. Another patient was lost to follow-up. Long-term administration of posaconazole (up to 10–15 days) was well tolerated (Negroni R).

Terbinafine

This antifungal was evaluated in a study (N'diaye B), where 20 patients with black grain eumycetoma (mainly *M. mycetomatis*) received a dose of 500 mg twice daily for 24 to 48 weeks, with good to moderate results: 5 were cured, 11 improved, 2 had no improvement, and the remaining 2 worsened.

Surgery

When the therapeutic response to surgery and antifungal treatment fails, a final solution may be amputation of the affected limb. Before surgical removal of eumycetomas,treatment with *terbinafine* (500–700 mg/kg daily) along with *itraconazole* (400 mg daily) for 6 to 12 weeks advised to be continued postoperatively to obtain cure of the disease or until adverse effects appear, or both.

The administration of these new antifungals is expensive. Patients with eumycetoma are most often located in countries where basic health services are limited with regard to drug therapy. This makes the continuous administration of expensive antifungals, for a suitable time and an appropriate dose, difficult.

Herein surgery is indicated for small, localized lesions and large lesions to reduce the mycetoma load and enable better response to medical treatment. The options include wide local surgical excisions, repetitive debridement, and amputation of the affected limb. Sungical treatment is associated with morbidity and deformations especially in advanced disease.

Bibliography

1. Ahmed AO, Van Leeuwen W, Fahal A, et al. Mycetoma caused by Madurellamycetomatis: a neglected infectious burden. Lancet Infect Dis 2004;4:566–74.
2. Estrada R, Chávez-López G, Estrada-Chávez G, López-Martínez R, Welsh O.
3. Eumycetoma. Clin Dermatol 2012 Jul-Aug;30(4):389–96.
4. Fahal AH. Management of mycetoma. Expert Rev Dermatol 2010;5: 87–93.
5. Gabhane SK, Gangane N Anshu. Cytodiagnosis of eumycotic mycetoma: a case report. Acta Cytol 2008;52:354–6.
6. N'diaye B, Dieng MT, Perez A, *et al*. Clinical efficacy and safety of oral terbinafine in fungal mycetoma. Int J Dermatol 2006;45:154–7.
7. Negroni R, Tobón A, Bustamante B, Shikanai-Yasuda MA, Patino H, Restrepo A. Posaconazole treatment of refractory eumycetoma and chromoblastomycosis. Rev Inst Med Trop S Paulo 2005;47:339–46.
8. Venugopal PV, Venugopal TV. Treatment of eumycetoma with ketoconazole. Australas J Dermatol 1993;34:27–9.

2. CHROMOBLASTOMYCOSIS
(Chromomycosis, Verrucous Dermatitis)

Veena Chandran

INTRODUCTION

Chromoblastomycosis is a chronic fungal infection of skin and subcutaneous tissue characterized by slow growing exophytic lesions. The causative agents are various types of pigmented fungi like *Fonsecaea pedrosoi, Phialophora verrucosa, Fonsecaea compacta, Cladosporium carrionii* and several other species. These fungi typically from clusters called muriform bodies (*copper penny* bodies /*sclerotic Medlar bodies*).

Geographical Distribution

The majority of cases have been reported from Central America, Indian subcontinent and Madagascar. In India, most of the cases are reported from areas with warm and humid climatic conditions. There are case reports from sub-Himalayan belt, Eastern and Western coasts. The central and North-Western arid zones of the country are relatively free of the disease.

Etiology

The causative fungi include *Fonsacea pedrosoi, Phialophora verrucosa, Fonsacea compacta, Cladosporium carrionii* and *Rhinocladiella aquaspersa*. *Fonsacea pedrosoi* is the most common causative organism worldwide and also in the humid tropical climates. The etiological agents of chromoblastomycosis have been discovered from soil, wood, vegetable debris, and similar substances. Usually the infection results from trauma such as puncture from a splinter of wood. This may be the reason the disease predominantly affects the extremities in male agricultural workers in rural areas.

CLINICAL FEATURES

The extremities are most commonly affected. Lesions have also been described on the face and neck. Unusual cutaneous sites afflicted are the penile shaft, vulva, and ala of the nose, and unusual extracutaneous spread was seen in the pleural cavity, ileocecal region, laryngotracheal area, and tonsils.

The lesions may be verrucous or hyperkeratotic slow growing plaques (Fig. 6.3) which may sometimes show atrophy or scaling. The brown sclerotic bodies may be visible on the surface of many of these lesions as black dots. Some lesions may show hypertrophy and enlarge

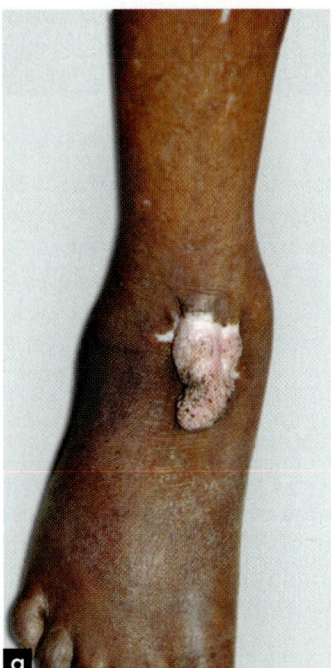

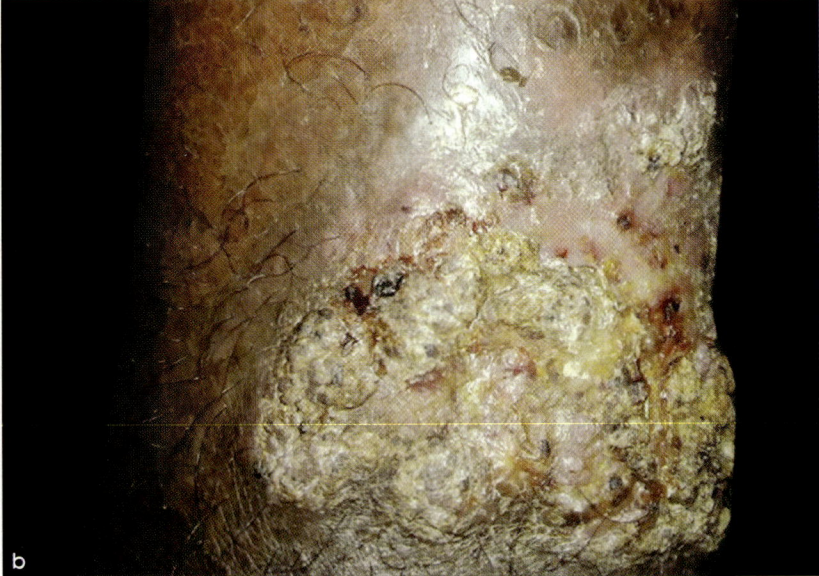

Fig. 6.3a and b: (a) Hyperkeratotic verrucous plaque with black dots on the surface; (b) Chromoblastomycosis: Verrucous cauliflower-like growth on the limbs

to form nodular lesions and cauliflower-like masses. Secondary infection in long standing lesions can lead to lymphatic stasis and elephantiasis. Squamous cell carcinoma can occur in long standing lesions.

Differential diagnoses include blastomycosis and other granulomatous conditions like lupus vulgaris, cutaneous leishmaniasis and tertiary syphilis.

INVESTIGATIONS

i. Skin scraping study of the surface black dots using 10% KOH is a simple test helpful in demonstrating the sclerotic bodies in many cases. Occasionally pigmented hyphae rather than sclerotic bodies may be seen.

ii. Skin biopsy shows granulomatous reaction and demonstrates the typical sclerotic bodies. The fungal cells are golden broun or chestnut in colour and can be easily identified in the infiltrate mainly within giant cells. Many cases show an organized mixed mycotic granuloma which contains many neutrophils. Pseudoepitheliomatous hyperplasia is also commonly observed. Transepidermal elimination of fungal cells may be seen.

iii. Fungal culture helps in isolation of the organism and identification of the fungal species. It is useful to identify the fungal species and correlate with treatment response as there is still a lot of variability in response to various treatment modalities. Culture is done at 15–30°C and is slow producing dark-grey-green to black and velvety colonies. The species can be identified by the type of conidial production.

TREATMENT

Different agents, combinations, and treatment modalities have shown immense variations in achieving success and may depend on the causative fungus and individual patient tolerance.

Antifungal therapy

Antifungals are the mainstay of treatment. The responses to itraconazole and terbinafine are found to be better if the causative agent is *Cladosporium carrionii*.

1. **Itraconazole** therapy either alone or in combination with other treatment modalities have been tried with good response.
   - Itraconazole *pulse therapy*: Itraconazole 400 mg daily for one week per month (1 week of therapy and 3 weeks off) for a total of 7 pulses has been shown to be very effective in some studies.

- Itraconazole 200 mg **daily** as monotherapy has also been found to be helpful.
- Itraconazole daily therapy or pulse therapy in combination with liquid nitrogen cryotherapy once in 2–4 weeks has been found to shorten duration of treatment and improve efficacy.

2. **Terbinafine:** 250 mg twice daily until complete resolution is another option.

3. **Potassium iodide therapy:** Potassium iodide has own therapeutic value in skin lesions in which neutrophils predominate in the early phases of the disease. It may also have a fungistatic action. Potassium iodide is now considered to be a cheap and cost effective drug for chromoblastomycosis especially in developing countries. Saturated solution of potassium iodide (1000 gm dissolved in 1000 ml of distilled water) is started at a rate of 1 drop thrice daily. The rate is increased by 1 drop per dose every day until a maximum of 40 drops thrice daily and maintained at that rate until complete clearance of the lesions. The dose is then tapered off at a rate of 1 drop per dose per day.

4. Use of heat therapy using heat retaining gas pack. This causes shrinkage of lesion but takes a longer time.

5. Surgery: Can be done only for very small lesions (but not with out antifungal therapy). In large plaques there is risk of autoinoculation and formation of satellite lesions.

Bibliography

1. Chandran V, Sadanandan SM, Sobhanakumari K. Chromoblastomycosis in Kerala, India. Indian J Dermatol Venereol Leprol 2012;78:728–33.

2. Kumarasinghe SP, KumarasingheMP. Itraconazole pulse therapy in chromoblastomycosis. Eur J Dermatol 2000 Apr-May;10(3):220–2.

3. Ranawaka RR, Amarasinghe N, HewageD.Chromoblastomycosis: combined treatment with pulsed itraconazole therapy and liquid nitrogen cryotherapy. Int J Dermatol. 2009 Apr;48(4):397–400. doi: 10.1111/j.1365–4632.2009. 03744.x.

4. Sharma NL, Sharma RC, Grover PS, Gupta ML, Sharma AK, Mahajan VK. Chromoblastomycosis in India.Int J Dermatol 1999;38:846–51.

5. Silva JP, de Souza W, Rozental S. Chromoblastomycosis: A retrospective study of 325 cases on Amazonic region (Brazil). Mycopathologia 1998;143:171–5.

3. SPOROTRICHOSIS (Rose Gardener's Disease)

Pooja Arora Mrig, Kabir Sardana

DEFINITION

Sporotrichosis is an acute or chronic subcutaneous fungal infection caused by dimorphic organism *Sporothrix schenckii* and closely related species. Both cutaneous and systemic forms can occur, though the latter is rare.

Epidemiology

Sporotrichosis is mainly seen in the tropical and subtropical regions in the world. The fungus grows on decaying vegetable matter. Hence the disease is more common in few occupational groups, e.g mine workers, forestry workers and gardeners. It is more common in adult males and has been rarely described in children. In the latter facial involvement is more frequent.

Etiology

Sporotrichosis is caused by *S. schenckii*. Other rare species include *S. braziliensis*, *S. mexicana*, *S. globosa* and *S. luree*. These have been collectively refuted to as *"Sporothrix schenckii* species complex".

Pathogenesis

The fungus enters the skin or mucous membrane through a breach caused by trauma (minor wound caused by thorn or insect bite). The source of infection is decaying vegetable matter. Incubation period is 8–30 days. The presentation and clinical course of disease depends on the immune status of the host and the size and virulence and thermotolerance of the inoculum. In patients who do not have prior exposure, lymphatics get involved whereas in patients without exposure, the disease remains localized to the skin ("fixed") type. Immunocompromised patients develop extensive disease with or without systemic involvement.

Clinical Features

The disease starts as a single papule that appears at a site of injury (usually the hand) weeks after inoculation. It can become ulcerated (Sportrichotic chancre) with discharge of purulent fluid. This is followed by appearance of several dermal and subcutaneous nodules and ulcers along the lymphatics (Fig. 6.4). This is called the **"sporotrichoid"** pattern. The nodules are connected by tender lymphatic cords. The regional lymph nodes may get enlarged. It is the most common variety and accounts for 70–80% of cases of cutaneous sporotrichosis.

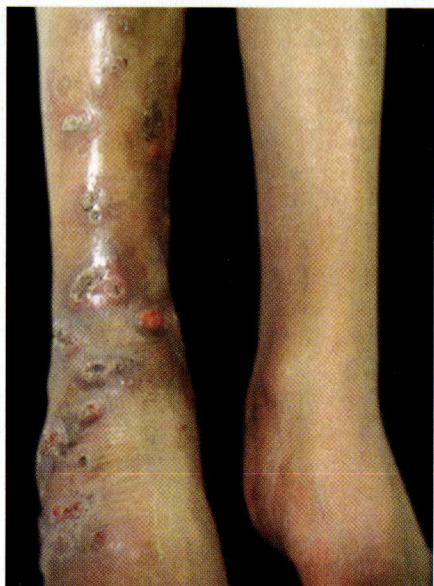

Fig. 6.4: Erythematous crusted oozy plaques over right lower limb

The **"fixed"** type is less common. The disease remains localized at the point of inoculation (Fig. 6.5). The lesions may be acneiform, nodular, ulcerated, verrucous or granulomatous. This type occurs due to high degree of host immunity.

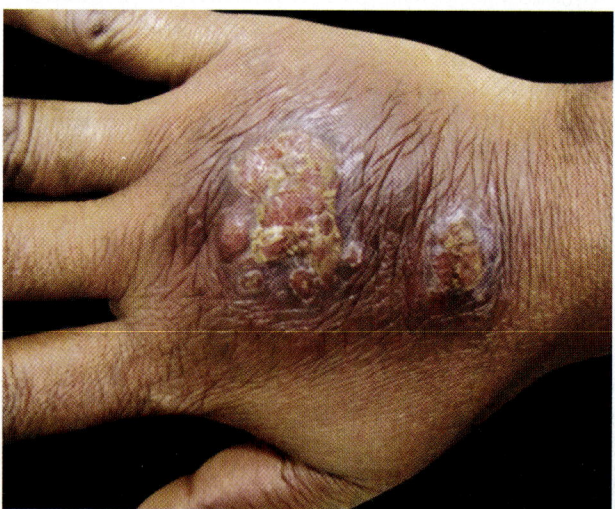

Fig. 6.5: A 'fixed' plaque with ulceration on the dorsum of the hand. A case of fixed sporotrichosis

Multifacial or disseminated cutaneous sporotrichosis: This is defined as >3 lesions involving 2 different anatomical sites. It may result from multiple traumatic implantation of the fingers or from hematogenous spread immunocompetent host.

Systemic forms are less common and occur due to inhalation. Lungs, joints, skin and meninges can get involved. No organ is immune to the disease. This variety occurs in immunocompromised patients.

Osteoarticular sporotrichosis is the most common systemic manifestation, and usually affects the knee wrist, elbow and ankle joints. It presents as tenosynovitis, joint effusion, bursitis and cyst formation. Pulmonary disease is characterized by cough, fever, weight loss, mediastinal lymphadenopathy, cavitation mimicking tuberculosis.

Differential Diagnosis

Differential diagnosis of "sporotrichoid" pattern is depicted in Box 6.1.

Investigations

i. Direct smear examination is insensitive due to scarcity of fungal cells. Fine needle aspiration cytology (FNAC) from lesions (especially extracutaneous or disseminated) show epithelioid cells granulomas, asteroid bodies and yeast cells.

ii. Histopathological examination: Concentric zones are seen in nodules of lymphocutaneous sporotrichosis: (a) *Central necrotic*

Box 6.1 Dermatoses distributed in a "Sporotrichoid" pattern

- Atypical mycobacterial infection (*M. marinum*)
- Sporotrichosis
- Nocardiosis
- Bacterial infections caused by *S. aureus* and *Strep. pyogenes*
- Leishmaniasis
- Tuberculosis
- Cat scratch disease
- Tularemia
- Anthrax
- Glanders
- Non-infectious causes: Lymphoma, Langerhans' cell histiocytosis, in-transit metastases, perineural spread of leprosy

zone containing polymorphonuclear leukocytes and amorphous debris (zone of chronic suppuration); (b) *Middle tuberculoid* zone composed of epithelioid cells, epithelial cells, giant cells (Langerhans' type); (c) *Syphiloid zone:* Comprising plasma cells, lymphocytes and fibroblasts with capillary hyperplasia and proliferation.

Pathology reveals a mixed granulomatous reaction with foci of neutrophils. The fungus appears as small (3–5 μm) cigar shaped or oval yeasts that may be surrounded by radiate eosinophilic substance. These are called asteroid bodies. Splendore-Hoeppli phenomenon (hyphae surrounded by an eosinophilic halo) may be seen.

iii. Culture: Fungus grows readily on common agar media. The colonies are initially leathery, moist and white in color that later become brown or black. Microscopy shows palmate or flower-like arrangement of conidia. Pigmentation increases with the addition of thiamine. Conversion to yeast phase can be done by incubation on brain-heart infusion agar supplemented with sheep's blood. The yeast is oval or cigar shaped.

iv. Intradermal tests: These detect delayed sensitivity using sporotrichin or peptide-rham-nomannan (PRM) antigen. It is insensitive and may be negative in disseminated sporotrichosis.

 v. Serology: ELISA, complement-fixation tests, immunofluorescence can be used but are not readily available.

vi. Detection of *S. schenkii* by PCR.

Treatment

An overview of treatment is given below:

First line	Second line
Itraconazole: 100–200 mg/day given until clinical recovery (at least 3 months)	Potassium iodide: Given as saturated solution started at five drops and increased slowly to 4–6 ml thrice daily. It should be continued for 3–4 weeks after clinical cure (Fig. 6.6).
Terbinafine: 250 mg/day given until clinical recovery	

Other Treatment Options

Thermotherapy: Hyperthermia directly damages the pathogen and also enhances the killing capacity of neurophils. Daily application of

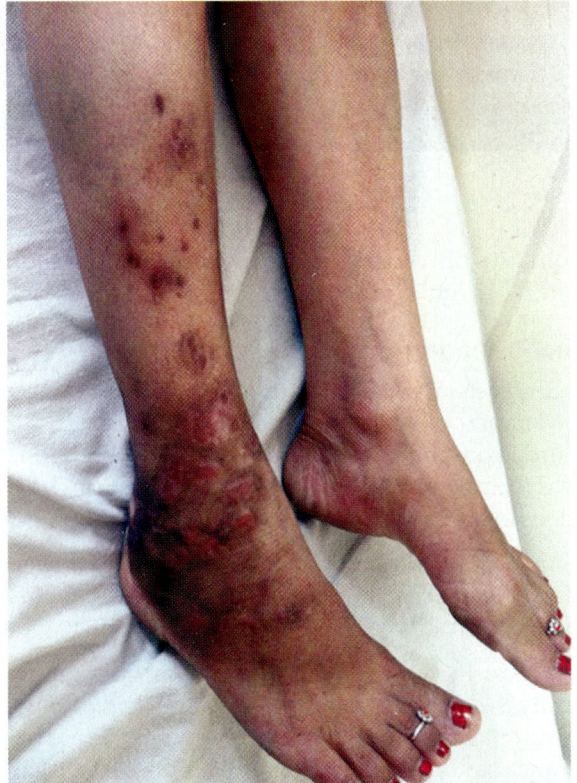

Fig. 6.6: Complete healing of lesions at 12 weeks of treatment

coal heat (42–43°C) to the lesion using heat compresses or in an infrared heater can be used to treat small lesions. In pregnant women heat is applied for 15–60 minutes several times daily until lesions heal.

Bibliography

1. CA Kaufmann. Old and new therapies for sporotrichosis. Clin Infect Dis 1995; 21:981–5.

2. da Rosa AC, Scroferneker ML, Vettorato R, *et al*. Epidemiology of sporotrichosis: a study of 304 cases in Brazil. J Am Acad Dermatol 2005; 52: 451–9.

3. Kauffman CA. Sporotrichosis. Clin Infect Dis 1999; 29: 231–6.

4. Restrepo A, Robledo A, Gomez I, *et al*. Itraconazole therapy in lymphangitic and cutaneous sporotrichosis. Arch Dermatol 1986; 122: 413–7.

4. SUBCUTANEOUS ZYGOMYCOSIS DUE TO BASIDIOBOLUS AND CONIDIOBOLUS
(Subcutaneous Zygomycosis, Basidiobolomycosis, Conidiobolomycosis, Rhinoentomophthoromycosis)

Pooja Arora Mrig, Kabir Sardana

DEFINITION

Subcutaneous zygomycosis is a localised subcutaneous mycosis characterized by chronic, woody swelling of subcutaneous tissue.

Etiology and Pathogenesis

The class Zygomycetes is divided into two orders; Mucorales and Entomophthorales. Members of the order Mucorales cause acute angioinvasive infection in immunocompromised patients that can be fatal (mucormycosis) whereas members of the Entomophthorales cause chronic subcutaneous infections in immunocompetent patients (entomophthoromycosis).

The order Entomophthorales comprises 3 important pathogenic species: Conidiobolus coronatus, Conidiobolus incongruus, Basidiobolus ranarum. These typically occur in immunocompetent patients.

Basidiobolomycosis: It is caused by *B. ranarum*. The organism occurs saprophytically in decaying plant material, soil, leaves from deciduous trees and intestines of amphibians and reptiles. The disease mainly occurs in tropical and subtropical countries and affects children. The vegetable matter is consumed by insects, frogs and other animals who in turn disseminate the fungus in the environment which then affects humans and other animals. It has also been described following intramuscular injection. Previous subclinical infection provides immunity to the disease hence the prevalence is low.

Basidiobolomycosis tends to affect the *limb girdle* region and *buttocks* in children whereas *conidiobolomycosis* affects the *rhinofacial region* in adult males and causes edema and infiltration of the central facial tissues in adult males. *C. coronatus* has been isolated from soil and decaying plant matter. Infection occurs by traumatic implantation or by inhalation. The fungus produces various enzymes such as collagenases, elastases, lipases, esterases which are involved in the pathogenesis of the disease.

Clinical Features

Basidiobolomycosis affects the limb or limb girdle area of children. Rarely other parts of the body may be involved. The disease presents as a single painless, subcutaneous swelling with a hard consistency that does not pit on pressure (Fig. 6.7). The smooth edge can be raised up by inserting the fingers underneath it. Satellite lesions may be present. The overlying skin is intact with a bluish or purple color at the active growing region. It may be normal or hyperpigmented. Ulceration does not occur.

The disease does not lead to functional impairment as the joints are not involved. Lymph nodes are not enlarged though a few cases of muscle and lymph node involvement have been reported. A case of basidiobolomycosis presenting with "saxophone penis" in a 2½-year-old boy has been described (Figs 6.8 and 6.9). This can occur due to involvement of lymphatics. Other organs, like lung and gastrointestinal tract, can rarely get involved.

Conidiobolomycosis (Fig. 6.10) causes subcutaneous inflammation of the submucosa in the central facial region. It is mainly seen in young adults. The disease starts from the inferior turbinates and spreads to involve the facial tissues. Nasal obstruction occurs first followed by infiltration and thickening of the skin over the nose with subsequent deformity. In later stages, pharynx, facial muscles and paranasal sinuses may also get affected.

Clinical classification of conidiobolomycosis is as below:

I: Limited to the nasal fossae, paranasal sinuses and pharynx
II: Infection spreads to the frontal region and lips
III: Muscles, bones and viscera are affected.

Differential Diagnosis

Basidiobolomycosis

- Lymphatic edema
- Subcutaneous malignant lymphoma.

Conidiobolomycosis

- Sarcoidosis
- Rhinosporidiosis
- Benign and malignant tumors of nasal cavity.

INVESTIGATIONS

i. *Direct examination with KOH:* It is done to demonstrate the fungus which appears as hyaline, wide, thin-walled aseptate or sparsely septate hyphae.
ii. *Histopathological examination:* Biopsy is taken from the active edge of the lesion and shows granulomatous infiltration with lymphocytes, histiocytes, multinucleate giant cells, plasma cells

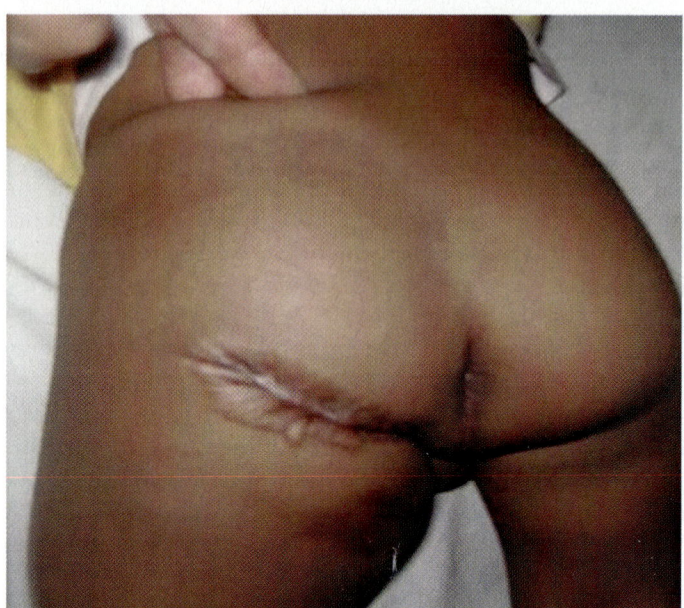

Fig. 6.7: Woody hard swelling over the left buttock in a 2-year-old boy. (The scar overlying the lesion is subsequent to incision and drainage)

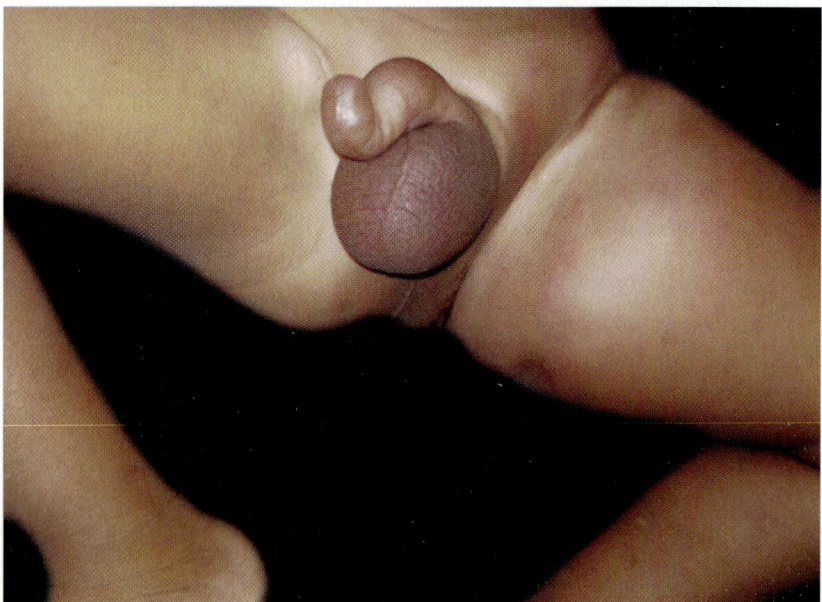

Fig. 6.8: Swelling of the scrotum and shaft of penis resembling "saxophone" penis

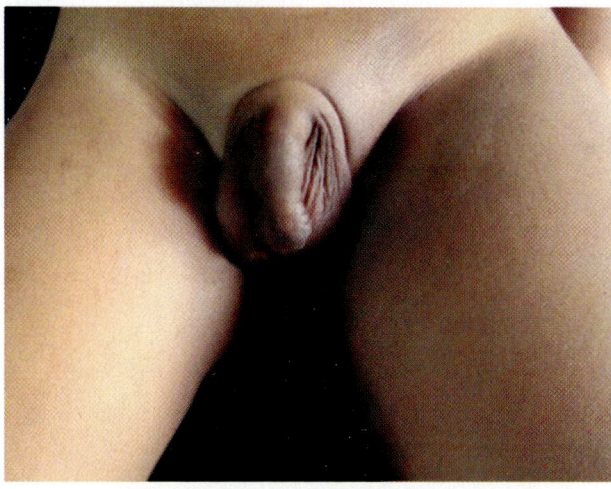

Fig. 6.9: Dramatic response to treatment with subsidence of swelling within days of starting potassium iodide

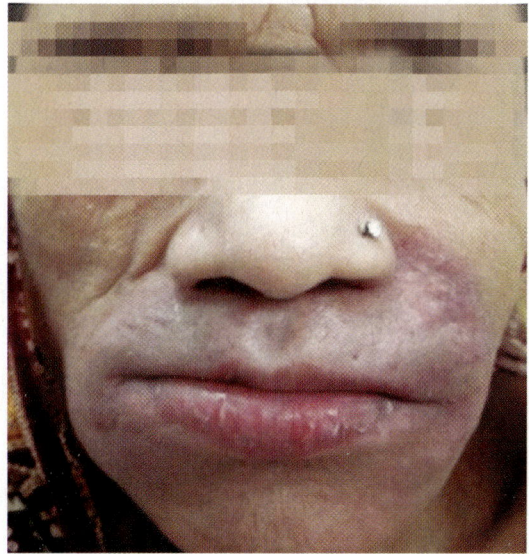

Fig. 6.10: Erythematous hard swelling over the lower half of face with thickening of lower lip

and eosinophils (Fig. 6.11). The fungal structures (4–10 µm) can be identified by hematoxylin and eosin or special stains like PAS and Grocott-Gomori (Figs 6.12 to 6.14). These may be surrounded by a thick eosinophilic sheath called the Splendore-Hoeppli phenomenon.

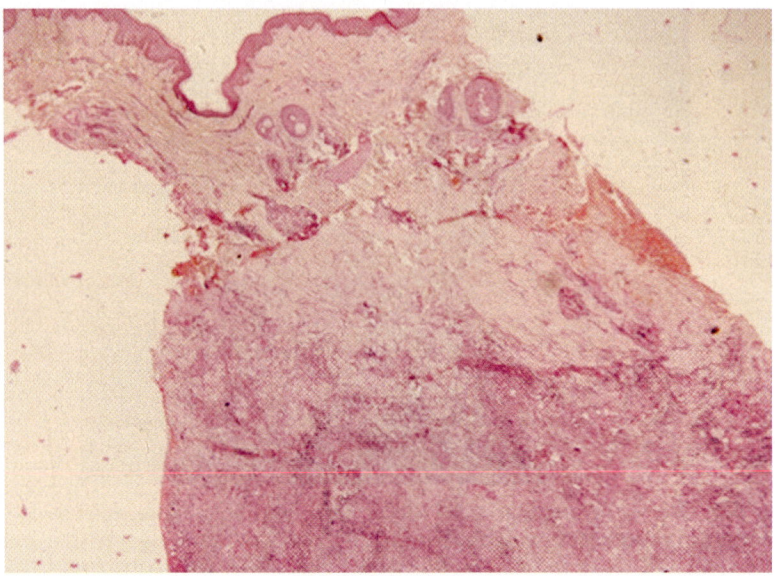

Fig. 6.11: Granulomatous inflammation in lower dermis (H & E, 40X)

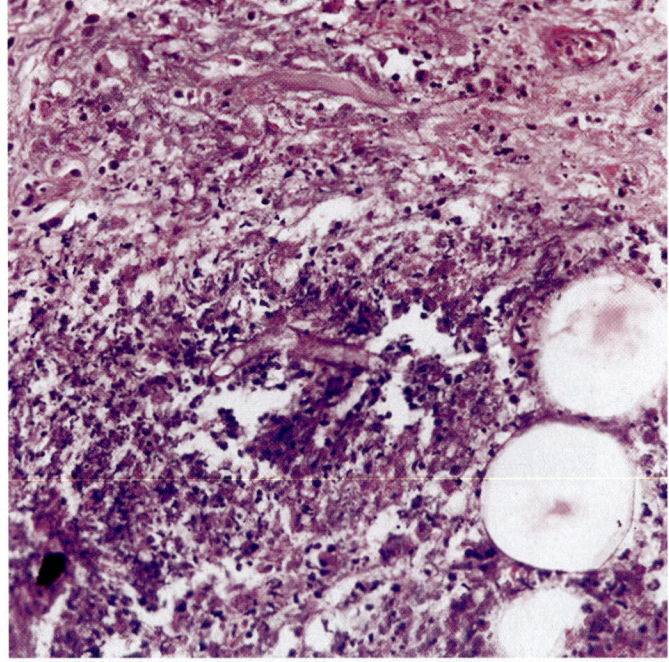

Fig. 6.12: Broad aseptate hyphae with scanty cytoplasm appearing as tube like structures seen within fungal granulomas (H & E stain, 40X)

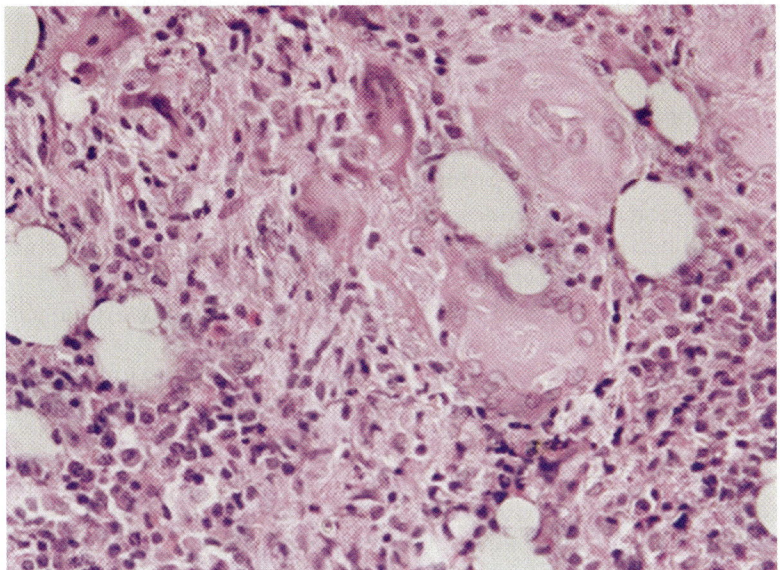

Fig. 6.13: Multinucleated giant cells with well defined tubular structures inside the giant cells (H & E, 40X)

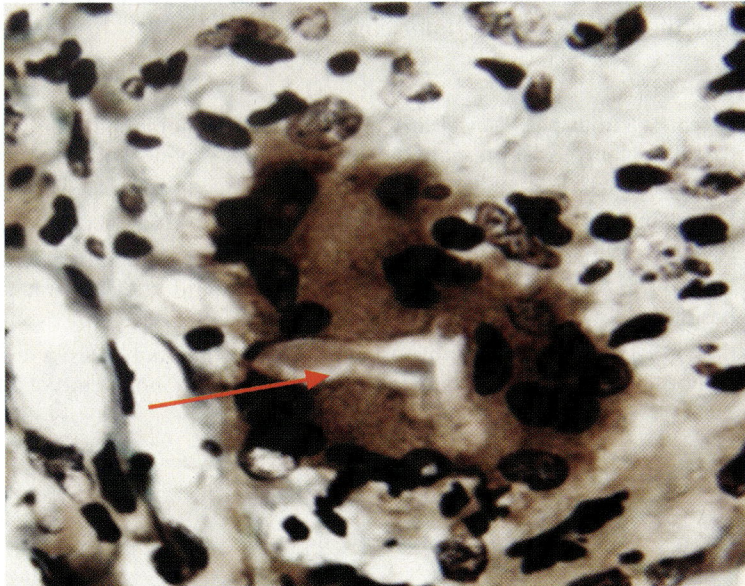

Fig. 6.14: Broad aseptate hyphae with scanty cytoplasm appearing as tube-like structures seen within fungal granulomas (methenamine silver stain, 100X)

iii. *Culture:* It is performed in SDA without cycloheximide or choloroamphenicol at 30–37°C.

B. *ranarum* grows very rapidly as waxy cream or yellow colonies with radial folds. Microscopy shows broad sparsely septate hyphae, 8–20 m in diameter. After 10–14 days, sexual zygospores with a prominent beak may be produced.

Colonies of ***Conidiobolus coronatus*** are waxy white to grey and become more powdery and beige later. Microscopy shows wide, sparsely septate hyphae and sporangiola.

iv. *Serology:* Serological tests to detect antibodies can be done using immunodiffusion and ELISA tests.

v. Leucocytosis, peripheral eosinophilia and raised erythrocyte sedimentation rate (ESR) may be present.

TREATMENT

Itraconazole is the treatment of choice and is used in a dose of 300 mg/day. Saturated solution of potassium iodide may be used in doses similar to sporotrichosis. Cotrimoxazole has been shown to be effective in conidiobolomycosis and may be added to first line treatment.

Other treatment options that have been tried include ketoconazole, fluconazole, dapsone, amphotericin and terbinafine.

Bibliography

1. Arora P, Sardana K, Bansal S, Garg VK, Rao S. Entomophthoromycosis (basidiobolomycosis) presenting with "saxophone" penis and responding to potassium iodide. Indian J Dermatol Venereol Leprol 2015;81:616–8.
2. Kamalam A, Thambiah AS. Basidiobolomycosis following injection injury. Mykosen 1982;25:512–6.
3. Kamalam A, Thambiah AS. Lymphedema and elephantiasis in basidiobolomycosis. Mykosen 1982;25:508–11.
4. Prabhu RM, Patel R. Mucormycosis and entomophthoramycosis: a review of the clinical manifestations, diagnosis and treatment. Clin Microbiol Infect 2004; 10 (Suppl. 1): 31–47.

5. PHAEOHYPHOMYCOSIS (Phaeomycotic Subcutaneous Cyst)

Pooja Arora Mrig, Kabir Sardana

DEFINITION

Phaeohyphomycosis designates fungal infections caused by pheoid or melanized fungi and characterized histopathologically by the presence of septate hyphae, pseudohyphae, and yeasts.

Epidemiology

The infection is seen in tropical countries. It may occur in immunocompromised host. The disease can be caused by a number of organisms, the major ones are listed below.

- *Exophiala jeanselmei* ⎤
- *Exophiala dermatitidis* ⎦ — Most common
- *Cladophiala phorabantiana*
- *Phialophora* spp.
- *Bipolaris* spp.
- *Exserohilum* spp.

All age groups and both genders be affected. It is more common in men due to occupational exposure. Immunocompromised patients are likely to have disseminated disease. *Cladosporium bantiana* is most commonly associated with CNS disease.

Pathogenesis

Phaeohyphomycosis results from trauma leading to inoculation of the causative organism.

Clinical Features

The clinical presentation depends on the immune status of the host: In immunocompetent patients superficial (tinea nigra and black piedra); cutaneous (scytalidiosis), corneal and subcutaneous (mycotic cyst). Systemic phaeohyphomycosis is seen in the immunocompromised host.

Rippon modified the classification proposed by McGinnisin 1988 and divided PHM into 5 types (Table 6.2).

Mycotic Cyst: Clinical Features

Mycotic cysts are subcutaneous cystic granulomas caused by pheoid (pigmented) and, rarely, nonpigmented fungi. A history of trauma or a wooden splinter injury weeks or months before the appearance of lesions is common.

Table 6.2: Classification of phaeohyphomycosis

1. Superficial: Black piedra and tinea nigra
2. Cutaneous: Dermatomycosis and onychomycosis
3. Mycotic keratitis
4. Subcutaneous or phaeohyphomycotic cyst
5. Invasive, system and cerebral type

The lesions appear as a single asymptomatic subcutaneous nodule or as asymptomatic erythematous plaques or nodular lesions (Fig. 6.15). In descending order of frequency, the most common locations are the feet, fingers, knee, toes, ankles, legs, and forearms. Lesions begin as small papules and evolve into larger subcutaneous cysts filled with pus.

The *differential diagnosis* of subcutaneous PHM includes lipomas, epidermal cysts, and foreign body granuloma. Early lesions may be similar to cutaneous leishmaniasis, lobomycosis, paracoccidioidomycosis, coccidioidomycosis, and sporotrichosis.

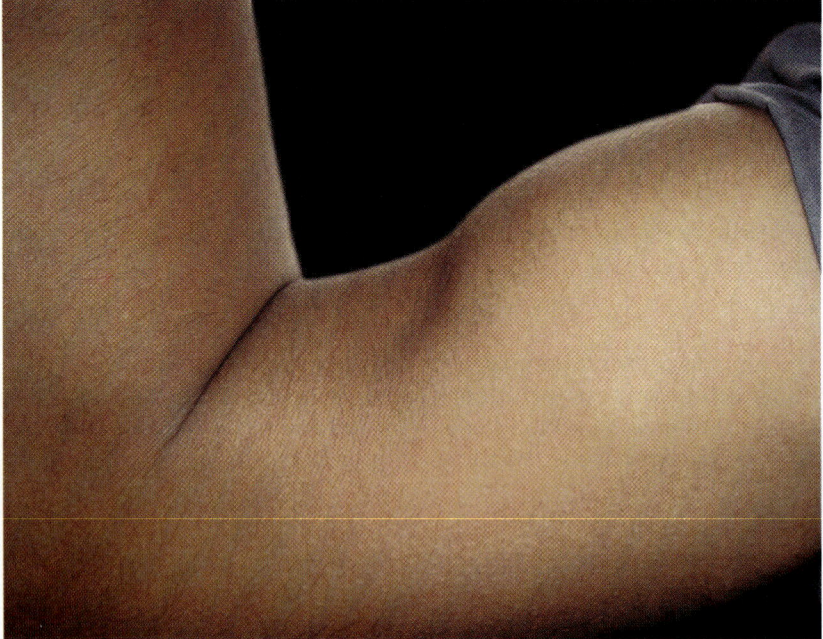

Fig. 6.15: A patient who was diagnosed as a case of lipoma, but excision revealed a encapsulated mass, histology revealed pigmented yeasts, pseudohyphae, and hyphae surrounded by a capsule. No other treatment was offered and the patient did not have a recurrence

Investigations

1. A KOH examination may show pigmented yeasts, pseudohyphae, and hyphae.

2. **Histopathological examination**

   Biopsy specimen shows an inflammatory cyst with a well defined wall that is surrounded by fibrosis. Mixed cellular infiltrate with multinucleate giant cells, macrophages, lymphocytes and neutrophils is seen around the cyst. Pigmented fungi may be seen on the inner aspect of the cyst.

3. **Culture**

   Exophiala jeanselmei: The colonies are initially moist and black but later become filamentous with a grey velvety mycelium. Microscopy shows septate brown hyphae with elliptical conidia.

   Bipolaris species: The colonies are pale grey in color and later become olive grey or black.

TREATMENT

Though excision is considered to be the preferred option, unfortunately, incision and drainage is usually followed by recurrence. Additionally, antifungal therapy is recommended for recurrent cases and for immunocompromised patients, but there are no standards in terms of agents or duration of therapy.

Case reports have documented the efficacy of flucytosine 150 mg/kg per day, itraconazole 200 mg per day, ketoconazole 200 mg per day, and IV or intralesional amphotericin B.

In vitro, the most effective agents are itraconazole, voriconazole, and amphotericin B. Combination therapy is useful for refractory cases, probably because of the combined mechanisms of action of various agents. *Synergy* has been demonstrated *in vitro* between amphotericin B and flucytosine, and itraconazole and flucytosine. Amphotericin B and itraconazole damage the fungal membrane, which might permit increased penetration of flucytosine. Once inside the cell, flucytosine inhibits DNA and RNA synthesis. Synergy leads to lower doses of each agent, increased antifungal effects, and decreased toxicity. But synergy between itraconazole and amphotericin has not been consistent. Itraconazole depletes ergosterol in the fungal membrane, which reduces the binding sites for amphotericin.

The best synergy and results are obtained with triple antifungal combinations. As mentioned before, the use of oral azoles is reserved for cases after incomplete excision or in which incision and drainage have been attempted.

Thus, the best response is obtained with itraconazole and voriconazole, followed by amphotericin B. Additionally, reduction of immunosuppressive medications should be attempted if at all possible. The prognosis in infections caused by pheoid fungi is generally good. Overall mortality is 28%, usually because of systemic infections. Brain infections carry the worse prognosis, with a mortality of at least 43%.

Bibliography

1. Agrawal A, Singh SM. Two cases of subcutaneous phaeohyphomycosis due to Curvularia pallescens. Mycoses 1995;38:301–3.

2. Ajello L. Hyalohyphomycosis and phaeohyphomycosis: two global disease entities of public health importance. Eur J Epidemiol 1986;2: 243–51.

3. Clancy CJ, Wingard JR, Nguyen MH. Subcutaneous phaeohyphomycosis in transplant recipients: review of the literature and demonstration of in vitro synergy between antifungal agents. Med Mycol 2000;38: 169–75.

4. deMonbrinson F, Piens MA, Ample B, Euvrad S. Two cases of subcutaneous phaeohyphomycosis due to Exophialajeanselmei, in cardiac and renal transplant patients. [letter]. Br J Dermatol 2004;150:596–624.

5. Fader RC, McGinnis MR. Infections caused by dematiaceous fungi: chromoblastomycosis and phaeohyphomycosis. Infect Dis Clin North Am 1988;2:925–38.

6. Fothergill AW, Rinaldi MG, Sutton DA. Antifungal susceptibility testing of *Exophiala* spp.: a head to head comparison of amphotericin B, itraconazole, posaconazole, and voriconazole. Med Mycol 2009;47: 41–3.

7. McGinnis MR. Chromoblastomycosis and phaeohyphomycosis: new concepts, diagnosis, and mycology. J Am Acad Dermatol 1983;8: 1–16.

8. Rallis E, Frangoulis E. Successful treatment of subcutaneous phaeohyphomycosis owing to Exophiala jeanselmei with oral tebinafine. [letter]. Int J Dermatol 2006;45:1369–70.

9. Ronan SG, Uzoaru I, Nadimpalli V, Guitart J, Manaligod JR. Primary cutaneous phaeohyphomycosis: report of seven cases. J Cutan Pathol 1993:223–8.

6. CUTANEOUS RHINOSPORIDIOSIS

Thurakkal Salim

INTRODUCTION

Rhinosporidiosis is a chronic granulomatous disorder of infective etiology. It is a disease caused by *Rhinosporidium seeberi* which primarily affects the mucosa of the nose, conjunctiva and urethra. It can rarely affect the skin. Though cutaneous lesions in rhinosporidiosis are rare, they may simulate many common dermatological conditions thus posing a diagnostic dilemma. The disease is more common in males and is usually seen between the second and fourth decade. Exposures to stagnant water, bathing in water in which cattle are also bathed, and repeated trauma have been blamed for its acquisition.

Geographical Distribution

The disease is endemic in India, Sri Lanka, South America, and Africa. There are isolated cases reported in other parts of the world including United States and Europe, as a result of the sociocultural phenomenon of the migration. Most cases of rhinosporidiosis occur in persons from or residing in the Indian subcontinent or Sri Lanka. In addition to humans, disease has been noted in cats, cattle, dogs, ducks, goats, horses, mules, parrots, and swan.

Etiology

Rhinosporidiosis has been known for over 100 years since its first description in Argentina by Guillermo Seeber in the year 1896 in an individual from Argentina. The etiological agent is *Rhinosporidium seeberi*, whose taxonomy has been debated in the last for decades since the microorganism is intractable to isolation and microbiological culture.

Rhinosporidium seeberi is closely related to several fish pathogens. It is an aquatic protozoan and recent taxonomy suggests it is in a new eukaryotic group of protists known as Mesomycetozoa. A few researchers have presented data that *R. seeberi* is a cyanobacterium. Ahluwalia et al suggested the cyanobacterium *Microcystis aeruginosa* as the causative agent for rhinosporidiosis, which has been isolated from clinical samples as well as from the water samples in which patients take bathing.

Mode of Spread

The presumed mode of infection from the natural aquatic habitat of *Rhinosporidium seeberi* is through the traumatized epithelium ('transepithelial infection') most commonly in nasal sites and rarely other mucosal epithelia or skin. The disease progresses with the local replication of *R. seeberi* and associated hyperplastic growth of host tissue and a localized immune response. The disease is prevalent in rural settings, particularly among individuals working or in contact with contaminated soil, stagnant water (ponds, or lakes) or sand. No immunodeficiency has been associated with infection.

The mode of spread of rhinosporidiosis to the skin can be by three means:

Autoinoculation: This explains the occurrence of satellite lesions adjacent to the nasal lesions and in the upper respiratory tract. Spillage of endospores from polyps after trauma or surgery is thought to be followed by 'autoinoculation' through the adjacent epithelium.

Hematogenous spread: The development of skin lesions distant to the nasal lesions could be due to a hematogenous spread of the infection.

Direct inoculation: Direct inoculation of the organism in traumatized skin, also known as the primary cutaneous type. The occurrence of disease at external urethral meatus without any lesions elsewhere is probably due to direct inoculation.

Clinical Features

Usually patients of cutaneous rhinosporidiosis present as poypoidal masses. Most of the cases will have associated mucosal lesions in the form of nasal or pharyngeal involvement (Fig. 6.16). Different reported variants of cutaneous rhinosporidiosis include; pedunculated or sessile growths, verruca vulgaris like lesions, friable nodular lesions, subcutaneous swellings, furunculoid lesions, cutaneous horn, shiny globular swellings, cutaneous ulceration, and cystic swellings.

Cutaneous lesions begin as tiny papules, and slowly evolve into large warty, poly-poidal masses. Nasal involvement can lead to nasal obstruction and bleeding, the masse can become quite large and tend to be very friable and vascular. The pedunculated or sessile polyp will have a purple-red surface studded with small white dots representing the sporangium within the epithelium (Fig. 6.17). This pattern gives the lesion, its characteristic strawberry-like appearance.

Cutaneous rhinosporidiosis can rarely present as non-healing ulcers (Fig. 6.18). We have earlier reported a case of rhinosporidiosis that presented as an as symptomatic ulcer over the anterior aspect of the leg.

Rhinosporidial granulomas in some isolated cases and disseminated cases occur as subcutaneous lumps with unbroken skin. These lesions may mimic a furuncle (Fig. 6.19).

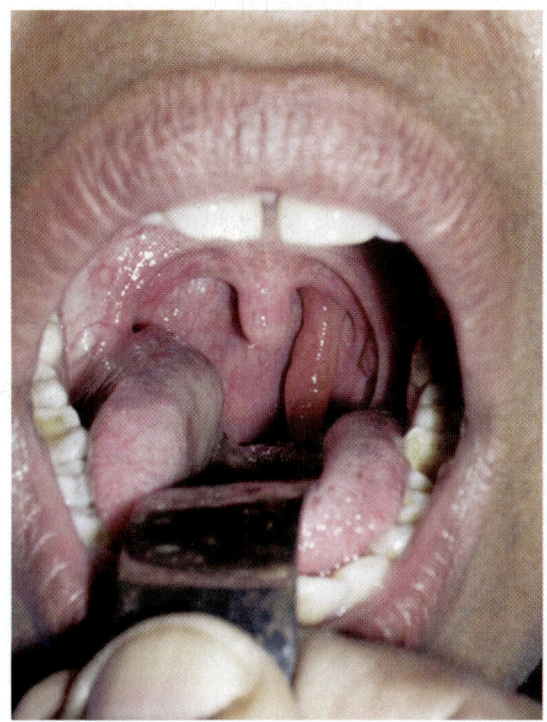

Fig. 6.16: Polypoidal mass hanging by the side of uvula

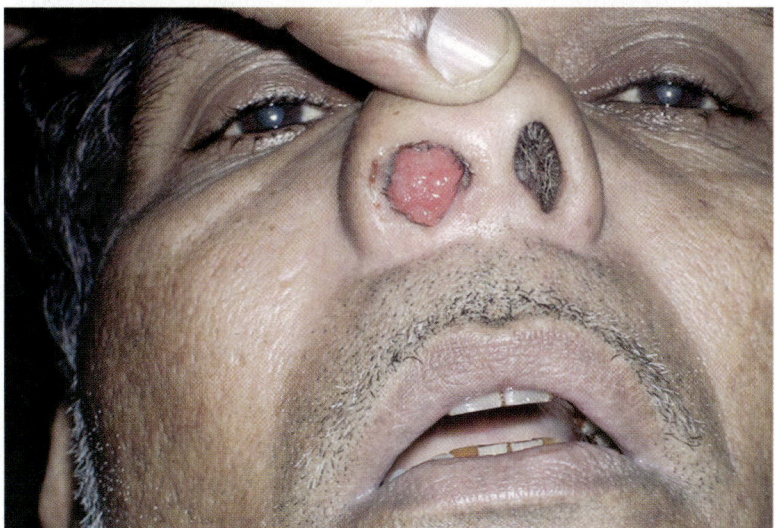

Fig. 6.17: Strawberry-like appearance of mass hanging from the right nostril

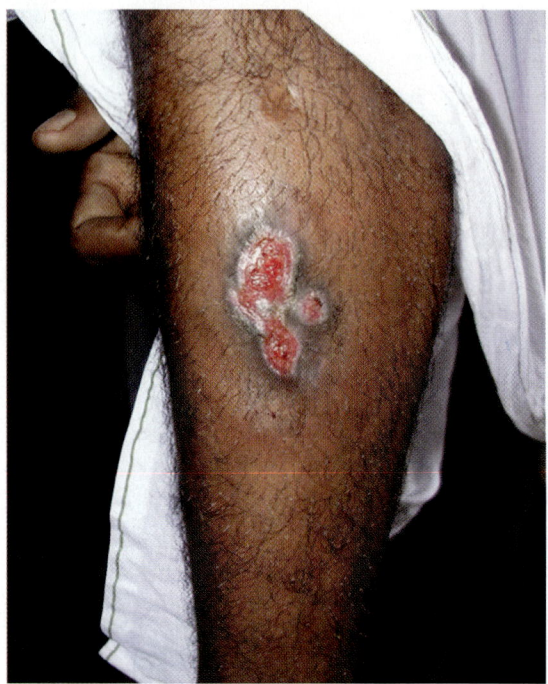

Fig. 6.18: Non-healing ulcer over the anterior aspect of leg

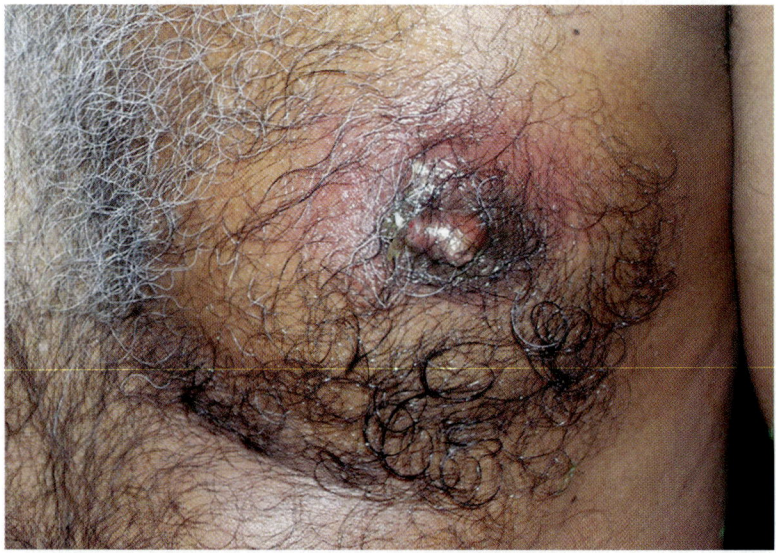

Fig. 6.19: Subcutaneous swelling over the left side of chest mimicking furuncle

Disseminated cutaneous rhinosporidiosis may occur with or without any evidence of immunosuppression. There are reports of disseminated cutaneous rhinosporidiosis presenting with polymorphic lesions, an asymptomatic subcutaneous giant mass, and a smaller painful pyogenic granuloma-like lesions. Sometimes the ulcerated lumps may mimic malignant lesions such as sarcomas and carcinomas.

Rhinosporiediosis may rarely present with pedunculated mass at the external urethral meatus (Fig. 6.20). The genitourinary tract is an extremely rare site of involvement, and only a few cases have been reported till date.

Differential Diagnosis

Because cutaneous rhinosporidiosis is so rare, a high degree of clinical suspicion and histopathological evaluation is required to differentiate the illness from other mimickers. It may manifest itself in a diverse manner mimicking several common dermatological conditions presenting with similar-appearing papules or masses including verruca vulgaris, coccidioidomycosis, bacillary angiomatosis, pyogenic granuloma, verrucous tuberculosis, donovanosis and ecthyma.

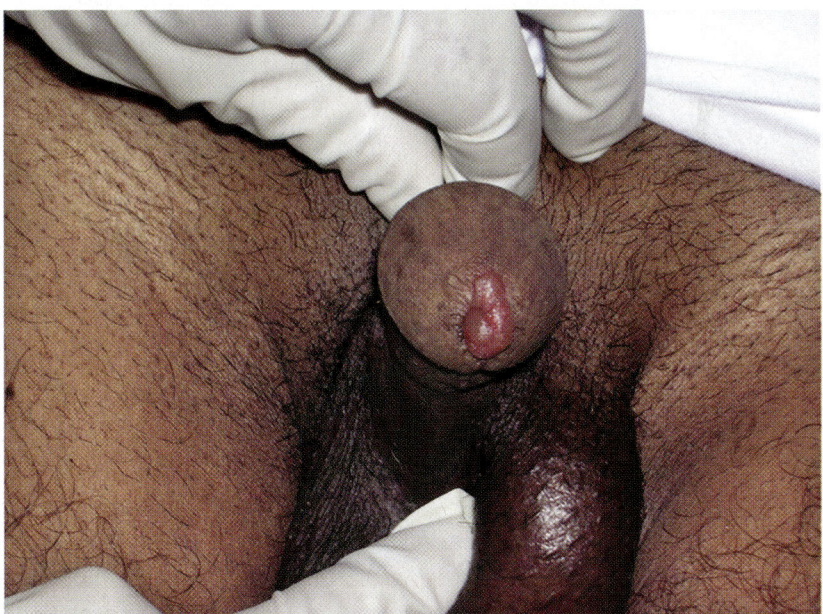

Fig. 6.20: Soft, pedunculated swelling at the external urethral meatus

Diagnosis

As the disease has a slow course, lesions may be present for many years before the patients become symptomatic and seek medical attention. There are chances of dissemination in long standing disease.

Many patients may reveal a history of contact with contaminated *water or bathing* in contaminated ponds. On close examination under magnification, small brownish *spots* representing sporangia, can be seen on a vascular and friable mass.

Diagnosis is made by identifying the typical structures of *R. seeberi* directly on microscopic examination. This includes examination of smears of macerated tissue or histology of prepared biopsy sample sections.

As the organism cannot be grown in culture, histopathology is the gold standard. Biopsy reveals a hyperplastic epithelium with a chronic inflammatory cell infiltrate composed of plasma cells, lymphocytes along with foreign body giant cells. Characteristic sporangia in various stages of maturation are seen as globular cysts of various sizes lined by well-defined wall containing endospores (Figs 6.21 and 6.22).

The organism can be observed with typical fungal stains (e.g. Gomori methenamine silver [GMS], periodic acid-Schiff [PAS]), as well as with standard hematoxylin and eosin (H & E) staining.

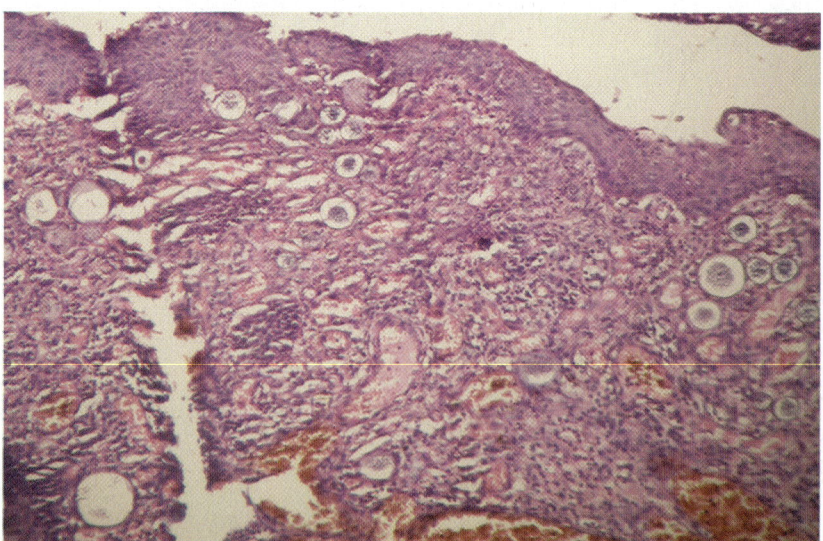

Fig. 6.21: Multiple thick walled sporangia at various levels of maturation

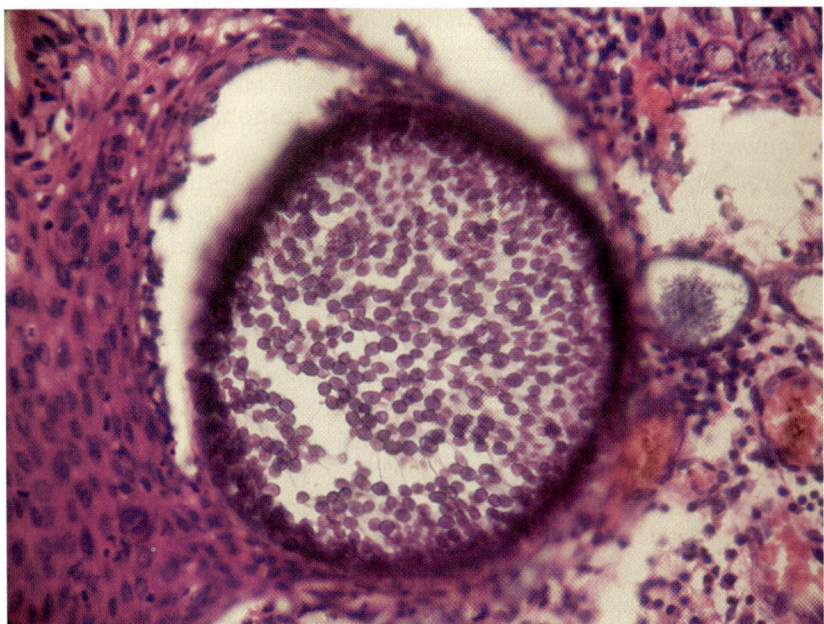

Fig. 6.22: Sporangia filled with endospores (H & E 40X)

An enzyme-linked immunosorbent assay (ELISA) test for identification of antirhinosporidial antibody has been developed and used for epidemiologic studies in endemic areas, but this testing is not available or routinely used in patient diagnosis.

Treatment

The cutaneous lesions should be treated early to prevent extension of lesions or dissemination. In general, the prognosis of cutaneous rhinosporidiosis is unfavourable due to its unrelenting behaviour and tendency to recur.

Rhinosporidiosis is treated with surgical excision because, generally, medical treatment has not been proven effective. The gold standard of rhinosporidiosis therapy is surgical excision with electrodesiccation. Recurrence has been reported with simple excision. Wide excision with electrocoagulation of the lesional base has been promoted to decrease recurrences.

Apart from cold steel surgeries, radiofrequenccy ablation and laser ablation can be tried as the chance of intraoperative bleeding and the spillage of spores are minimal.

Currently, dapsone is the only effective drug used as a surgical adjunct. Dapsone is believed to arrest the maturation of the sporangia and induce fibrosis in the stroma. It also prevents any post-surgery colonization or adjacent inoculation that may occur as a result of endospore release from traumatized polyps.Hence, it remains an adjunct to surgical removal and electrodesiccation which remain the treatment of choice.

Adjuvant medical therapies, including trimethoprim/sulfadiazine, sodium stibogluconate and antifungals (such as griseofulvin and amphotericin B), ciprofloxacin, have been attempted with limited success.

Bibliography

1. Ahluwalia KB, Maheshwari N, Deka RC. Rhinosporidiosis: A study that resolves etiologic controversies 1997;11:479–83.

2. Arseculeratne SN. Recent advances in rhinosporidiosis and *Rhinosporidium seeberi*. Indian J Med Microbiol 2002;20:119–131.

3. Das S, Kashyap B, Barua M, *et al*. Nasal rhinosporidiosis in humans: new interpretations and a review of the literature of this enigmatic disease. Med Mycol. 2011;49(3):311–5.

4. Fredricks DN, Jolley JA, Lepp PW, Kosek JC, Relman DA. *Rhinosporidium seeberi*: A human pathogen from a novel group of aquatic protistan parasites. Emerg Infect Dis 2000;6:273–82.

5. Ghorpade A, Ramanan C. Verrucoid cutaneous rhinosporidiosis. J Eur Acad Dermatol Venereol 1998;10:269–70.

6. Ghorpade A. Giant cutaneous rhinosporidiosis. J Eur Acad Dermatol Venereol 2006;20:88–9.

7. Kaushal S, Mathur SR, Mallick SR, Ramam M. Disseminated cutaneous, laryngeal, nasopharyngeal, and recurrent obstructive nasal rhinosporidiosis in an immunocompetent adult: a case report and review of literature. Int J Dermatol 2011;50(3):340–2.

8. Kumari R, Laxmisha C, Thappa DM. Disseminated cutaneous rhinosporidiosis. Dermatol Online J 2005;11:19.

9. Nayak S, Acharjya B, Devi B, Sahoo A, Singh N. Disseminated cutaneous rhinosporidiosis. Indian J DermatolVenereolLeprol 2007;73:185–7.

10. Salim T, Komu F. Varied presentations of cutaneous rhinosporidiosis: A report of three cases. Indian J Dermatol 2016;61:209–12.

11. Shenoy MM, Girisha BS, Bhandari SK, Peter R. Cutaneous rhinosporidiosis. Indian J DermatolVenereolLeprol. 2007;73(3):179–181.

12. Sudasinghe T, Rajapakse RP, Perera NA, Kumarasiri PV, Eriyagama NB, Arseculeratne SN. The regional seroepidemiology of rhinosporidiosis in Sri Lankan humans and animals. Acta Trop 2011 Oct-Nov. 120(1-2):72–81.

7. LOBOMYCOSIS
(Keloidal Blastomycosis, Lacaziosis, Lobo's Disease)

Pooja Arora Mrig, Kabir Sardana

DEFINITION

It is a chronic subcutaneous fungal infection caused by *Lacazia loboi* characterised by keloidal skin lesions.

Epidemiology

Lobomycosis has been described in Central and South America. The disease has been linked to contact with marine environment (especially dolphins), soil and vegetation. It usually occurs in men.

Etiology

Lobomycosis is caused by *Lacazialoboi*. This fungus cannot be isolated in culture.

Pathogenesis

The causative agent enters the skin through a wound and might be associated with water. It spreads via autoinoculation.

Clinical Features

The disease is characterised by presence of keloidal skin lesions on exposed parts of the body, i.e distal extremities, face (Fig. 6.23a and b). It can affect the trunk also. The plaques enlarge over time to form multi-nodular plaques that may have a smooth or verrucous surface. Ulceration can occur. The disease remains localised to the skin. There is no lymphadenopathy. The general health of patient is not affected.

Differential Diagnosis

Chromoblastomycosis.

Complications

Squamous cell carcinoma may develop in chronic cases.

Investigations

  i. KOH mounts of epidermal crusts to identify fungal cells
  ii Histopathological examination
    There is diffuse infiltrate of lymphocytes, macrophages and giant cells. Fungal cells can be identified within the giant cells and appear as short chains of oval or round cells joined by short tubular structures ("brass knuckles")
  iii. Culture
    The organism cannot be cultured

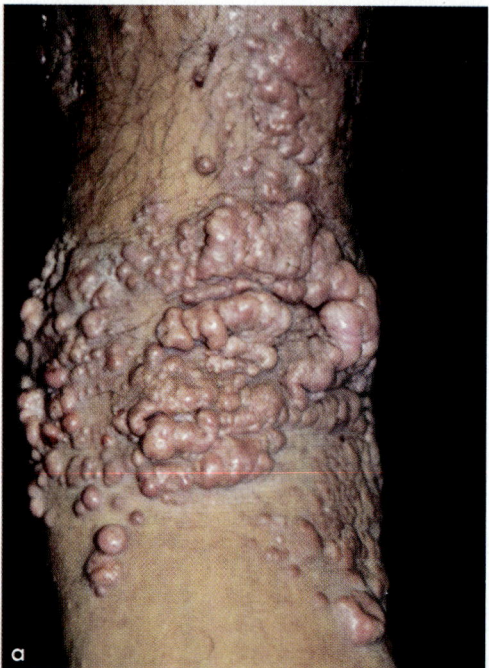

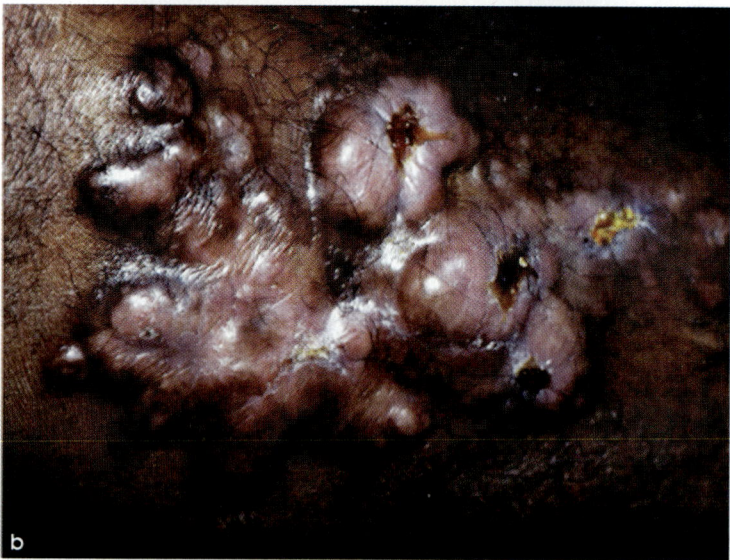

Fig. 6.23a and b: (a) Isolated and confluent papules, plaques, and nodule on the left calf of a patient with lobomycosis. (b) Nodules, plaques, and ulcerative lesions caused by local trauma on the left calf. (Dr Sinésio Talhari, PhD, Faculty of Medicine, Nilton Liins University, Amazonas, Brazil)

Treatment

Surgical excision is the treatment of choice. Antifungals are ineffective. Patients with widespread disease may benefit from clofazimine and itraconazole.

Bibliography

1. Carneiro FP, Maia LB, Moraes MA, *et al*. Lobomycosis; diagnosis and management of relapsed and multifocal lesions. Diag Microbiol Infect Dis 2009;65:62–4.

2. Paniz-Mondolfi AE, Reyes Jaimes O, Dávila Jones L. Lobomycosis in Venezuela. Int J Dermatol 2007; 46: 180–5.

3. Talhari S, Talhari C. Clin Dermatol 2012;30:420–4.

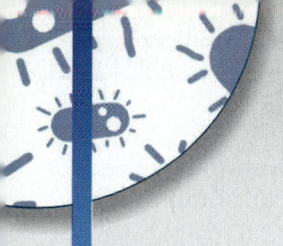

CHAPTER 7

Systemic Fungal Infections

The classification of this class of infections is detailed in Chapter 1. Though rare, in the era of HIV and related causes of immunosuppression, a large number of cases are being seen of systemic fungal disorders.

1. HISTOPLASMOSIS
(Darlina's Disease, Cave Disease, Ohio Valley Disease, Reticuloendotheliosis)

Pooja Arora Mrig, Kabir Sardana

DEFINITION

Histoplasmosis is a systemic mycosis caused by dimorphic fungus *Histoplasma capsulatum*. The fungus infects the reticuloendothelial cells where it is lives intracellularly.

Epidemiology

There are two varieties of the fungus *H. capsulatum* and *H. capsulatum* var. *duboisii*. The former causes small-form histoplasmosis that occurs throughout the world whereas the latter causes large form or African histoplasmosis that is seen only in Africa. The disease is usually seen in male agricultural workers. Certain factors predispose to histoplasmosis. These are immunocompromised states (e.g. AIDS), leukemia, lymphoma, corticosteroid treatment.

Pathogenesis

H. capsulatum is a saprophyte that is found in soil in warm, moist climates. It is found in the feces of birds, fowl and bats which act as reservoirs for infection.

The disease occurs due to inhalation of spores of *H. capsulatum* causing primary cutaneous disease with regional lymph node enlargement. It can rarely occur by direct cutaneous inoculation of the fungus causing primary cutaneous disease with regional lymph node enlargement (Fig. 7.1).

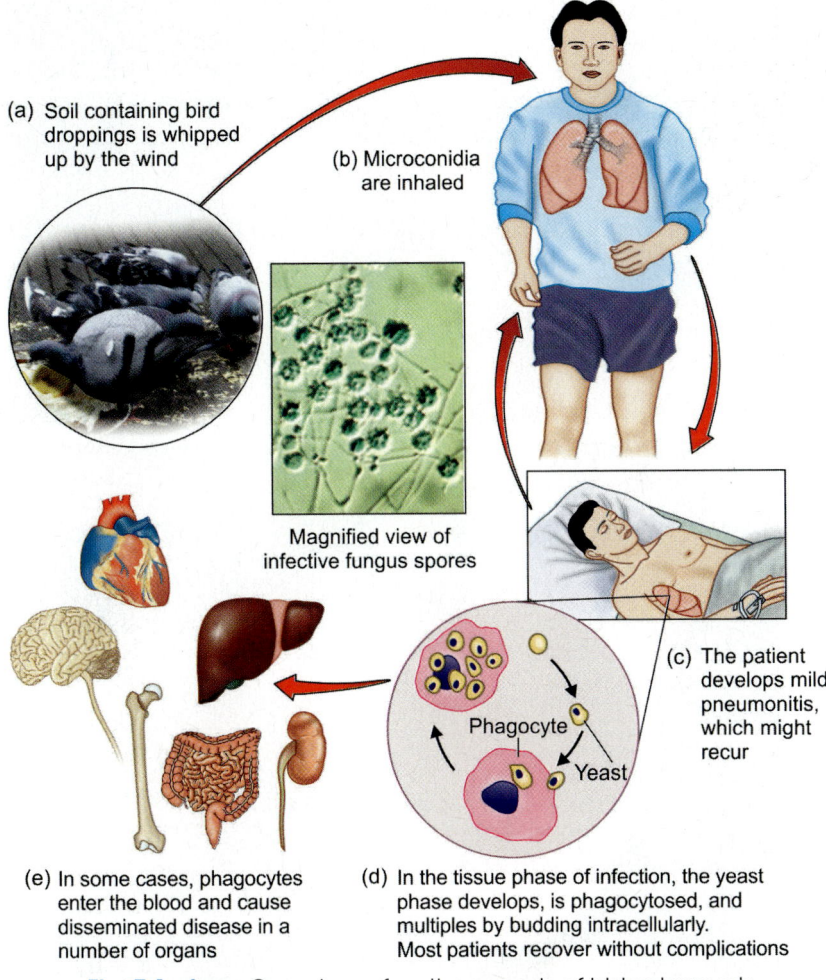

(a) Soil containing bird droppings is whipped up by the wind

(b) Microconidia are inhaled

Magnified view of infective fungus spores

Phagocyte

Yeast

(c) The patient develops mild pneumonitis, which might recur

(e) In some cases, phagocytes enter the blood and cause disseminated disease in a number of organs

(d) In the tissue phase of infection, the yeast phase develops, is phagocytosed, and multiples by budding intracellularly. Most patients recover without complications

Fig. 7.1a to e: Overview of pathogenesis of histoplasmosis

Clinical Features

Skin lesions are more common in African histoplasmosis.

Primary cutaneous Histoplasmosis is rare and arises due to direct inoculation of organism into the skin leading to formation of a local granuloma or ulcer with local lymphadenopathy.

Skin lesions in histoplasmosis arise due to dissemination from *primary pulmonary lesion* and can have varying manifestations in the form of *papules, nodules, abscesses, fistulae and scars* (Fig. 7.2). Pigmentary changes may occur.

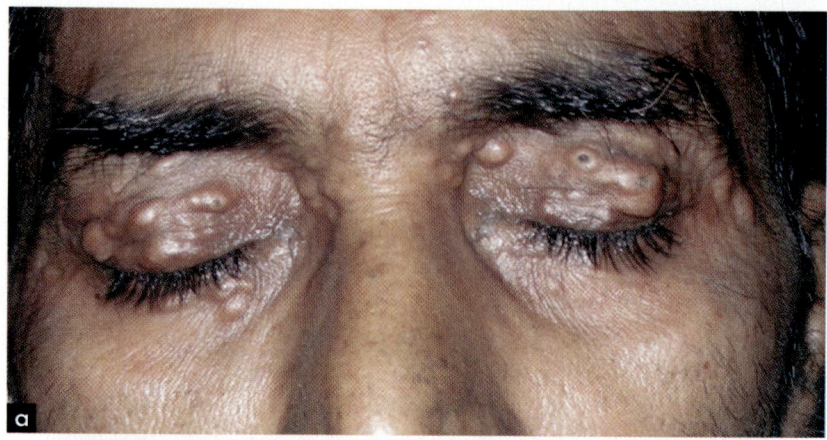

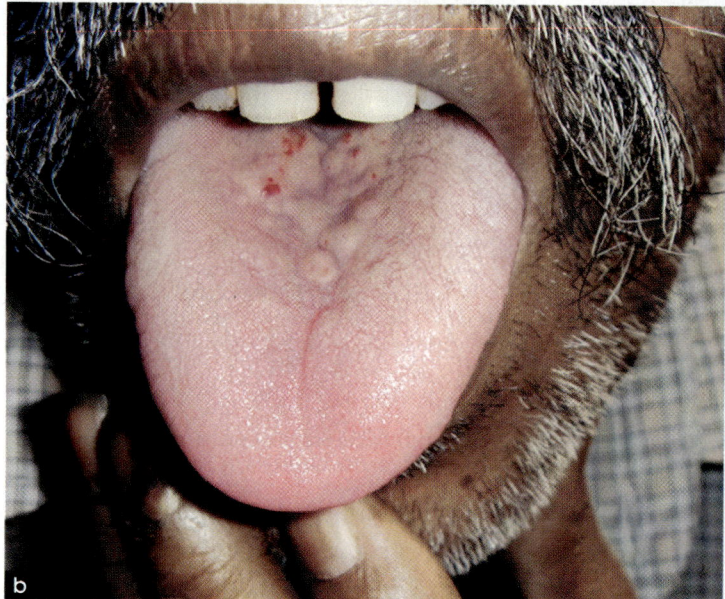

Fig. 7.2a and b: Multiple papules and nodules in a case of histoplasmosis HIV. The patient was put on amphotericin B but died after 2 weeks due to pulmonary complications

Clinical variants of histoplasmosis are:

i. **Asymptomatic histoplasmosis:** This is seen in endemic areas. There is no evidence of infection except positive skin test reactivity.

ii. **Acute pulmonary histoplasmosis:** It is uncommon. Patient has symptoms suggestive of an acute infection of the lungs. This may be accompanied by skin changes in the form of erythema nodosum or erythema multiforme. Chest radiograph shows localized infiltration or diffuse mottling.

iii. **Acute disseminated histoplasmosis:** This is also an uncommon variant. There is involvement of lungs along with other organs— enlargement of liver and spleen, fever, anemia, loss of appetite and generalized lymphadenopathy. Clinical features are variable though pulmonary signs are prominent and may simulate miliary tuberculosis. Skin involvement manifests as cutaneous or mucocutaneous granulomas and is more common in AIDS patients. Multiple papules and nodules with central softening may be seen. The disease has a poor prognosis and is fatal.

iv. **Chronic pulmonary histoplasmosis**: This variant resembles tuberculosis and is usually seen in adults.

v. **Chronic disseminated histoplasmosis**: This usually presents with chronic oral ulceration and Addison's disease that occurs due to infiltration in adrenal glands. Laryngeal involvement, ulceration or granulomas may occur.

Factors affecting severity of disease are:

- AIDS
- Leukemia, lymphoma
- Corticosteroid treatment
- Connective tissue diseases.

African Histoplasmosis

The disease is confined to a few regions of Africa. It is rarely seen in AIDS patients. Skin and bone are the common sites of involvement. Lungs and lymph nodes may also be affected. Skin involvement can manifest in the form of molluscum contagiosum like papules, abscesses or ulcers. The disease has a chronic course. Serology is often negative in this clinical type.

Differential Diagnosis

- Molluscum contagiosum
- Cryptococcosis
- Talaromyces infections

  Lung involvement can mimic tuberculosis

Diagnosis

i. *Identification of Histoplasma* in biopsy specimens, sputum, peripheral blood, bone marrow, lymph node aspirate. It appears as small intracellular yeast cells (2–5 µm) that can be seen clearly using fungal stains like methenamine silver and PAS (Fig. 7.3). Initially there is a little tissue reaction. Granulomatous changes, necrosis and fibrosis occur later. *H. duboisii* is much larger and giant cells predominate in its tissue reaction.

ii. *Culture*: Can be done from skin biopsy, bone marrow, blood, sputum, body fluids. Culture should be done at 25°C and 37°C. Growth appears in 4–6 weeks. However, culture should be maintained for 12 weeks before reporting negative results. Tuberculate microconidia develop at 25°C.

iii. *Histoplasmin skin testing*: It should be done only in non-endemic areas. It is not useful in diagnosis and is utilized only as an epidemiological tool. It can be negative in patients with disseminated disease.

iv. *Serology:* It can be done using complement fixation test and immunodiffusion test. A rising complement fixation titre indicates disseminated disease.

v. *Polymerase chain reaction*: It can be done in blood and tissue to identify histoplasmosis. It is highly sensitive and specific.

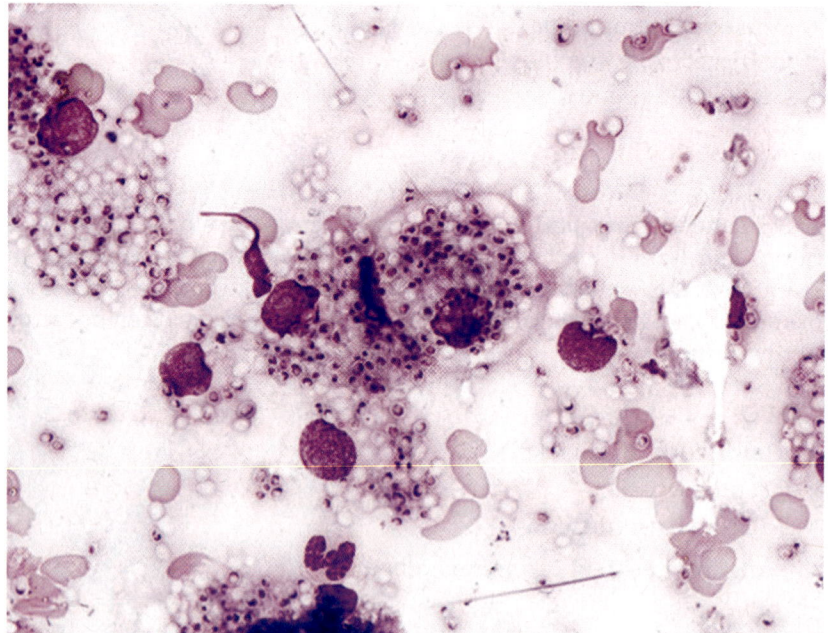

Fig. 7.3: Small intracellular yeast cells (2–5 µm) that can be seen clearly using fungal stains like methenamine silver and PAS

Management

An overview is given here and detailed listing is given on page 262.

First Line

- Itraconazole: 100 mg daily until clinical remission
- Amphotericin B: Used in patients with severe disease in a dose of 0.5–1 mg/kg/day (liposomal amphotericin B 3 mg/kg/day) for 2 weeks followed by itraconazole 200 mg OD/BD.

Second Line

Fluconazole: 800 mg daily for 3 months then 400 mg daily until clinical remission.

Posaconazole: Insufficient evidence

- HIV patients with disseminated disease require lifelong treatment with itraconazole as maintenance therapy after initial treatment with amphotericin
- HAART may reduce the requirement for maintenance therapy in some cases
- Those with solitary skin lesions may respond to excision alone.

Bibliography

1. Chang P, Rodas C. Skin lesions in histoplasmosis. Clin Dermatol 2012;30:592–8.
2. Kauffman CA. Histoplasmosis: a clinical and laboratory update. Clin Microbiol Rev 2007; 20: 115–32.
3. Wheat LJ, Azar MM, Bahr NC, et al. Histoplasmosis. Infect Dis Clin North Am 2016;30:207–27.

2. BLASTOMYCOSIS

G. Raghu Rama Rao

INTRODUCTION

Blastomycosis is one of the rare deep *mycotic* infections caused by inhalation of spores of *Blastomyces dermatitidis*. It was commonly known as North American blastomycosis and was initially thought to be restricted to areas around Great lakes—Mississippi, North America. But cases have been reported from all over the world including India. There are three clinical forms of the disease: *Pulmonary, disseminated* and *primary cutaneous*. Cutaneous blastomycosis is almost always secondary to lung involvement.

EPIDEMIOLOGY

B. dermatitidis, a dimorphic fungus, exists as a mould in soil. In human and animal tissues, it forms large, round budding yeast cells. Increase in soil temperatures and rainfall accelerates the growth of the fungus. In addition, decaying wood and other organic materials such as bird and animal excreta, water ways, ponds and river banks act as a natural source of *B. dermatitidis*. The disease often occurs in individuals who engage in outdoor activities such as construction or farming or recreational activities or playing in the dusty atmosphere. Men and woman are equally prone to blastomycosis. Majority of reported cases are in the age group varying from 20 to 70 years. Childhood blastomycosis constitutes 3–10% of cases. *B. dermatitidis* is a true pathogen and often affects immunocompetent individuals.

TRANSMISSION

Inhalation of *B. dermatitidis* spores is the usual mode of infection in humans. Very rarely direct accidental cutaneous inoculation may also result in primary blastomycosis. Transplacental infection of newborn and venereal transmission are some of the less common transmission routes.

INCUBATION PERIOD

Incubation period for pulmonary blastomycosis ranges from 30 to 40 days and for primary cutaneous blastomycosis is 14 days.

PATHOGENESIS

Inhalation of conidia is the most common route of infection. Once the conidia reaches the alveoli, they transform into yeast and induce an inflammatory response. Macrophages are the first to inhibit the transformation. Cell-mediated immunity Th1 is mainly responsible for control of infection and humoral immunity does not play a significant role. Yeasts are resistant to host's immunological response. Blastomycosis adhesion (BAD-1) cell wall protein mediates cellular adhesion and is the main virulence factor and target for cellular and humoral immunity. BAD-1 suppresses phagocyte release of TNF-α. Melanin, another virulence factor, protects the fungus from influx of leukocytes. Dissemination to other organs can occur via blood or lymphatics.

CLINICAL FEATURES

Clinical features range from a transient pulmonary infection to chronic pulmonary infection or to more widespread disseminated disease. Skin is the most frequent site (40–80%) of dissemination of pulmonary blastomycosis followed by bones (10–50%), genitourinary tract (10–30%) and central nervous system (1–5%). The mortality is very high with CNS involvement.

Pulmonary blastomycosis is asymptomatic or mild and usually goes unrecognized and resolves without treatment. Lung involvement usually manifests as acute or chronic pneumonia. This is very similar to pulmonary tuberculosis with cavity formation and lung abscess. There may be low grade fever, chest pain, cough and hemoptysis. If untreated, the disease may frequently disseminate to other organs like skin, bones, genitourinary and central nervous system.

Cutaneous blastomycosis: In most cases, cutaneous lesions develop after secondary dissemination from the primary focus in the lung and rarely after primary accidental inoculation of spores. The lesions are painless, papulonodules with heaped up borders. These lesions slowly enlarge to form verrucous plaques (Figs 7.4 to 7.6). They appear on the face, neck, chest, back and extremities. Mucous membranous may be involved in the form of ulcerative lesions seen on the mucosa of the nose, mouth and throat. Regional lymphadenopathy is an uncommon feature.

Primary cutaneous blastomycosis is very rare. Direct cutaneous inoculation manifests as a chancre at the site of inoculation. Local lymph nodes are involved in 65% cases. A mixture of verrucous lesions, ulcers, nodules and papules may be seen in primary cutaneous blastomycosis.

Other symptoms: Osteomyelitis occurs in about 30% of cases. The spine, ribs and long bones are the commonest sites of infection. Arthritis is less common, affects knee, ankle, elbow and wrist. The prostate, epididymis or testis are involved in 15–35% of cases.

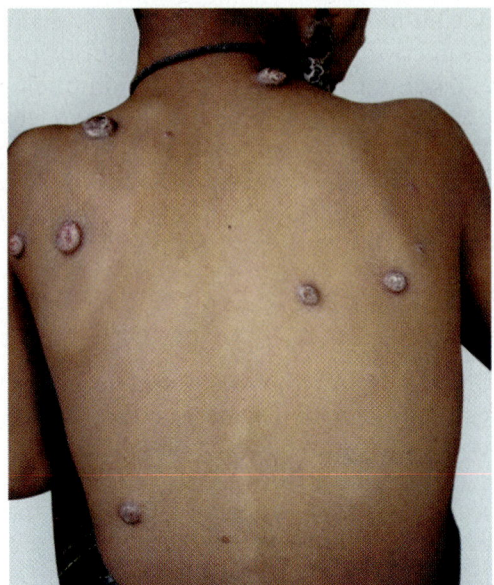

Fig. 7.4: Multiple annular hyperkeratotic lesions of blastomycoses on the back

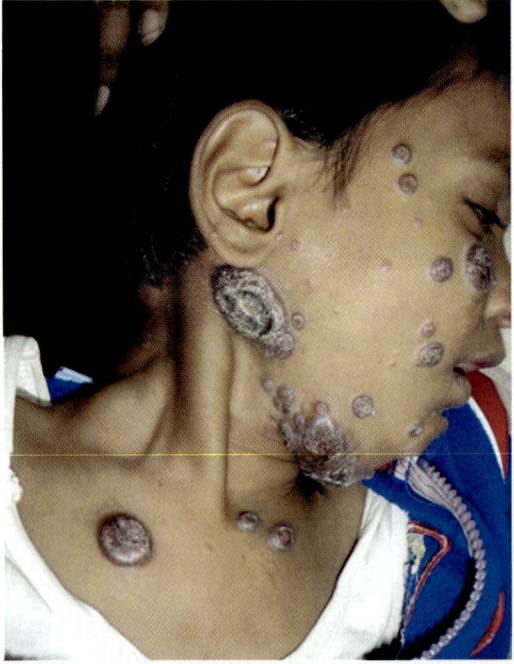

Fig. 7.5: Hyperkeratotic verrucous lesions of blastomycoses

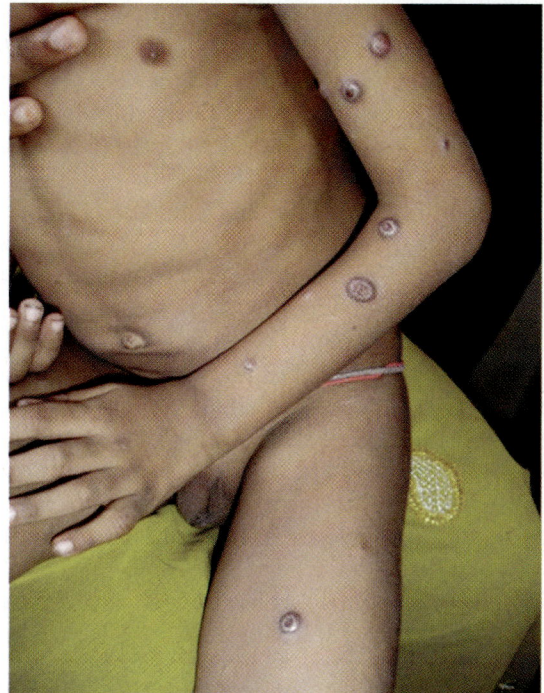

Fig. 7.6: Annular lesions of blastomycoses

Self- limited genital ulceration and endometrial infection in woman are reported after venereal transmission of *B. dermatitidis*. Meningitis and spinal brain abscess rarely develop after hematogenous spread of the fungus and may be fetal.

Adrenal glands, thyroid, liver and spleen are sometimes involved. Choroidoretinitis and endophthalmitis have been reported. Blastomycosis in immunocompromised patients particularly HIV patients carries a high mortality.

DIFFERENTIAL DIAGNOSIS

In india, tuberculosis of lung, skin, bone or genital tract can be confused with blastomycosis. Other systemic fungal infections like coccidio-idomycosis, histoplasmosis, mucocutaneous paracoccidiomycosis and chronic infections should be considered in the differential diagnosis.

DIAGNOSIS OF BLASTOMYCOSIS

1. **Direct microscopy:** Microscopic examination is a standard method of identifying the fungus in potassium hydroxide (KOH) wet mounts of the sputum and exudates.

2. **Culture:** This is the gold standard method for isolation and identification of the fungus *B. dermatitidis*. Brown wrinkled yeast colonies are observed at 37°C and mycelia forms at room temperature (25°C), producing white fluffy colonies on Sabouraud's dextrose agar (SDA) after 1–3 weeks. Culture is negative in 1/3 of cases.

3. **FNAC:** Diagnosis may also be confirmed by FNAC. On FNAC, rounded structures of yeast measuring 8–15 µm with refractile cell wall are observed. PAS and Gomori methenamine silver stains help in identifying *B. dermatitidis*.

4. **Histopathology:** Skin biopsy specimens from cutaneous blastomycosis show pseudoepitheliomatous hyperplasia with ill-defined granuloma with multi-nucleated giant cells in the dermis. Broad based yeast forms are seen within the giant cells. Occasional intraepidermal blastomycetic cells are also seen in Fig. 7.7.

5. **Serological tests:** ELISA tests are available to detect *B. dermatitidis* antibodies in blood, urine or body fluids of patients and their sensitivity is of 93%.

6. **PCR assays:** These are also available for rapid detection of *B. dermatitidis* in clinical and soil samples.

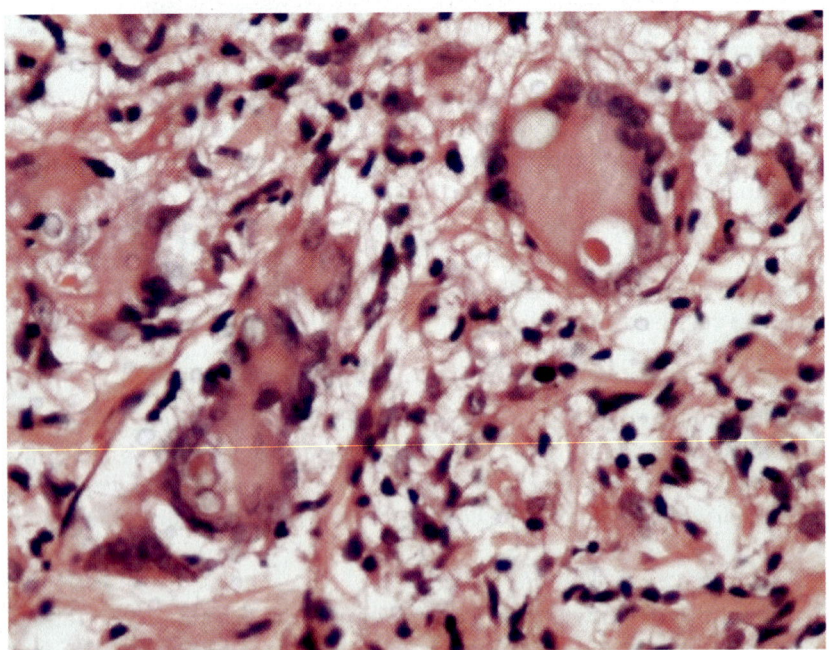

Fig. 7.7: Fungal yeast forms within giant cells (H& E, 400X)

TREATMENT

Mild to moderate blastomycosis: Oral itraconazole is the recommended drug. The dosage is 10 mg/kg/day (to a maximum of 400 mg orally per day) for 6 months. Serum levels should be measured after administering itraconazole for 2 weeks to confirm adequate drug exposure. The ideal serum level is greater than 500 µg/dl.

Severe blastomycosis: Amphotericin B 0.7–1 mg/kg/day, or lipid formulation of amphotericin B at a dosage of 3–5 mg/kg/day is recommended for 1–2 weeks or until improvement is noted, followed by oral itraconazole 10 mg/kg/day (up to 400 mg/day) in reducing doses, not exceeding 1 year.

Blastomycosis in pregnant women: Azoles should be avoided during pregnancy and amphotericin B (lipid formulation) is recommended.

Blastomycosis in newborns: For newborns, amphotericin B is the preferred drug (1 mg/kg daily).

PROGNOSIS

Excellent clinical responses (>90%, with a few relapses) are achieved with itraconazole at 200 mg/day for 6 months in immunocompetent patients. Amphotericin B affords cure rates of 97% in uncomplicated disease.

PREVENTION AND CONTROL

As there is no effective vaccine, early diagnosis and prompt treatment are imperative in decreasing mortality.

Bibliography

1. AR Mason, GY Cortes, J Cook, JC Maize, BH Thiers. Cutaneous blastomycosis: A diagnostic challenge. IJD 2008; 47: 824–30.
2. Chapman SW, Dismukes WE, Proia LA, *et al*. Clinical practice guidelines for the management of blastomycosis: 2008 update by the Infectious Diseases Society of America. Clin Infect Dis 2008;46:1801–12.
3. HS Randhavva, A Chowdhary, S Kathuria, Pradip Roy, Deepti S Misra, Sarika Jain, Tulsi D Chugh. Blastomycosis in India: Report of an imported case and current status. Medical Mycology, 2013; 51: 185–92.
4. Rao GR, Narayan BL, Durga Prasad BK, *et al*. Disseminated blastomycosis in a child with a brief review of the Indian literature. Indian J Dermatol Venereol Leprol 2013;79:92–6.
5. Richardson MD, Warnock DW. Blastomycosis. In: Fungal Infection: Diagnosis and Management. 3rd edn. USA: Blackwell 2003: 241–48.

3. COCCIDIOIDOMYCOSIS

Vikram Narang, Bhavna Garg, Neena Sood, Harpreet Kaur

DEFINITION

Coccidioidomycosis (commonly known as valley fever or San Joaquin fever) a fungal disease endemic in Western hemisphere is caused by the dimorphic soil dwelling fungus *Coccidioides*. Most human infections are caused by *Coccidioides immitis*. Coccidioidomycosis may vary from a clinically inapparent infection to a severe or fatal mycosis. Coccidioidomycosis is extremely rare in India, however, with an increase in international travel some travellers may acquire infection indigenous to the regions travelled that may pose clinical problems thus determining a history of exposure is critical for diagnosis.

Geographical Distribution

The fungus is endemic to a geographically delineated area within the United States known as the Lower Sonoran Life Zone. In recent years, the incidence of the disease has increased in California and Arizona, which is due to the rapid immigration of previously unexposed persons from states outside the endemic areas. The disease in the nonendemic areas like India is usually imported and suspected based on the evidence of endemic exposure.

Etiology

Coccidioidomycosis is caused by the dimorphic soil-dwelling fungus *Coccidioides immitis*. The disease transmission is either through direct contact or indirect exposure to contaminated secretions (Fig. 7.8). The incubation period for primary pulmonary or cutaneous coccidioidomycosis is usually 1–3 weeks, however, disseminated disease or chronic pulmonary coccidioidomycosis can occur months or years after the initial infection.

The reason for the disease not being prevalent in India might be attributed to the lack of optimum conditions such as the semi-arid climate and the flora for the fungus to thrive. Exposure to soil containing spores is the only risk factor for acquiring the disease. High inoculum exposures during windstorms, digging, farming, and construction are more likely to result in symptomatic disease.

Clinical Features

After being exposed to the infecting agent, majority of the individuals remain asymptomatic, while around 40% develop "valley fever," which is a self-limiting flu-like illness, 5% of people develop pulmonary

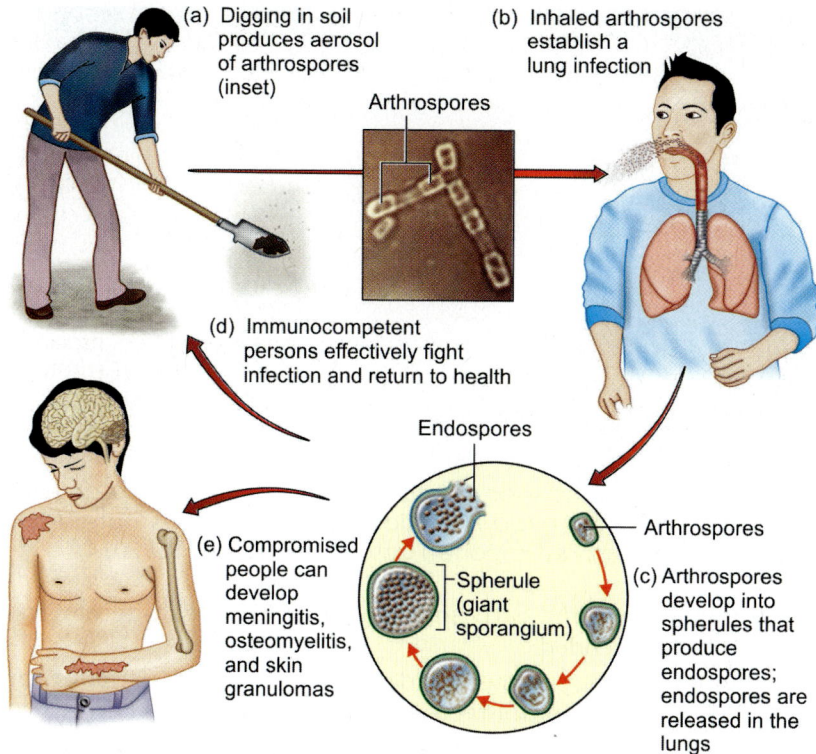

Fig. 7.8a to e: An overview of the pathogenesis of coccidioidomycosis

disease, and only 0.5% people develop a disseminated disease involving skin, bones, and central nervous system. Isolated cutaneous involvement is rare (Fig. 7.9a).

Investigation
Serological Tests
Serological tests are the most widely used method of diagnosis and are used in combination with clinical symptoms and other laboratory tests. Tests for *Coccidioides* spp. include enzyme immunoassay (EIA), immunodiffusion, and complement fixation (CF) tests. CF and immunodiffusion tests are designed to identify tube precipitin antibodies.

IgM or complement-fixing antibodies (IgG) are primarily performed at large reference laboratories using commercial immunodiffusion kits. Qualitative detection of *Coccidioides* spp. IgM and IgG can be performed using the enzyme-linked immunoassay. Serological tests may be

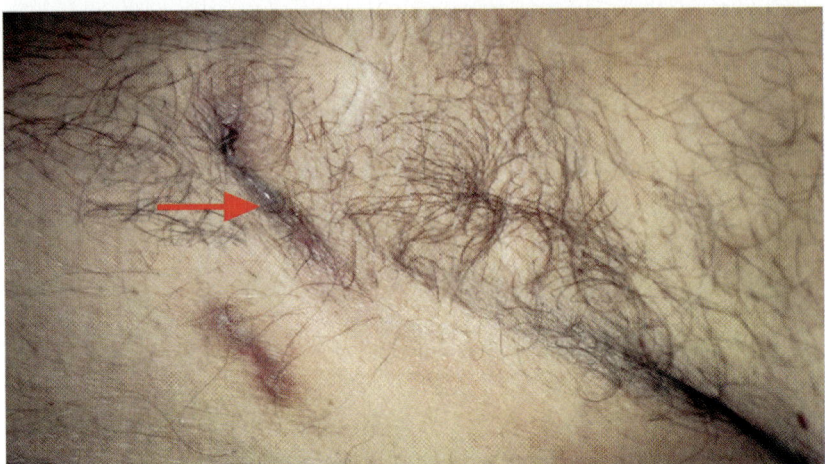

Fig. 7.9a: Skin lesions seen as discharging sinuses in cutaneous coccidioidomycosis (*cited from* Narang, *et al.* Primary cutaneous coccidioidomycosis: First imported case in North India. IJD, 2014)

insensitive in detecting early infection, therefore, serial serological testing is recommended.

Although serology is most widely used, the gold standard for diagnosis of coccidioidomycosis remains a positive culture or histopathological/cytopathological identification of the organism in clinical specimens.

Histopathological Examination

Histopathological examination of the lesion at tissues is considered to be more valuable and easier to perform as culture and molecular diagnostic modalities are not routinely available in laboratories in the nonepidemic regions. Identification of endospore-containing spherules differing in diameter from 20 to 200 μm without budding under microscopy is definitely diagnostic of coccidioidomycosis (Fig. 7.9b). Commonly used histological stains such as the hematoxylin and eosin and PAS distinguish typical morphological structures of coccidioidomycosis spherules and can also differentiate it from budding yeast forms of *Blastomyces, Histoplasma, Cryptococcus*, or *Candida*.

Culture

In tissue culture, *C. immitis* is identified by large globular sporangia, which contain sporangiospores or endospores. The spores enlarge to form spherules and rupture of the spherules leads to the release of

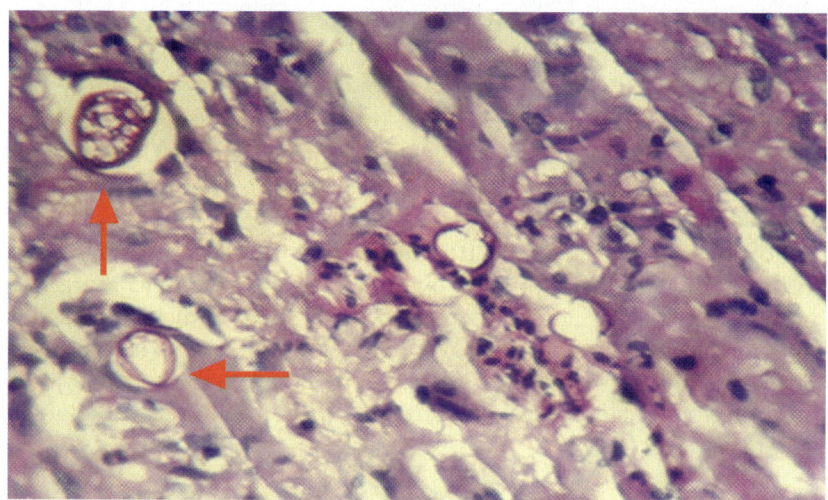

Fig. 7.9b: Microphotograph showing granulomas with endospores of *Coccidioides immitis* (*cited from* Narang, *et al.* Primary cutaneous coccidioidomycosis: First imported case in North India. IJD, 2014)

endospores, which elicit a suppurative reaction as evidenced in our case. Intact sporangia usually elicit a granulomatous reaction of histiocytes, epithelioid cells, and giant cells of the foreign body or of Langhans' type.

Treatment

Coccidioidomycosis encompasses a broad spectrum of illness and severity varies widely, from mild respiratory syndrome to severe pulmonary and extrapulmonary lesions, the optimal management strategies also vary widely among individual patients. Although the vast majority of patients who present with early infections will resolve without specific antifungal therapy, patients who present with severe pneumonia soon after infection warrant antifungal therapy. Patients who develop chronic pulmonary or disseminated disease also warrant antifungal therapy (prolonged—potentially lifelong especially in patient with overt immune-deficient conditions).

Specific antifungal drugs and their usual dosages for treatment of coccidioidomycosis include amphotericin B deoxycholate (0.5–1.5 mg/kg per day or alternate day administered intravenously), lipid formulations of amphotericin B (2.0–5.0 mg/kg or greater per day administered intravenously), ketoconazole (400 mg everyday administered orally), fluconazole (400–800 mg/day administered orally or intravenously), and itraconazole (200 mg twice per day or 3 times per day administered orally).

Newly available antifungal agents of possible benefit for the treatment of refractory coccidioidal infections are voriconazole and caspofungin. Voriconazole has not been approved by the United States Food and Drug Administration (FDA) for the treatment of coccidioidomycosis.

Combination therapy with members of different classes of antifungal agents has not been evaluated in patients, and there is a hypothetical risk of antagonism. However, some clinicians feel that outcome in severe cases is improved when amphotericin B is combined with an azole antifungal. If the patient improves, the dosage of amphotericin B can be slowly decreased while the dosage of azole is maintained.

Bibliography

1. Desai SA, Minai OA, Gordon SM, *et al*. Coccidioidomycosis in non-endemic areas: A case series. Respir Med 2001;95:305–9.

2. Galgiani JN, Ampel NM, Blair JE, Catanzaro A, Johnson RH, Stevens DA, *et al*. Coccidioidomycosis. Clinical Infectious Diseases 2005; 41:1217–23.

3. Gildardo JM, Leobardo VA, Nora MO, Jorge OC. Primary cutaneous coccidioidomycosis: Case report and review of the literature. Int J Dermatol 2006;45:121–3.

4. Malo J, Monjagatta LC, Wolk DM, Thompson R, Hage CA, Knox KS. Update on the Diagnosis of Pulmonary Coccidioidomycosis Annals ATS 2014; 11:243:53.

5. Narang V, Garg B, Sood N, Goraya SK. Primary cutaneous coccidioidomycosis: First imported case in North India. Indian J Dermatomolgy 2014;59:422–4.

4. MUCORMYCOSIS

Sumit Mrig, Vineet Narula

Fungal sinusitis is the inflammation of lining mucosa of paranasal sinuses caused due to the presence of fungal elements in nose and paranasal areas. It comprises 6–9% of all rhinosinusitis. It is broadly classified into invasive and noninvasive types. The noninvasive form is generally seen in immunocompetent patients and includes allergic fungal sinusitis and mycetoma. Invasive fungal sinusitis is mostly caused by saprophytic fungi of the order mucorales (*mucor, rhizopus, absidia*).

Rhinocerebral mucormycosis is a rare opportunistic infection affecting sinus, nasal cavity, oral cavity and brain. It is caused by saprophytic fungus belonging to *Phycomycetes genera*. There are different manifestations of mucormycosis; rhinocerebral being the most common type. Others include gastrointestinal, pulmonary, cutaneous, disseminated and lingual forms.

Etiopathogenesis

Saprophytic aerobic fungi of the class Phycomycetes (order Mucorales) cause rhinocerebral mucormycosis, also known as phycomycosis. The 3 genera responsible for most cases are *Rhizopus, Absidia,* and *Mucor*. Researchers have also reported cases of rhinocerebral mucormycosis caused by *Rhizomucor, Saksenaea, Apophysomyces,* and *Cunninghamella* species.

The fungus is ubiquitous in nature mostly found in soil and decaying vegetation. The infection occurs via airborne spores and colonise the nose, paranasal sinus, throat and oral mucosa. The fungus then spreads into the walls of blood vessels (angioinvasion), nerves, cartilage, bone and meninges as well as the perineural space. It can erode bone through sinus and spread into orbit and retroorbital area extending into the brain. Pterygopalatine fossa has been thought to be the possible reservoir of organisms. Advanced infection leads to cavernous sinus thrombosis, purulent arteritis, tissue ischemia and infarction.

Risk Factors

An underlying risk factor is recognized in most of the cases of mucormycosis. This has emerged as an increasingly important pathogen during the past decade particularly evident in hematopoietic stem cell transplant recipients and hematological malignancies.

Seventy percent of mucormycosis cases occur in patients with diabetes mellitus. *Rhizopus* species have an active ketone reductase system that enables them to thrive in an acidic pH and glucose-rich medium. Hyperglycemia enhances fungal growth and impairs neutrophil chemotaxis, therefore, individuals with diabetic ketoacidosis are commonly affected. *Rhizopus* species also favor an iron-rich environment and are frequently isolated in patients receiving deferoxamine therapy (an iron-chelating agent).

Other predisposing factors include: Burns, immunodeficiency due to HIV/AIDS, immunosuppression in chronic steroid use, chemotherapy, post-transplantation, and IV drug use. However, no underlying condition is recognized at the time of diagnosis in 15–20% of the patients.

Clinical Presentation

1. Rhinocerebral disease may manifest as unilateral, retro-orbital headache, facial pain, numbness, fever, hyposmia, and nasal stuffiness, which progresses to black discharge (Figs 7.10a and b). Initially, mucormycosis may mimic sinusitis. Late symptoms that indicate invasion of the orbital nerves and vessels include diplopia and visual loss.

   Orbital swelling and facial cellulitis are progressive. Black pus discharges from the necrotic palatine or nasal eschars. Necrotic eschars can be noted in the nasal cavity, on the hard palate, or as facial lesions; although these lesions are suggestive of mucormycosis, their absence does not exclude the possibility of this disease. Proptosis, ptosis, chemosis, and ophthalmoplegias indicate retro-orbital extension. Cranial nerves V and VII are the most commonly affected. Loss of vision can occur with retinal artery thrombosis.

   Cerebral symptoms include altered mental status and seizures. Neurological findings may be observed such as cranial nerve palsies and cerebral edema.

2. *Pulmonary mucormycosis:* This form of mucormycosis is most commonly seen in neutropenic cancer patients undergoing remission induction treatment. The clinical presentation is non-specific. Patients often present with an unremitting fever (greater than 38°C) that fails to respond to broad-spectrum antibacterial treatment. Cough is a common presenting symptom. The radiological signs are also non-specific, but infiltrates and nodules are more frequent than consolidation or cavitation. Pleural effusion is uncommon.

3. *Cutaneous mucormycosis:* Although inhalation is the usual route of infection in patients with mucormycosis, traumatic inoculation of spores can lead to extensive necrotic cutaneous infections. This form of disease is most often seen in patients with burns or other forms of local trauma.

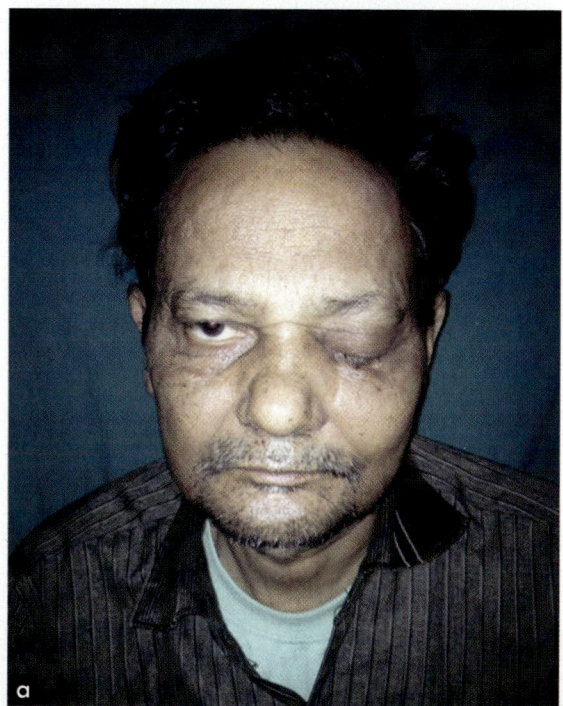

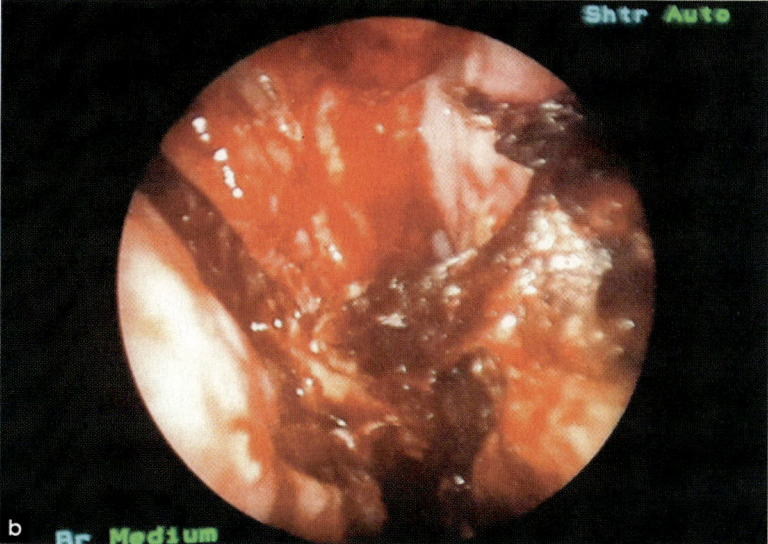

Fig. 7.10a and b: (a) A patient showing left eye drooping of eyelids because of complete ophthalmoplegia due to mucormycosis; (b) Nasal endoscopic picture showing black necrotic crusts in the nasal cavity

Cutaneous mucormycosis is an aggressive disease, even in the face of surgical debridement and antifungal treatment. It can lead to necrotizing fasciitis or to widespread disseminated infection. The initial signs include cutaneous erythema and subcutaneous swelling. The margins of the lesion become raised and indurated, and the central region becomes necrotic and evolves into an ulcer covered with a black eschar (Fig. 7.11). The lesions are indistinguishable

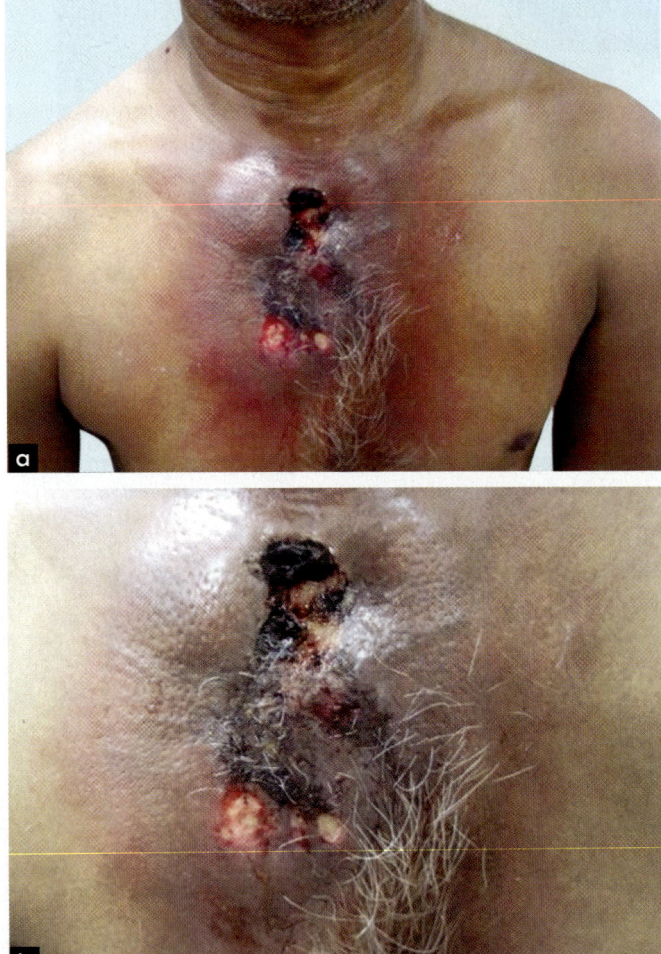

Fig. 7.11a and b: (a) Woody hard tender swelling with ulceration seen over the chest in a 56-year-old non-diabetic male; (b) Ulceration with black necrotic eschar and seropurulent exudate. Surrounding skin has erythema and peau d' orange appearance

from those caused by *Aspergillus* species and can resemble ecthyma gangrenosum. The lesions are painful and the patient can be febrile. The development of severe underlying necrosis and infarction in a burn should suggest the diagnosis.

Investigations

Diagnosis requires high index of clinical suspicion. Laboratory studies are often nonspecific and may reflect the underlying metabolic acidosis and hyperglycemia. Blood culture is often negative. CSF findings may be normal even in the presence of brain involvement.

Imaging studies are helpful to determine the extent of the disease. CT scan demonstrates sinus opacification and bony destruction of the sinus and orbit. Bone erosion is a late finding. Cavernous sinus thrombosis and CNS lesions are also evident on CT scan (Fig. 7.12).

MRI with contrast is more accurate in determining the soft tissue extension, early vascular intracranial invasion and infection among peripheral nerves before clinical signs develop. Sinus X-ray reveals opacification of the involved sinus.

Histology remains the mainstay of tissue diagnosis which demonstrates typical nonseptate broad fungal hyphae with right-angled branching (Fig. 7.13). Hyphae can be identified by hematoxylin and eosin stain technique, but are more clearly seen in PAS Grocott-Gromori methenamine silver nitrate. Also observed is evidence of angioinvasion and subsequent thrombosis and tissue necrosis. Tissue culture provides further confirmation but is positive in only 15–25% of cases.

Differential Diagnosis

Rhinocerebral mucormycosis resembles bacterial or allergic fungal sinusitis clinically. Other mimics include sinonanasal or orbital malignancies, chronic sinusitis, granulomatous disorders, Graves' disease, pseudotumor or cavernous sinus thrombosis. A high index of clinical suspicion as well as histological evidence of mucormycosis on special stains clinches the diagnosis.

Complications

Rhinocerebral mucormycosis progresses rapidly and can result in carotid artery occlusion, cavernous sinus thrombosis, and CNS infarction secondary to fungal thrombosis, leading to hemiparesis, hemiplegia, coma, and death. Other complications of rhinocerebral mucormycosis include CNS hemorrhage, abscess, and cerebritis,

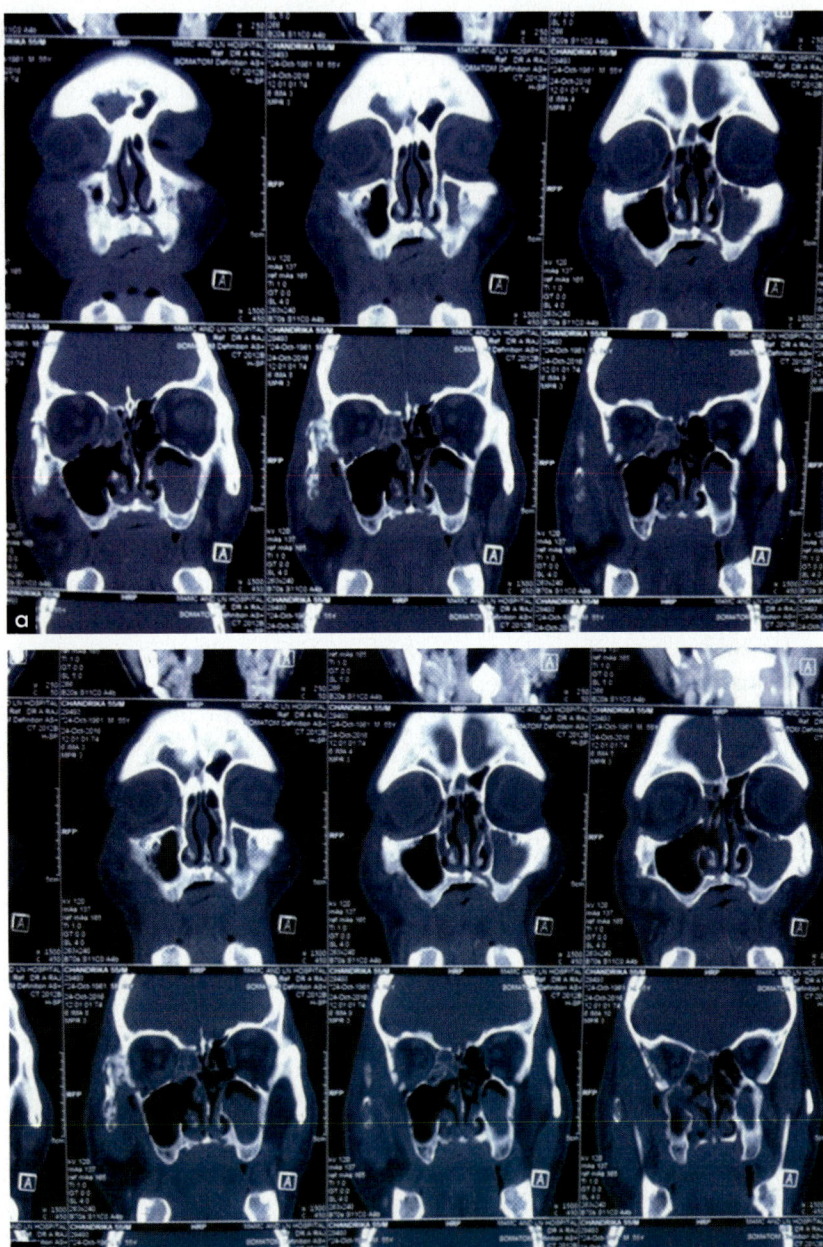

Fig. 7.12a and b: Contrast enhanced CT scan of nose and paranasal sinuses suggestive of mass involving left maxillary sinus and nasal cavity eroding the hard palate

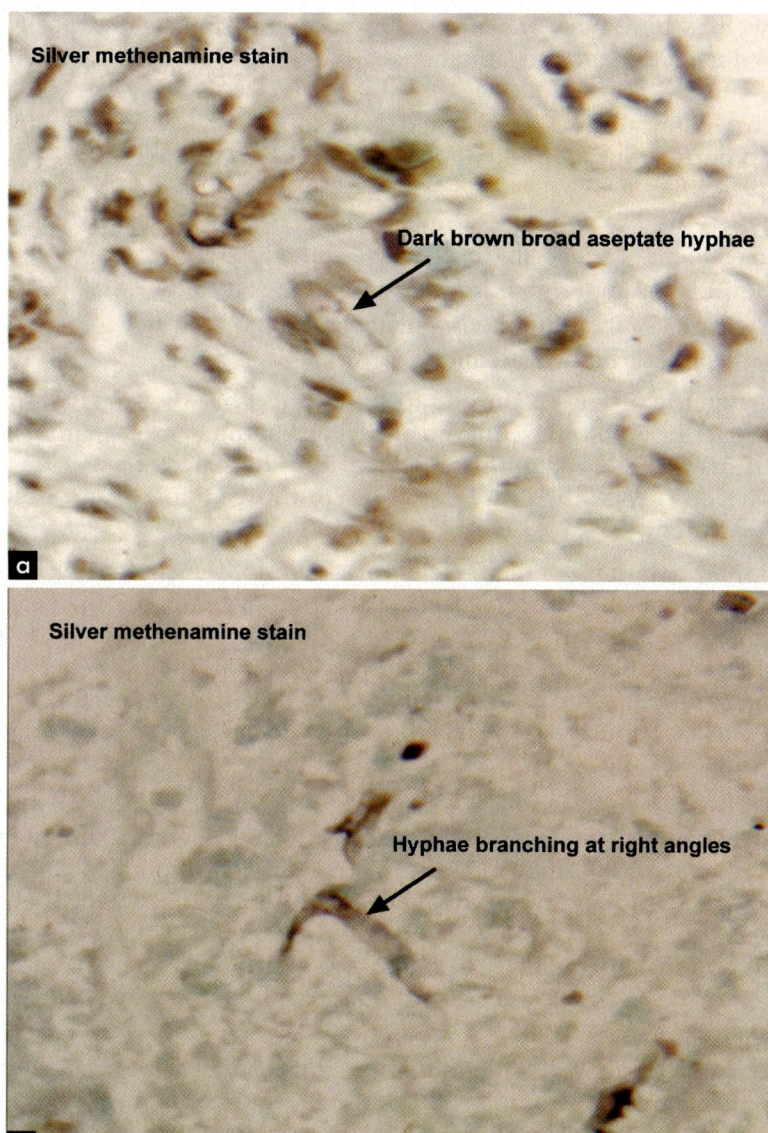

Fig. 7.13a and b: (a) Dense acute on chronic inflammation with multiple epithelioid cell granulomas admixed with lymphocytes, plasma cells and eosinophils with focal areas of necrosis. A few broad thin-walled aseptate hyphae branching at right angles are seen within the granulomas and necrotic material (H & E, 100X); (b) Silver methenamine stain showing the dark brown aseptate fungal hyphae branching at right angles

as well as blindness and airway obstruction from head and neck infections. Permanent residual effects of the disease occur up to 70% of the time.

Neurological function can be recovered if no irreversible damage has occurred, but morbidity is very common.

Management

Management of mucormycosis is three-tiered:
1. Reversal of underlying immunocompromised state
2. Prompt administration of systemic antifungal
3. Urgent surgical debridement

When the disease is limited to sinus and orbit, the survival rate approaches 50 to 80% and surgical debridement in combination with systemic antifungal and local amphotericin irrigation is curative. The fatality rate escalates to more than 80% in brain involvement.

Amphotericin B is the only reliable systemic antifungal approved for the treatment of mucormycosis. At the present time, the liposomal formulation is the drug of choice based on efficacy and safety data. Lipid preparations of amphotericin B are used at 5 mg/kg/d. Some have used doses of up to 7.5–10 mg/kg/d to treat mucormycosis, especially CNS disease. The total dose given over the course of therapy is usually 2.5–3 g.

Posaconazole, a triazole, is currently considered a second-line drug for treatment of mucormycosis and the typical dose is 400 mg twice daily (total of 800 mg/d). Administration with a high-fat meal/ food and acidic beverages enhances absorption of the drug. Patients on posaconazole should avoid antacids, especially proton pump inhibitors. Isavuconazole is effective in treatment of rhinocerebral mucormycosis that is refractory to amphotericin B and posaconazole.

Surgical debridement is the mainstay of treatment with drainage of all sinus and abscess fluid collections. It is required to move as much devitalized tissue as possible. Orbital exenteration with removal of the affected sinus may be required in orbital invasive cases.

Prompt control of diabetes mellitus and discontinuation of immunosuppressive therapy is warranted. G-CSF can be administered to reconstitute host immune defence.

As chronic presentation with late sequelae have been observed, patient require long-term follow-up to detect recurrence and residual infection.

Bibliography

1. Chakrabarti, *et al*. Fungal Rhinosinusitis: A categorisation and definitional Schema addressing Current Controversies. Laryngoscope 2009;119(9): 109–18.

2. Eva M. Guti_errez-Delgado, Jos_e Luis Trevi~no-Gonz_alez, Adolfo Montemayor-Alatorre, Luis Angel Cece~nas-Falc_on, *et al*. Chronic rhinoorbitocerebral mucormycosis: A case report and review of the literature. Annals of Medicine and Surgery 2016;6:87–91.

3. Hosseini S, Borghei P. Rhinocerebral Mucormycosis: Pathways of spread. Eur Arch Otorhinolaryngol 2005;262:932–8.

4. Mallis A, Mastronikolos S, Naxakis S, *et al*. Rhinocerebral mucormycosis: an update. European Review for medical and pharmacological sciences. 2010; 14:987–92.

5. Roden M, Zacutis T, Buchanon W *et al*. Epidemiology and outcome of zygomycosis: A review of 929 reported cases. Clin Inf Dis 2005;41:634–6.

5. CRYPTOCOCCOSIS

Pooja Arora Mrig, Kabir Sardana

DEFINITION

Cryptococcosis is a systemic fungal infection caused by *Cryptococcus neoformans*, that is an encapsulated yeast.

Brain and meninges are the major organs affected, though it can affect other parts of the body also especially the lungs and skin.

Epidemiology

Cryptococcosis occurs throughout the world and has no geographic predilection. The disease is common in adults. Predisposing factors include:

- AIDS
- Malignant lymphomas especially Hodgkin disease
- Sarcoidosis
- Collagen diseases
- Cancers
- Systemic corticosteroid therapy
- Immunosuppressant therapy following organ transplantation.

Use of ART has led to decrease in incidence of cryptococcosis.

Etiology

It is caused by *C. neoformans* and *C. gattii* organism.

New variety	Previous serotype	Geographical distribution
C. neoformans var. *grubii*	A	Common in Europe, USA
C. neoformans gattii	B, C	Tropical countries (Africa)
C. neoformans var. *neoformans*	D	Europe, USA

The neoformans and grubii varieties are saprophytes and can be found in soils enriched with pigeon droppings. Whereas the *C. gattii* has been isolated from bark debris and leaves from red gum trees.

Bird droppings act as reservoir of infection. Animal-human or human-human transmission has not been described.

Pathogenesis

The portal of entry is the respiratory tract resulting in a primary pulmonary infection with subsequent dissemination to CNS, bone and skin.

The skin can get involved in two ways:

- Primary cutaneous crytococcosis: Due to direct inoculation into skin, which is rare in the absence of systemic infection
- Secondary cutaneous cryptococcosis: Where skin gets involved due to dissemination after a primary pulmonary infection. It can occur in immunocompetent hosts.

Clinical Features

CNS is the main organ of involvement and can present as chronic meningitis or may simulate a brain tumor. This may be accompanied by fever. Pulmonary or urinary tract crytococcosis have a favorable prognosis if they occur in the absence of CNS involvement.

Cutaneous lesions (that occur due to dissemination) may occur before or after the appearance of CNS or pulmonary symptoms. Skin is involved in 10% of cases. The presentation is variable and can range from multiple papulonodules (around the nose and mouth) to ulcers (punched out with rolled edge) and abscesses, molluscum contagiosum like lesions (Fig. 7.14). Most frequent type of cutaneous lesions are subcutaneous erythema nodosum-like swellings.

In AIDS patients, CNS symptoms are minimal. Skin is more frequently involved (paules with central softening) and blood culture may be positive.

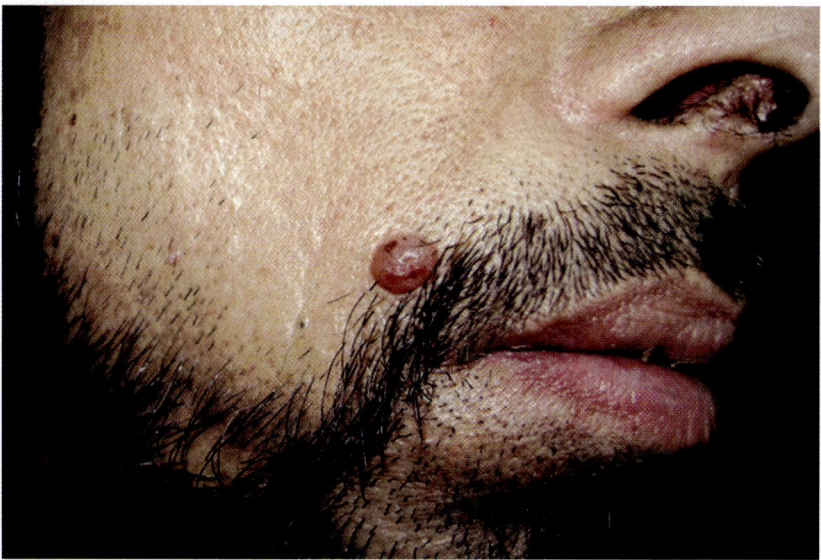

Fig. 7.14: Cryptococcosis. Single nodule in a patient who was HIV positive with meningitis

Differential Diagnosis of Skin Lesions in Cryptococcosis

- Molluscum contagiosum
- Folliculitis
- Cellulitis
- Ecthyma gangrenosum
- Vasculitis
- **Systemic fungal infections:** Histoplasmosis, infections caused by *Talaromyces marneffei*

Investigations

i. *Histopathological examination*

Histopathological examination of infected tissues range from a minimal inflammatory reaction to a frank granulomatous reaction without caseation. Encapsulated budding cells (5–15 μm) can be seen in tissue sections or in direct microscopy of CSF or pus. PAS stain can be used to visualize the yeast form whereas mucicarmine or alcian blue stain helps to visualise the capsule. India ink preparations can also be used.

ii. *Culture*

Media should not contain cycloheximide as it inhibits the growth. Culture plates should be kept at 30°C for 4 weeks. The growth appears as soft, mucoid, cream to pale brown colonies. Addition of various melanin precursors (e.g. caffein acid media) can lead to formation of characteristic brown colonies. Microscopy and physiological tests (urease and phenoloxidase production, carbohydrate utilisation tests) can be used to identify the fungus.

iii. *Serology*

It is rapid, specific and useful test that depends on the detection of crytococcal capsular antigen using latex agglutination test, ELISA assay. Titres are high in AIDS patients. However, serology may be negative in localised cutaneous lesions in non-HIV patients.

Management

A detailed overview is given in Page 261.

First Line

Amphotericin B: 0.5–1 mg/kg daily for 4–6 weeks or amphotericin B 0.2–1 mg daily (or liposomal amphotericin B 3 mg/kg daily) for 2 weeks followed by fluconazole 400 mg daily for 4 weeks or until remission.

Second Line

High dose fluconazole 800 mg daily for 6–8 weeks. It is less effective.

Bibliography

1. Chayakulkeeree M, Perfect JR. Cryptococcosis. Infect Dis Clin North Am 2006;20:507–44.

2. Christianson JC, Engber W, Andes D. Primary cutaneous cyrptococcosis in immunocompetent and immunocompromised hosts. Med Mycol 2003;41:177–88.

3. Hay RJ. *Cryptococcus neoformans* and cutaneous cryptococcosis. Semin Dermatol 1985;4:252–9.

6. HYALOHYPHOMYCOSIS

Pooja Arora Mrig, Kabir Sardana

The term "hyalohyphomycosis" is used to refer to infections due to colourless (hyaline) moulds that adopt a septate hyphae form in tissue.

Fusarium Infection

Fusarium species have long been recognized as a cause of nail and corneal infection in immunocompetent patients and are now believed to be the second most frequent cause of invasive fungal infection (after aspergillosis) among immunocompromised individuals, particularly in neutropenic cancer patients and haematopoietic stem cell transplant (HSCT) recipients.

Epidemiology

The mechanisms by which human infection is acquired are not well understood and several suggested routes of transmission, including inhalation, implantation following trauma, and acquisition via contaminated intravascular devices have been implicated. In some cases, it has been found that the source of disseminated Fusarium infection in an immunocompromised individual was a nail infection or a localized skin infection. The isolation of *Fusarium* species from hospital water distribution systems has led some specialists to suggest that inhalation of bioaerosols generated during showering could be an important source of invasive infection in HSCT recipients and other immunocompromised individuals

Clinical Features

Fusarium species cause a broad-spectrum of human disease ranging from superficial infection of the nail and cornea in immunocompetent persons to disseminated invasive infection in immunocompromised patients.

Localized deep infections, including cases of endophthalmitis, osteomyelitis, arthritis, brain abscess and dialysis-associated peritonitis, have also been reported.

Like aspergillosis and mucormycosis, *Fusarium* species have a predilection for *vascular invasion*, resulting in thrombosis, infarction and tissue necrosis. The lungs and paranasal sinuses are the most common initial sites of damage.

The usual initial presentation in the neutropenic patient is a persistent fever (> 38°C) that is unresponsive to antibacterial and antifungal treatment. Other presenting signs include pleuritic chest pain, non-productive cough and hemoptysis. The radiological findings range from non-specific infiltrates to nodular or cavitating lesions, depending on the timing of the investigation.

Fusarium infection often leads to the development of cutaneous lesions, either as the initial site of involvement or as a metastatic site and has been reported in about 70% of reported cases.

Among immunocompetent individuals, cutaneous Fusarium infections typically are localized and develop after skin breakdown at the site of infection. These infections most commonly present as necrotic lesions that complicate extensive burns or trauma, cellulitis adjacent to onychomycosis, or chronic ulcers and abscesses.

Treatment

Isolates of *Fusarium* are often resistant to amphotericin B and breakthrough infection has been reported during empirical treatment with this agent. Nonetheless, most specialists still regard amphotericin B as the drug of choice for patients with Fusarium infection. It should be given at the maximum tolerated dosage of 1.0–1.5 mg/kg per day. If the disease fails to respond to the conventional formulation, treatment should be changed to one of the lipid-based formulations of the drug at dosages of at least 5 mg/kg per day. Even with high-dose amphotericin B treatment, the prognosis is dismal unless the neutrophil count recovers.

Itraconazole and fluconazole are not active against *Fusarium* species, but limited animal data and some anecdotal clinical reports suggest that the new triazole antifungal agent voriconazole is effective against these moulds. The definitive assessment of this agent awaits more experience.

Bibliography

1. Anaissie, EJ, Kuchar, RT, Rex, JH, *et al*. Fusariosis associated with pathogenic Fusarium species colonization of a hospital water system: a new paradigm for the epidemiology of opportunistic mold infections. Clinical Infectious Diseases 2001:33:1871–78.

2. Bodey, GP, Boktour, M, Mays, S. *et al*. Skin lesions associated with Fusarium infection. Journul of American Academy of Dermatology 2002;47:659–66.

3. Boutati, EI, Anaissie, EJ. Fusarium, a significant emerging pathogen in patients with hematologic malignancy: ten years' experience at a cancer center and implications for management. Blood 1997;90:999–1008.

4. Castiglioni, B, Sutton, DA, Rinaldi, MG, *et al*. *Pseudalles-cheria boydii* (anamorph *Scedosporium apiospermum*) infection in solid organ transplant

recipients in a tertiary medical center and review of the literature. Medicine (Baltimore) 2002;81:333–48.

5. Gutikrrez-Rodero, F, Moragbn, M, Ortiz de la Tabla, V, *et al.* Cutaneous hyalohyphomycosis caused by *Paecilomyces lilacinus* in an immuno-compromised host successfully treated with itraconazole: case report and review. European Journal of Clinical Microbiology and Infectious Diseases 1999;18:814–8.

6. Marr, KA, Carter, RA, Crippa, F, *et al.* Epidemiology and outcome of mold infections in hematopoietic stem cell transplant recipients. Clinical Infectious Diseases 2002;34:909–17.

7. OTHER OPPORTUNISTIC INFECTIONS

Pooja Arora Mrig, Kabir Sardana

SYSTEMIC CANDIDIASIS

Definition

It is a systemic fungal infection caused by *Candida* species.

Etiology

Systemic candidosis is caused by yeasts belonging to the genus Candida. *C. albicans* is the most common species. *C. tropicalis* the causative species in patients with leukemia is most likely to cause cutaneous lesions.

Pathogenesis

The organism usually originates in the patient's own gastrointestinal tract. Factors favoring dissemination are leukemia, neutropenia, patients on long term corticosteroid therapy or broad spectrum antibiotics. Candida may invade the skin along intravenous infusion lines.

Candida evades the host defences due to its ability to exist as pseudohyphae in tissue and blastoconidia in blood.

Clinical Features

Lesions start as macules and papules with a pale center on the trunk or extremities. The lesions become nodular and hemorrhagic. Lesions resembling ecthyma gangrenosum may be seen. Pustules, abscesses and purpuric lesions may be seen. The latter is seen in patients with thrombocytopenia. Unlike cutaneous candidiasis, subcorneal pustules are not seen.

Sites of involvement include liver, spleen, kidney, muscle, retina and heart valves. Septicemia may occur with fever, tachycardia, dyspnea and hypotension.

Investigations

i. *Histopathology*

Budding yeast cells and pseudohyphae can be seen in the dermis (and not stratum corneum as is seen in mucocutaneous candidiasis)

ii. *Blood Culture*

Treatment

- Intraveous amphotericin B
- Azole drugs
- Caspofungin

INFECTIONS CAUSED BY TALAROMYCES MARNEFFEI
(Penicilliosis, Talaromycosis)

Talaromyces marneffei is a dimorphic fungus that causes systemic fungal infection in both immunocompetent and immunocompromised patients especially in AIDS.

Epidemiology

T. marneffei is endemic in South-East Asia and China. It has also been reported in the US. The reservoir is thought to be in Bamboo rats which are underground dwelling rodents. The disease affects adults of both sexes and is rare in children.

Pathogenesis

The fungi is found in the soil and causes disseminated infection in immunocompromised patients.

Clinical Features

Patients generally present with fever, cough and chest infection. *P. marneffei* infects the liver, spleen and lymph nodes. Signs of dissemination like anemia and hepatospelinomegaly are present. Skin is involved in 50% of cases in the form of umbilicated paules (resembling molluscum contagiosum), necrotic nodules, acne form lesions and ulcers. The most common sites of involvement are the face (especially the forehead), arms and trunk. Ulcers may be seen over mucosal surfaces.

Differential Diagnosis

Other disseminated fungal infections like histoplasmosis and crytococcosis.

Investigations

i. Histopathology of tissue sections, smears and blood films show the characteristic cells that appear as small, oval structures that are divided by a septum, seen inside macrophages and giant cells. Leishmanin stain can be used to identify the cells. *T. marneffei* appears similar to histoplasmosis.

ii. Culture: *T. marneffei* is a dimorphic fungus. It grows rapidly on glucose-peptone agar at 25°C producing green or greyish colonies with a red pigment. At 37°C the organism produces yeast-like colonies.

iii. Serology: Western blot can be used but is available in a few centers only.

Management

- Amphotericin B is required in severe cases
- Itraconazole 200–400 mg/day shows good response and is given until clinical remission.

Bibliography

1. Blot SI, Vandewoude KH, Hoste EA, Colardyn FA. Effects of nosocomila candidemia on outcomes of critiically ill patients. American Journal of Medicine 2002; 113: 480–5.

2. Blumberg HM, Jarvis WR, Soucie JM, *et al*. Risk factors for candidal bloodstream infections in surgical intensive care unit patients: the NEMIS prospective multicenter study. Clinical Infectious Diseases 2001; 33: 177–86.

3. Calderone RA (ed). Candida and candidiasis. Washington, DC: ASM Press, 2002.

4. Drouhet E. Penicilliosis due to Penicillium marneffei: a new emerging systemic mycosis in AIDS patients travelling or living in Southeast Asia. Journal of Medical Mycology 1993; 3: 195–224.

5. Nittayananta W. Penicilliosis marneffei: another AIDS defining illness in Southeast Asia. Oral Disease 1999; 5: 286–93.

6. Ungpakorn R. Cutaneous manifestations of Penicillium marneffei infection. Current Opinion in Infectious Diseases 2000; 13: 129–34.

8. APPROACH TO DIAGNOSIS AND TREATMENT OF SYSTEMIC FUNGAL INFECTIONS

Pooja Arora Mrig, Kabir Sardana

Though most dermatologists may not encounter systemic fungal infections, fever in a neutropenic patient should warrant an investigation of fungal infections.

Though the intricacies may be beyond the purview of this book, an overview is provided as follows.

Box 7.1: Definitions of fungal infections

Endemic fungal infections (histoplasmosis, blastomycosis, coccidioidomycosis, and paracoccidioidomycosis)

Either systemic or only confined to lungs, must be proven by culture from the site affected, in a host with symptoms attributed to the fungal infection. If cultures are negative or unattainable, histopathological demonstration of the appropriate morphological forms must be combined with serological support.

Box 7.2: Criteria for probable and possible invasive fungal infections

Host factors

1. **Neutropenia:** Neutrophils <500/mm^3 for more than 10 days
2. Persistent **fever** for >96 h refractory to appropriate broad spectrum antibacterial treatment
3. Body temperature either >38 C or <36 C and any of the following predisposing conditions:
   a. Prolonged neutropenia (>10 days) in the previous 60 days
   b. Recent or current use of significant immunosuppressive agents in the previous 30 days
   c. Invasive fungal infection in a previous episode
   d. Coexistence of AIDS
4. Signs and symptoms indicating GVHD
5. Prolonged use of corticosteroids (>3 weeks)

Microbiological criteria

1. Positive culture of a mold (including *Aspergillus* species, *Fusarium* species, zygomycetes, *Scedosporium* species) or *C. neoformans* from sputum, BAL
2. Positive culture or cytology/direct microscopy for molds from sinus aspirate
3. Positive cytology/direct microscopy for a mold or *Cryptococcus* from sputum, BAL

(Contd.)

Box 7.2: Criteria for probable and possible invasive fungal infections (*Contd.*)

4. Positive *Aspergillus* antigen in BAL, CSF or ≥ 2 blood samples
5. Positive cryptococcal antigen in blood
6. Positive cytology/direct microscopy for fungal elements other than *Cryptococcus* in sterile body fluids
7. Two positive urine cultures of yeasts in the absence of urinary catheter
8. *Candida* casts in urine in the absence of urinary catheter
9. Positive blood culture of *Candida* species
10. Pulmonary abnormality and negative bacterial cultures of any possible bacteria from any specimen related to lower respiratory tract infection, including blood, sputum, BAL, etc.

1. Essential **clinical examination** in neutropenic and solid organ transplant patients with suspected invasive fungal infection (Box 7.3).

Box 7.3*

Organ/system	Features	Likely infection
Skin	Scattered lesions, often on limbs; maculopapular, progressing to pustular lesions with central necrosis	Acute disseminated candidosis, disseminated aspergillosis, or Fusarium infection
Sinus	Upper respiratory tract symptoms with necrotic or ulcerated areas	Invasive aspergillosis or mucormycosis
Palate	Ulceration, including the hard palate	Rhinocerebral mucormycosis
Chest	Signs are few and non-specific: all should be investigated	Invasive pulmonary aspergillosis, PCP, or other fungal pneumonia
Eyes	Funduscopy may reveal 'cottonwool ball' lesions of *Candida* choroidoretinitis— rare in neutropenic patients	Acute disseminated candidosis
Central nervous system	Headache, altered mental state, seizure, focal neurologic signs, and neck stiffness	Cryptococcal or candidal meningitis

*Denning DW, *et al*. Guidelines for the investigation of invasive fungal infections in haematological malignancy and solid organ transplantation. European Journal of Clinical Microbiology and Infectious Diseases 1997; 16: 424–36.

2. Essential *investigations* for the laboratory diagnosis of systemic fungal infections (Box 7.4).

Box 7.4

Aspergillosis
- Microscopy of sputum, BAL fluid (enhanced by calcofluor white), and stained biopsy material
- Culture of respiratory secretions and biopsy material
- Twice weekly EIA for galactomannan (platelia *Aspergillus*, Bio-Rad, FDA approval 2003) in 'high risk' and 'intermediate risk' patients (variable results between laboratories)
- Detection of β-1,3-D-glucan (glucatel, associates of Cape Cod Inc)
- PCR screening twice weekly on whole blood in high/intermediate risk hematology patients (if available locally)

Blastomycosis
- Microscopy of pus, sputum, bronchial washings, and urine
- Culture of pus, sputum, bronchial washings, and urine
- Detection of antibody by immunodiffusion

Candidiasis
- Microscopy of body fluids (enhanced by calcofluor white) and stained biopsy material
- Culture of blood and other body fluids
- Culture of respiratory secretions
- Culture of biopsy material
- Detection of precipitins by CIE
- ELISA for *Candida* mannan (Bio-Rad) (variable results between laboratories)
- ELISA for *Candida* anti-mannan (limited value in immunocompromised patients)
- Detection of β-1,3-D-glucan (glucatel)
- PCR on whole blood (if available locally)

Coccidioidomycosis
- Microscopy of sputum, joint fluid, pus, and CSF sediment
- Culture of sputum, joint fluid, CSF sediment, and pus
- Coccidioidin or spherulin skin test
- Detection of IgM in serum by latex agglutination, tube precipitin test, or immunodiffusion test
- Detection of IgG in serum by classical complement fixation test or immunodiffusion
- Detection of antibody in CSF if meningitis is suspected

(Contd.)

Box 7.4 (*Contd.*)

Cryptococcosis
· Microscopy of CSF or other body fluids and secretions
· Culture of CSF, blood, sputum, urine, and prostatic fluid
· Detection of antigen in CSF, urine, and blood by latex agglutination (e.g. Immuno-mycologics Inc; Meridian Diagnostics Inc; Bio-Rad) and ELISA (Meridian Diagnostics Inc)

Histoplasmosis
· Microscopy of stained smears of peripheral blood, sputum, bronchial washings, and pus
· Culture of blood, sputum, bone marrow, pus, and tissue
· Detection of antibody by immunodiffusion and complement fixation
· Detection of antigen by radioimmunoassay in blood, urine, CSF, and BAL

Mucormycosis
· Microscopy of material from necrotic lesions, sputum, and BAL
· Culture of nasal and palatal scrapings, biopsy material, and sputum
· PCR on whole blood (if available locally)

Paracoccidioidomycosis
· Microscopy of pus, sputum, and crusts from granulomatous lesions
· Culture of pus, sputum, and crusts from granulomatous lesions
· Detection of antibody by complement fixation

Penicillium marneffei infection
· Microscopy of Wright-stained bone marrow smears, touch smears of skin, or lymph node biopsies
· Culture of skin biopsies, lymph node biopsies, blood, pus, bone marrow
· Aspirates, sputum, and BAL
· Detection of antibody by ELISA (under development)

Sporotrichosis
· Microscopy of stained pus and tissue
· Culture of pus and tissue

Unusual fungal infections
Hyalohyphomycosis
· *Fusarium*
  – Culture of blood and biopsies of cutaneous lesions
· *Scedosporium*
  – Culture of respiratory secretions and CSF

Phaeohyphomycosis
· Paranasal infection (*alternaria, bipolaris, curvularia, exserohilum*)
  – Microscopy of sinus mucus, pus, scrapings, and stained tissue sections
  – Culture of sinus mucus, pus, and scrapings

(*Contd.*)

Box 7.4 (*Contd.*)

· Cerebral phaeohyphomycosis (*Cladophialophora* [*Xylohypha*] *bantiana*)
  – Culture of sinus material and respiratory secretions

Yeast Infections

· Trichosporonosis
  – Microscopy of smears and histopathologic sections of cutaneous lesions
  – Culture of blood and biopsies of cutaneous lesions
· Systemic Malassezia (Pityrosporum) infection
  – Microscopy of stained blood smears
  – Culture of blood, with subculture onto lipid-rich media
  – Culture of catheter tip in lipid-containing broth

3. Therapy of specific infections
   a. Aspergillosis (Box 7.5)

	Box 7.5
Disease type	*Therapies*
Allergic (ABPA)	Designed for acute asthmatic exacerbations and for avoiding end-stage fibrosis
	Mild disease may not require treatment
	Indications for steroids: Increasing serum concentrations, new or worsening infiltrates on chest radiographs
	Prednisolone 1.0 mg/kg per day until radiographs are clear, then 0.5 mg/kg per day for 2 weeks followed by alternate day dosing for 3–6 months
	Bronchodilators and postural drainage may help to reduce mucus plugging
	Itraconazole 200 mg/day 16 weeks
Aspergilloma	Surgical resection with perioperative amphotericin B
	Intracavitary instillation of amphotericin B 10–20 mg in 10–20 ml distilled water
Chronic necrotizing	Surgical resection
	Itraconazole 200–400 mg per day
	Parenteral and local amphotericin B
Sinonasal	
· Allergic sinusitis	Surgical debridement to remove polyps and allergic mucous
	Conservative surgical drainage plus antibiotics
	Amphotericin B solution
	Itraconazole oral solution (single cases)
	Frequent recurrence

(*Contd.*)

Box 7.5 (*Contd.*)

Disease type	*Therapies*
· Chronic indolent invasive in immunocompetent	Surgical debridement and drainage combined with amphotericin B 1.0 mg/kg/day. Long-term suppressive treatment with itraconazole may prevent recurrence In chronic granulomatous sinusitis surgical removal of paranasal granuloma

b. Blastomycosis (Box 7.6)

Box 7.6

Type of disease	*Treatment*
Pulmonary: Mild/moderate disease	Itraconazole, oral, 200 mg per day up to 6 months, or up to 3 months if lesions resolve; if no improvement, increase to 400 mg per day
	Oral ketoconazole 400 mg per day, increasing to 600–800 mg/kg as required
	Fluconazole 400–800 mg/kg if itraconazole not absorbed
Pulmonary: Life threatening	Amphotericin B 0.7–1.0 mg/kg/d. If good response itraconazole 200–400 mg/d. Little experience with lipid formulations of amphotericin B
Disseminated: Mild/moderate disease	If no CNS involvement: – Itraconazole 200–400 mg/d for at least 6 months – Fluconazole 400–800 mg/d if itraconazole not tolerated CNS involvement: Amphotericin B 0.7–1.0 mg/kg/d to a total dose of 2 g
Disseminated: Life threatening	Amphotericin B 0.7–1.0 mg/kg per day to a total dose of 1.5–2.5 g
Disseminated: Osteomyelitis	Amphotericin B 0.5–0.7 mg/kg per day Itraconazole 12 months

c. Candidosis (Box 7.7)

Box 7.7

Type of disease	*Treatment*
Mucosal	Reversal of known risk factors Antifungals · Topical · Nystatin suspension 4–6 ml 4 times daily, 7–14 days

(Contd.)

Box 7.7 (*Contd.*)

Type of disease	Treatment
	• Nystatin pastilles 4–5 times daily, 7–14 days • Clotrimazole troches, one 10 mg troche 5 times daily • Itraconazole oral solution 200 mg per day, 7–14 days • Amphotericin B oral suspension 1 ml 4 times daily, 100 mg/ml suspension in azole-refractory disease • Systemic: Fluconazole, itraconazole
Oropharyngeal	Improvement of host defenses Topical antifungals • Nystatin suspension • Clotrimazole troche • Fluconazole 100–200 mg, two divided doses, or 3 mg/kg, two divided doses in children • Itraconazole oral solution 200 mg/day, preferably in two intakes for 1 week. If no response, continue for further week • Amphotericin B 0.5 mg/kg, 3–7 days Antifungal susceptibility testing not generally indicated but useful in refractory infections
Esophageal	Fluconazole 200 mg per day orally, 14–21 days Itraconazole oral solution 200 mg per day Fluconazole-refractory disease: Itraconazole oral solution ≥ 200 mg/day, or amphotericin B iv 0.3–0.7 mg/kg per day Caspofungin 50 mg/d 7–21 days Antifungal susceptibility testing not generally indicated but useful in refractory infection

Candidemia
• Non-neutropenic
	Removal of all existing central venous catheters
	Fluconazole 800 mg loading dose, followed by 400 mg per day for 2 weeks
	Amphotericin B 0.5 mg/kg per day, 2 weeks
	Amphotericin B 0.75–1 mg/kg per day–less sensitive yeasts
	    Abelcet® 5 mg/kg per day
	    AmBisome® 1–3 mg/kg per day or higher
	    Amphotec® 2–6 mg/kg per day
	Caspofungin 70 mg loading dose, followed by 50 mg/day. Infuse over 1 h

(Contd.)

Box 7.7 (*Contd.*)

Type of disease	Treatment
· Persistent neutropenia	Catheter removal Amphotericin B 1 mg/kg per day plus flucytosine AmBisome® 1.3 mg/kg per day or higher neonates amphotericin B
· *Candida glabrata* infection	Amphotericin B ≥ 0.7 mg/kg per day
· *Candida krusei* infection	Amphotericin B 1.0 mg/kg per day
· *Candida lusitaniae* infection	Fluconazole 400 mg per day

d. Cryptococcosis (Box 7.8)

Box 7.8

Meningitis in normal hosts
· Amphotericin B 0.7–1.0 mg/kg, plus flucytosine 37.5 mg/kg every 6 h for 4 weeks, or for 6.10 weeks in patients with risk factors that correlate with a high frequency of relapse
· Amphotericin B 0.7–1.0 mg/kg per day, plus flucytosine 100 mg/kg per day for 2 weeks, followed by fluconazole 400 mg per day for a minimum of 10 weeks, then fluconazole maintenance for 6–12 months
· Lipid formulations of amphotericin B

Meningitis in AIDS
· Amphotericin B 0.7–1.0 mg/kg per day plus flucytosine 100 mg/kg per day for 2–3 weeks, followed by fluconazole 400 mg per day for a minimum of 10 weeks, then fluconazole 200 mg per day for life
· Liposomal amphotericin B (AmBisomeR) 4 mg/kg per day or itraconazole 200–400 mg/kg per day
· Maintenance therapy with fluconazole 200 mg per day for life
· Combination of fluconazole 400–800 mg/day plus flucytosine 100 mg/kg per day but high incidence of side effects
· If CD4 T-lymphocyte count increases above 100–200 cells per l following highly active antiretroviral therapy (HAART), maintenance treatment can be discontinued

Pulmonary-normal hosts
· Usually none, observation only
· Asymptomatic: If treatment considered fluconazole 200–400 mg per day for 3–6 months
· Symptomatic infection:
  – Fluconazole 200–400 mg per day for 3–6 months
  – Itraconazole 200–400 mg per day for 6–12 months
  – Amphotericin B 0.4–0.7 mg/kg per day up to a total dose of 1000–2000 mg

(*Contd.*)

Box 7.8 (*Contd.*)

Maintenance
- Fluconazole 200–400 mg po 4 times daily, lifelong
- Itraconazole 200 mg po 2 times daily, lifelong
- Amphotericin B 1 mg/kg iv 1–3 times per week, lifelong

e. Histoplasmosis (Box 7.9)

Box 7.9

Type of disease	*Treatment*
Acute pulmonary	Spontaneous improvement in most cases, observe; where required, amphotericin B 0.5–0.7 mg/kg per day with steroids, or oral itraconazole 200 mg per day for 6–12 weeks If hypoxic, amphotericin B 0.7 mg/kg/d, or lipid formulation 3 mg/kg/d followed by itraconazole 200–400 mg/d for 12 weeks
Chronic pulmonary	Oral itraconazole 400 mg per day for 12–24 months Amphotericin B 0.7 mg/kg per day for 10 weeks or AmBisome® 3 mg/kg per day in renal impairment 12 months follow-up after discontinuation of treatment
Disseminated	
• Non-immunosuppressed	Oral itraconazole 200–400 mg per day for 6–18 months, but fluconazole 400 mg/d if itraconazole not tolerated Amphotericin B 0.7–1.0 mg/kg per day for 10 weeks in severe disease, infants 1.0 mg/kg for minimum of 6 weeks
• AIDS	For severe disease: Amphotericin B 0.7–1.0 mg/kg per day induction treatment, followed by itraconazole 400 mg/d to complete 12 weeks total induction period. In itraconazole intolerance, fluconazole 800 mg/d. Relapse common once drug discontinued For milder disease: Oral itraconazole 600 mg per day for 3 days, then 200 mg twice daily

(*Contd.*)

Box 7.9 (*Contd.*)

Type of disease	Treatment
	For maintenance: Amphotericin B 50 mg weekly or twice weekly highly effective but inconvenient; itraconazole 200–400 mg per day, or fluconazole 100–400 mg per day if itraconazole not absorbed, for life
Focal infections	**CNS:** Amphotericin B 0.7–1.0 mg/kg/d, total dose 35 mg/kg over 3–4 months, followed by fluconazole 800 mg/d for another 9–12 months. In amphotericin B failure or intolerance, liposomal amphotericin B 3–5 mg/kg/d for 3–4 months
	Bone/joint/skin: Itraconazole 200 mg 4 times daily for variable periods
	Mediastinal fibrosis Itraconazole 200 mg 4 times daily for 6 months. Surgical resection if progressive life threatening obstruction. Surgical mortality is 20%

f. Mucormycosis (Box 7.10)

Box 7.10

Type of disease	Treatment
Rhinocerebral	Control of diabetic acidosis
	Aggressive surgical debridement of all necrotic tissue
	Amphotericin B 1.0–1.5 mg/kg per day, total dose 30–40 mg/kg, if contraindicated
	AmBisome® 5 mg/kg per day or higher
	Optimal duration and total dose of amphotericin B not determined
Pulmonary	Reversal of predisposing conditions
	Restitution of neutrophils–spontaneously or with colony-stimulating factors–and reduction of glucocorticosteroid dose
	Amphotericin B: Rapid escalation to 1.0–1.5 mg/kg per day
	Following stabilization, resection of necrotic lung tissue

g. Sporotrichosis (Box 7.11)

Box 7.11

Type of disease	Preferred therapy
Pulmonary	Difficult to treat, relapse common
	Clinical outcome improved by lobectomy and concomitant amphotericin B 1 mg/kg per day, substituted by itraconazole 400 mg per day upon improvement
	For less severe disease, itraconazole 400 mg per day from outset
CNS	Refractory to antifungal therapy
Osteoarticular	Itraconazole 400 mg per day for 12 months or longer: Shorter courses lead to relapse
	Fluconazole 400–800 mg per day is less effective; use where there is itraconazole intolerance
Disseminated	Amphotericin B 1 mg/kg per day, continue until total dose of 1–2 g administered
	For less acute disease, itraconazole 400 mg per day
	For AIDS patients, lifelong itraconazole to prevent relapse

h. Miscellaneous infections (Box 7.12)

Box 7.12

Disease	Therapy
Fusariosis	Correct neutropenia
(*Fusarium* species)	Amphotericin B 1.0–1.5 mg/kg per day, or liposomal amphotericin B 5 mg/kg per day
	Flucytosine 25 mg/kg every 6 h for non-responders (reversal of neutropenia necessary for recovery)
Pseudallescheriosis	Surgical removal if possible
(*Pseudallescheria boydii*,	Miconazole 600 mg every 6 h iv usually best
Scedosporium	initial treatment for seriously ill patients
apiospermum)	(amphotericin B not effective)
	Itraconazole 400 mg per day for other patients
Phaeohyphomycosis	Skin and subcutaneous tissue disease
	Occasional dissemination: surgical excision
	Itraconazole (oral solution) 400 mg per day
Trichosporonosis	Correct neutropenia
(*Trichosporon* species)	Amphotericin B 1.0–1.5 mg/kg per day
Paecilomyces lilacinus	Itraconazole 200 mg per day 3 months
Malassezia	Remove intravascular catheter
(*Pityrosporum*) septicemia	Fluconazole 1 g iv per day if fungemia exists

Bibliography

1. Ascioglu S, Rex JH, dePauw B, *et al*. Defining opportunistic invasive fungal infections inimmunocompromised patients with cancer and hematopoietic stem cell transplants: an international consensus. Clinical Infectious Diseases 2002; 34: 7–14.

2. Caillot D, Casasnovas O, Bernard A, *et al*. Improved management of invasive pulmonaryaspergillosis in neutropenic patients using early thoracic, computed tomographic scan and surgery. Journal of Clinical Oncology 1997; 15: 139–147.

3. Calderone RA (ed). Candida and candidiasis.Washington, DC: ASM Press, 2002. Perfect JR, Casadevall A. Cryptococcosis. Infectious Diseases Clinics of North America 2002; 16:837–874.

4. Centers for Disease Control and Prevention. Guidelines for prevention of nosocomial pneumonia. Morbidity and Mortality Weekly Report 1997; 46 (RR-01): 1–79.

5. Chapman SW, Bradsher RW, Campbell GD. Practice guidelines for the management of patients with blastomycosis. Clinical Infectious Diseases 2000; 30: 679–683.

6. Clancy CJ, Wingard JR, Hong Nguyen M. Subcutaneous phaeohyphomycosis in transplant recipients: review of the literature and demonstration of in vitro synergy between antifungal agents. Medical Mycology 2000; 38: 169–175.

7. Denning DW, *et al*. Guidelines for the investigation of invasive fungal infections in hematological malignancy and solid organ transplantation. European Journal of Clinical Microbiology and Infectious Diseases 1997;16: 424–436.

8. Erer B, Galimberti M, Lucarelli G, *et al*. Trichosporon beigelii: a life-threatening pathogen in immunocompromised hosts. Bone Marrow Transplantation 2000; 25: 745–749.

9. Eucker J, Sezer O, Graf B, Possinger K. Mucormycoses. Mycoses 2001; 44: 253–260.

10. Ferguson BJ. Mucormycosis of the nose and paranasal sinuses. Otolaryngologic Clinics of North America 2000; 33:349–365.

11. Fleming RV, Walsh TJ, Anaissie EJ.Emerging and less common fungal pathogens. Infectious Disease Clinics of North America 2002; 16:915–933.

12. Garcia-Diaz JB, Baumgarten K. Phaeohyphomycotic infections in solid organ transplant patients. Seminars in Respiratory Infections 2002; 17: 303–309.

13. Kauffman CA, Hajjeh R, Chapman SW. Practice guidelines for the management of patients with sporotrichosis. Clinical Infectious Diseases 2000; 30: 684–687.

14. Kauffman CA. Management of histoplasmosis. Expert Opinion in Pharmacotherapy 2002; 3: 1067–1072.

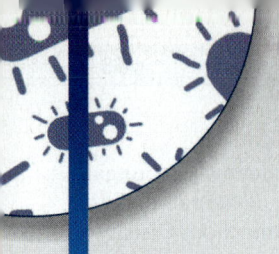

CHAPTER 8

Antifungal Drugs

1. INTRODUCTION

Kabir Sardana

The introduction of early precursors of the modern approach to the development of antibiotics through the work of the new chemical and dyeing industries in the late nineteenth century provided a number of different chemicals, some of which had an antifungal effect. These included *brilliant green, gentian violet,* and *magenta paint,* the last of which, when combined with resorcinol, was known as Castellani's paint after its inventor Aldo Castellani. Gentian violet, is less effective in *Dermatophyte* infections, but has a therapeutic effect in *Candida* infections.

A further advance was the combination of *salicylic acid* with *benzoic acid,* with the action being a combination of descaling fungal infected skin and inhibiting the growth of the organisms. It was used in an ointment called **Whitfield's ointment** and is composed of 3% salicylic acid and 6% benzoic acid.

After 1945, developments in treatment (Box 8.1) focused on antifungals with specific antifungal activity and multiple mechanisms of action as depicted in Fig. 8.1. The first of these, mainly used for superficial infections, were derivatives of undecylenic acid such as zinc undecenoate which inhibits the growth of *Dermatophytes* or thiocarbamates, tolnaftate, and tolciclate which were the first inhibitors of squalene epoxidase which plays a key role in the biosynthesis of ergosterol in the fungal cell membrane. Another early specific antifungal was haloprogin, an acetylenic compound, which was thought to inhibit oxygen uptake; haloprogin had a broader spectrum of activity, affecting yeasts as well as *Dermatophyte* fungi.

In 1950, a new family of antifungal agents, the **polyenes**, also derived from microorganisms (*Streptomyces* species, such as *S. nodosus*),

Box 8.1: History of antifungal therapy

- The first antifungal, amphotericin B deoxycholate, was introduced in 1958. It offers potent, broad spectrum antifungal activity but is associated with significant renal toxicity and infusion reactions.
- Flucytosine, a pyrimidine analogue introduced in 1973, is active against *Candida* and *Cryptococcus*. Its use is limited by emergence of drug resistance and toxicity.
- Thr first-generation azole drugs, including fluconazole and itraconazole, became available in the 1990s. These agents offer the advantage of oral administration and have good activity against yeast pathogens. Due to CYP450 interactions, there are many drug-drug interactions.
- Lipid-based amphotericin B formulations were introduced in the 1990s and maintain the potent, broad spectrum activity of the deoxycholate formulation with less toxicity.
- The echinocandin drugs became available in the 2000s and offer excellent activity against *Candida* with a few drug-drug interactions; however, they are available in parenteral form only.
- The second-generation of azole drugs, including voriconazole, posaconazole and isavuconazole were brought to market beginning in the 2000s. The major advantage of these agents is the extended spectrum of activity against filamentous fungi and oral formulations.

evolved. These include the topically active compounds nystatin and natamycin as well as amphotericin B which when stabilized with bile salts, provided an intravenous means of treatment. Other polyene drugs, such as hamycin, were not developed further for human use. Nystatin is still used in the treatment of superficial mycoses, and *amphotericin B*, although usually nowadays given in a lipid-associated form, remains a first-line drug in the management of systemic mycoses. A topical preparation is licensed in India for candidiasis but is effective against dermatophytes and nondermatophyte infection also.

In 1958 *griseofulvin*, a compound synthesized from the mold fungus *Penicillium griseofulvum*, was found to be active orally in the treatment of dermatophytosis in humans, and its rapid development led to the rapid elimination of tinea capitis in much of Europe and the United States. It was only active orally although many attempts have been made to produce a topically active version; yet none have been commercially viable. The drug works through inhibition of the formation of microtubules in the fungal cell.

The early 1970s saw the introduction of the first **azole antifungals** whose mode of action was the inhibition of 14α demethylase. The first products miconazole and econazole have been followed by other imidazoles and then by a subbranch of this group called triazoles. Ketoconazole was the first of these compounds to be found to have activity after oral absorption. This was followed by fluconazole and

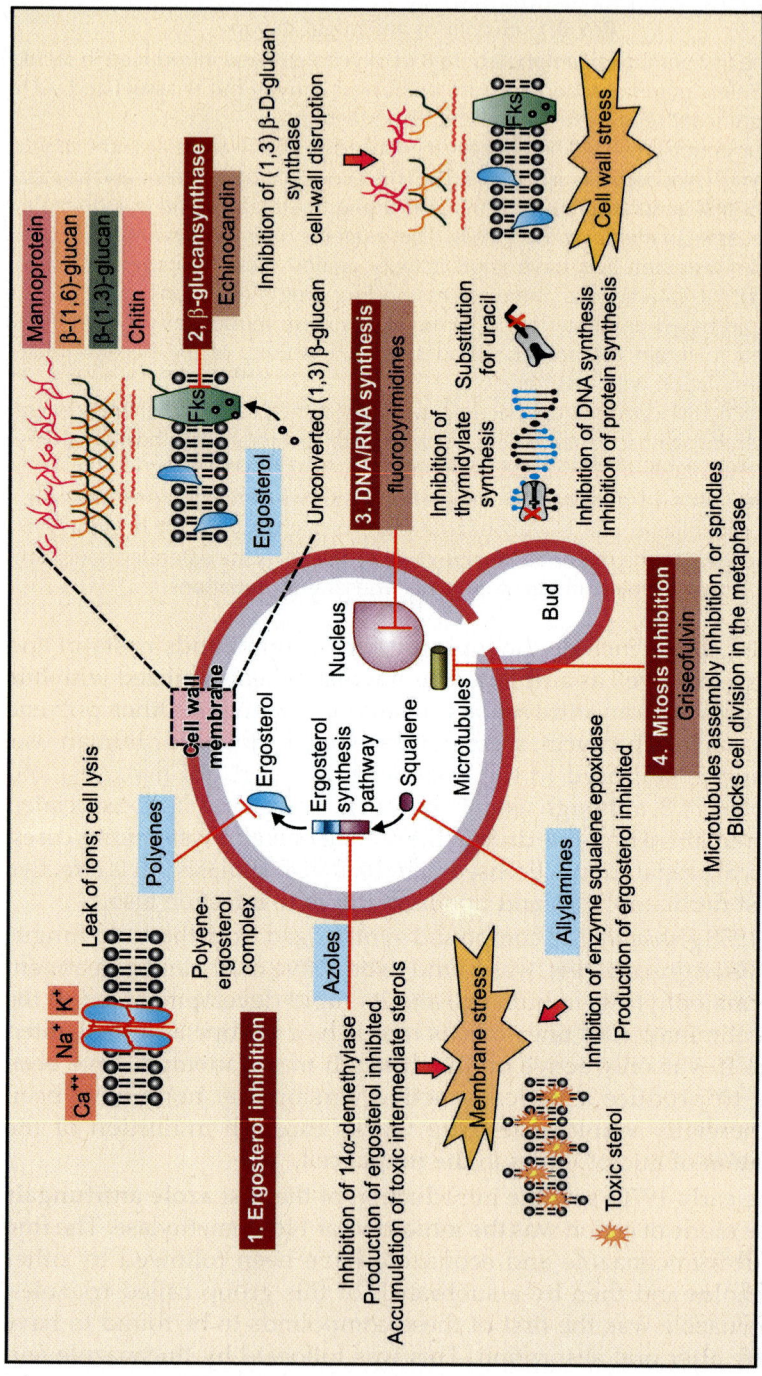

Fig. 8.1: Target of action of common antifungal drugs

(*From* Clinical Approach to Fungal Infections)

then by newer triazoles such as itraconazole, posaconazole, and voriconazole, all of which are absorbed after oral administration. The triazole antifungals have also expanded (albaconazole, isavuconazole, ravuconazole, terconazole, and pramiconazole) although at the time of writing no new drugs have been licensed. A further topical thiazole agent, abafungin has also been assessed in clinical trials, mainly against dermatophytes, but has not yet been licensed. The reformulation of azoles such as **itraconazole** to overcome variations in absorption, e.g. **Lozanoc** has also been attempted.

Another family of antifungal agents, the **allylamines**, was developed which had both topical (terbinafine, butenafine, and naftifine), and terbinafine oral activities. These are all potent inhibitors of squalene epoxidase. Ciclopirox olamine, a hydroxypyridone antifungal which disrupts the cell membrane structure, and the morpholine derivatives amorolfine which inhibits two stages of the formation of ergosterol, D14 reductase and D7-D8 isomerase activity, were later additions.

Other recent developments have been the introduction of the **echinocandins** such as caspofungin, anidulafungin, and micafungin, all available as intravenous compounds used in the treatment of Candida and other systemic infections. They act by inhibition of the formation of the fungal cell wall through interaction with 1, 3 β-glucan synthase.

FUTURE OF ANTIFUNGAL THERAPY

Antifungal therapy has become progressively more effective since second-generation azoles, echinocandins, and lipid formulations of amphotericin B were introduced. But since 2006, no new classes of antifungals have been approved.

Voriconazole is now the agent of choice for invasive aspergillosis, allowing patients to survive leukemia and transplantation who would otherwise have died. Nevertheless, even now about ~30 to 50% of invasive aspergillosis patients still die, for reasons that include late diagnosis, infection of sites such as the brain that are not effectively treated with drugs, and drug resistance. The mortality from candidemia, a fungal infection mainly treated with echinocandins and fluconazole, also remains high at ~50%.

Drug Resistance in Fungi

Many fungi are *intrinsically resistant* to certain anti-fungals; notably, *Candida krusei* (to fluconazole), *Aspergillus terreus* (to amphotericin B), *Cryptococcus* spp. (to the echinocandins), and *Scedosporium* spp. (to all current antifungals). While about 20 years ago, azole-sensitive

Candida albicans was common this is not the case now. *C. glabrata* is particularly problematic: It is the second-most-commonly isolated *Candida* species in the European Union (EU) (>10%) and United States (>20%) and has high rates of resistance to fluconazole and voriconazole, as well as (more recently) to echinocandins. Azole- and echinocandin-resistant *C. glabrata* can only be treated with intravenous amphotericin B.

Intrinsically resistant mold infections are also being observed, including, zygomycetes and *Fusarium* spp. Zygomycetes only respond to posaconazole and amphotericin B, and there are no drugs for Scedosporium.

The emergence of azole resistance is a growing problem, particularly in the Netherlands, where azole-resistant *Aspergillus fumigatus* is now commonplace. Unlike bacteria, fungi are not known to transfer resistance genes between them, nor is patient-to-patient transmission common. The rural and other commercial uses of azole fungicides are the likely, but not yet proven, culprit for the emergence of these resistant strains (E. Snelders et al., 2012). Restriction of azole fungicide use has been proposed but is challenging for multiple reasons, notably, the lack of alternative fungicides for many key crops.

In India there is widespread use of weedicides and fungicides for crops, specially wheat, and it can be theorized that this may be the possible cause of rising resistance in India.

Newer Drug Discovery

A long list of drugs (Fig. 8.2) have been added to antifungal basket, but there have been a number of failures in antifungal development, notably the antibody against HSP90 (heat shock protein 90), Mycograb and the histone deacetylase inhibitor MGCD290, both of which were insufficiently active in patients. Searches of current literature, conference reports, and drug company pipeline reports suggest that only four compounds are in active clinical development for the treatment of systemic disease, with a further two agents (entered clinical development in 2015).

A few other compounds are in preclinical development, many with modes of action that differ from the currently marketed agents (Fig. 8.2). Difficulties in identifying new broad-spectrum compounds and a chronic lack of investment in novel antifungal agents are both responsible for the limited drug development pipeline. Most major pharmaceutical companies are not investing in antifungals, preferring to focus on other apparently more lucrative areas. This is true in India where the so called research is in combining various antifungals in esoteric and illogical combinations and copying molecules which top in the ORG rating.

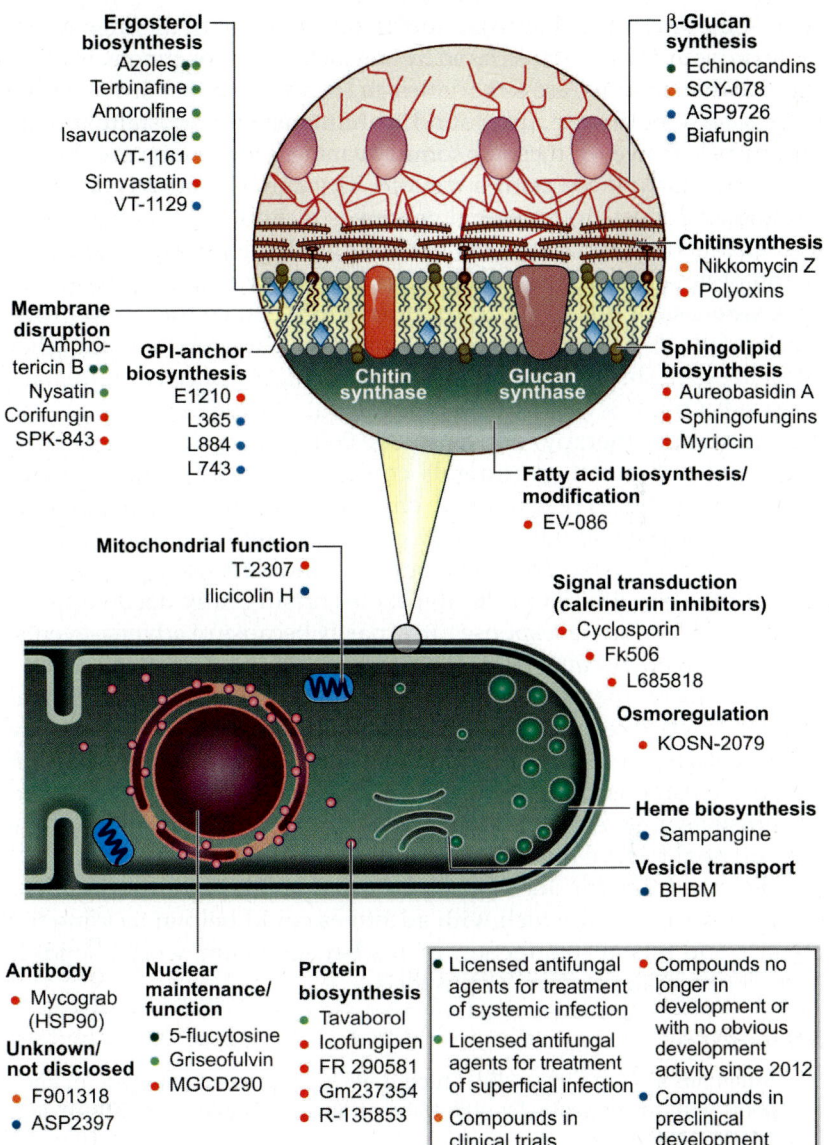

Ergosterol biosynthesis
- Azoles ••
- Terbinafine •
- Amorolfine •
- Isavuconazole •
- VT-1161 •
- Simvastatin •
- VT-1129 •

β-Glucan synthesis
- Echinocandins
- SCY-078
- ASP9726
- Biafungin

Chitinsynthesis
- Nikkomycin Z
- Polyoxins

Membrane disruption
- Amphotericin B ••
- Nysatin •
- Corifungin •
- SPK-843 •

GPI-anchor biosynthesis
- E1210 •
- L365 •
- L884 •
- L743 •

Chitin synthase

Glucan synthase

Sphingolipid biosynthesis
- Aureobasidin A
- Sphingofungins
- Myriocin

Fatty acid biosynthesis/ modification
- EV-086

Mitochondrial function
- T-2307 •
- Ilicicolin H •

Signal transduction (calcineurin inhibitors)
- Cyclosporin
- Fk506
- L685818

Osmoregulation
- KOSN-2079

Heme biosynthesis
- Sampangine

Vesicle transport
- BHBM

Antibody
- Mycograb (HSP90)

Unknown/ not disclosed
- F901318
- ASP2397

Nuclear maintenance/ function
- 5-flucytosine
- Griseofulvin
- MGCD290

Protein biosynthesis
- Tavaborol
- Icofungipen
- FR 290581
- Gm237354
- R-135853

- Licensed antifungal agents for treatment of systemic infection
- Licensed antifungal agents for treatment of superficial infection
- Compounds in clinical trials
- Compounds no longer in development or with no obvious development activity since 2012
- Compounds in preclinical development

Fig. 8.2: An overview of approved and in-trial antifungal drugs. The pipeline of antifungal development is sparse, but it is promising that two compounds currently in clinical development are active against novel targets (nikkomycin Z, which targets chitin synthesis, and F901318, the novel target of which remains undisclosed) and that a number of preclinical agents target functions other than cellular integrity

In some ways, the challenges to the development of antifungals are more pronounced than those faced by antibacterial development. Because fungi, like mammals, are eukaryotes, many proteins that are potential targets for therapy are also found in humans,with substantial drug toxicity risk. However, there are some advantages to working in eukaryotes, particularly those with a diploid lifestage. Chemically induced haploinsufficiency, a functional genomics technology, has been used in *C. albicans* and *Saccharomyces cerevisiae* to identify the mechanism of action of novel antifungal agents, yielding many new drug targets.

Awareness of the spectrum of fungal diseases continues to grow. For example, *Aspergillus* may have an important and treatable amplifier effect in cystic fibrosis (CF), asthma, and chronic obstructive pulmonary disease (COPD). Severe asthma with fungal sensitization responds to oral antifungal therapy, and with 350,000 asthma deaths annually, approved and novel antifungals could play an important part in reducing deaths. Treatment of chronic pulmonary aspergillosis (including aspergilloma) probably reduces death rates, and certainly reduces morbidity. No drug development candidates exist yet for these indications, but alternatives to the azoles are urgently needed-partly because of inadequate response rates, partly because of adverse events, and definitively because of resistance.

Cryptococcal meningitis is another important target for antifungal drug research. It responds poorly to fluconazole, with >60% mortality at 10 weeks in sub-Saharan Africa; the combination of amphotericin B and flucytosine is better, but not widely available and difficult to administer safely. A new potent agent for cryptococcal meningitis has the potential to save many lives.

It is hoped that for dermatophytes a proper and effective delivery system is discovered which with additives could help in tackling the menace and this in conjunction with a barrier cream, would be ideal to target recalcitrant dermatophytosis.

Bibliography

1. Brugmans JP, Van Cutsem JM, Thienpont DC. Treatment of long-term tinea pedis with miconazole. Double-blind clinical evaluation. Arch Dermatol. 1970;102:428–32.
2. Castellani A. Carbol fuchsin paints in the treatment of certain cases of epidermophytosis. Amer Med. 1928;34:351–6.
3. E Snelders, *et al*. PLOS ONE 7, e31801, 2012.
4. GD Brown, *et al.*, Sci. Transl. Med. 4, 165rv13, 2012.
5. Gooskens V, Pönnighaus JM, Clayton Y, Mkandawire P, Sterne JA. Treatment of superficial mycoses in the tropics: Whitfield's ointment versus clotrimazole. Int J Dermatol 1994;33:738–42.

6. Hay RJ. Lipid amphotericin B combinations; 'la crème de la crème'? J Infect 1999;39:16–20.

7. Hempel M. Clinical experiences in the local treatment of dermatomycoses with Econazole lotion. Mykosen 1975;18:213–9.

8. JM Valdez, et al. Clin. Infect. Dis. 2011;52, 726.

9. Katragkou A, Tsikopoulou F, Roilides E, Zaoutis TE. Posaconazole: when and how? The clinician's view. Mycoses 2012;55:110–22.

10. Lozanoc 50 mg hard capsules (itraconazole)-UK/H/4345/001/DC; PL 37190/0001.

11. M. Slavin, et al. Clin. Microbiol. Infect. 10.1016/j.cmi.2014.12.021 (2015).

12. Maley AM, Arbiser JL. Gentian violet: a 19th century drug re-emerges in the 21st century. ExpDermatol 2013;22:775–80.

13. Mikulska M, Novelli A, Aversa F, Cesaro S, de Rosa FG, Girmenia C, et al. Voriconazole in clinical practice. J Chemother 2012;24:311–27.

14. Narat JK. Brilliant green: a clinical study of its value as a local antiseptic. Ann Surg. 1931;94:1007–12.

15. Petranyi G, Ryder NS, Stütz A. Allylamine derivatives: new class of synthetic antifungal agents inhibiting fungal squaleneepoxidase. Science. 1984;224:1239–41.

16. Polak A. Mode of action of morpholine derivatives. Ann N Y Acad Sci. 1988;544:221–8.

17. S Perkhofer, et al. Int. J. Antimicrob. Agents: 2010;36:531.

18. Sehgal VN. Ciclopirox: a new topical pyrodoniumantimycotic agent. A double-blind study in superficial dermatomycoses. Br J Dermatol 1976;95:83–8.

19. Stevens DA. Advances in systemic antifungal therapy. Clin Dermatol 2012;30:657–61.

20. T. Vos, et al. Lancet. 2012;380:2163.

2. SYSTEMIC ANTIFUNGAL DRUGS

Pooja Agarwal, Surabhi Sinha, Suchita Gawde, C Srinivas

Systemic antifungal drugs aim to provide a brief overview of the mechanism of action and indications of antifungal drugs. Superficial dermatophytoses usually respond to topical antifungal agents, which rarely have serious side effects. Fungal infections of the hair and nails as well as systemic mycoses generally necessitate treatment with systemic antifungal medications. Furthermore, fungal infections in patients who are immunocompromised or who have extensive skin involvement often require systemic treatment. Systemic antifungal therapy is also occasionally necessary for superficial infections resistant to topical treatments in immunocompetent individuals.

The antifungal drugs can be classified as under:

1. Polyenes—amphotericin B, nystatin, natamycin
2. Heterocyclic benzofuran—griseofulvin
3. Azoles
   a. Imidazoles—clotrimazole, miconazole, ketoconazole
   b. Triazoles—fluconazole, itraconazole, posaconazole, voriconazole, ravuconazole
4. Allylamines—terbinafine, naftifine
5. Echinocandins—caspofungin, micafungin, anidulafungin
6. Antimetabolites—flucytosine
7. Chitin synthesis inhibitor—nikkomycin
8. Protein synthesis inhibitors—sordarins, azasordarins
9. Thiocarbamate—tolnaftate

The mode of action of the antifungal drugs is listed in Table 8.1 and is depicted in Fig. 8.2. The pharmacokinetics of the most commonly used antifungals are listed in Table 8.2.

Here it is important to appreciate that in dermatology, it is the skin pharmacokinetics that is important as dermatophytoses is localized to the stratum corneum and this has been detailed in Table 8.3 which summarises the distribution of commonly used antifungals in skin, hair and nails.

Ketoconazole has largely fallen out of use due to side effects. The commonly used antifungals are discussed one by one and their indications are summarised in Table 8.4. Table 8.5 gives a brief encapsulation of the important drug interactions of common antifungals.

Though in dermatology, systemic and deep fungal infections are uncommon, a summary of the dosimetry for them is given in Table 8.6.

Table 8.1: Summary of common antifungal drugs

Class of drug	Mode of action	Effect
Azoles	Interfere with cell membrane synthesis via inhibition of the fungal 14α-demethylase which is necessary in synthesis of ergosterol, an important component of the fungal cell membrane. These drugs may also impair fungal triglyceride/phospholipid synthesis and inhibit fungal oxidative/peroxidase enzymes (resulting inaccumulation of toxic levels of hydrogen peroxide)	Fungistatic
Allylamines	Interferes with cell membrane synthesis via inhibition of squalene epoxidase, which is required for lanosterol formation	Fungicidal
Griseofulvin	Disrupts mitotic spindle by interacting with microtubules, thereby inhibiting mitosis in dermatophytes	Fungistatic
Polyenes	Bind irreversibly to cell membrane sterols (e.g. ergosterol) and increase membrane permeability	Fungistatic at low concentration, fungicidal at higher concentration
Echinocandins	Interfere with cell wall synthesis/permeability via inhibition of β(1,3)-D-glucan synthesis	Fungistatic

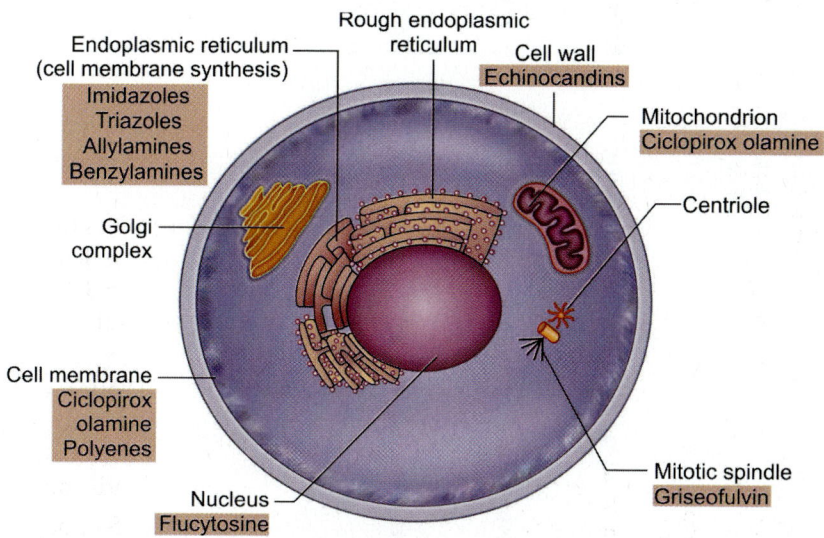

Fig. 8.3: Sites of action of antifungal drugs

Table 8.2: Pharmacokinetics of most commonly used antifungal drugs

	Half life	Peak post dosing levels	Bioavailability	Metabolism	Excretion
Fluconazole	30 hr	1–2 hr	>90%	Little first-pass hepatic metabolism	Renal 80% as parent drug, 11% metabolites; 2% faeces
Itraconazole	21 hr	3–5 hr	55%	Extensive hepatic metabolism by CYP3A4; active metabolite: hydroxyl-itraconazole	Renal 40% inactive metabolites; fecal 3–18% parent drug
Griseofulvin	10–22 hr	2–4 hr		Hepatic, major metabolites are 6-demethyl-griseofulvin and its glucuronide conjugate	Renal 50%, 1% excreted unchanged in urine; 36% in faeces
Terbinafine	36 hr	2 hr	40%	Significant first-pass hepatic metabolism	Renal 70%; clearance decreased 50% in renal impairment or hepatic cirrhosis

Table 8.3: Distribution of common antifungals in skin, hair and nail*

Skin

Drug	First detection	Mode of delivery	Detection after last dose
Terbinafine	Within 24 hours	Passive dermo-epidermal diffusion, through **sebum** and through incorporation of drug from migrating **basal keratinocytes**	2–3 weeks after oral therapy
Fluconazole	7 hours	Through **sweat** and by **direct diffusion** through the dermis and epidermis	
Itraconazole	24 hours	Passive diffusion from the **plasma** to the keratinocytes	3–4 weeks

Nails

Terbinafine	1 week	Via both the nail matrix and the nail bed	(= 7 to 9 months)
Fluconazole	1 day	Diffusion from the nail bed	6 months
Itraconazole	1 week-finger nail 2 weeks-toe nails	Via both the nail matrix and the nail bed	9–11 months

Hair

Terbinafine	1 week	Via the sebum	50 days (7 weeks)
Fluconazole	—	—	4–5 months
Itraconazole	1 week	Via the sebum, and by incorporation into the hair follicle	9 months

*It is important to note that the secretion of terbinafine and itraconozole is via the sebum, griseofulvin is via the sweat and fluconazole is by direct diffusion across the dermis and this drug achieves the highest levels in the skin but on a daily dose. Hence, griseofulvin is ideal for patients who either sweat profusely or do not have sebum excretion. Thus, systemic drugs should take into acount the skin type age and other factors that dermine the secretion of the drug into the skin. Probably fluconazole may be the ideal antifungal drug for difficult cases of dermatophytoses, in a dose of 50 to 100 mg daily for 14 to 20 days.

Table 8.4: Indications of antifungal drugs

Drug	Antifungal spectra	Indication category	Pregnancy
Griseofulvin	Trichophyton, Microsporum, Epidermophyton spp.	1. Tinea capitis and onychomycosis 2. Superficial fungal infections: Widespread, severe or resistant to topical antifungals	C
Terbinafine	Epidermophyton floccosum, Trichophyton mentagrophytes, T. rubrum, T. tonsurans	1. Onychomycosis 2. Superficial fungal infections caused by Trichophyton , Microsporum canis and Epidermophyton floccosum: Widespread, severe or resistant to topical antifungals	B
Itraconazole	Dermatophytes Blastomyces dermatitidis, Histoplasma capsulatum and Candida parapsilosis at concentrations similar to MIC values, but is only fungistatic against C. albicans.	1. Onychomycosis 2. Oropharyngeal and esophageal candidiasis 3. Superficial fungal infections: Widespread, severe or resistant to topical antifungals 4. Blastomycosis, histoplasmosis and aspergillosis	C
Fluconazole	Candida spp.,T. tonsurans, T. rubrum, Microsporum canis	1. Oropharyngeal, esophageal, vaginal and systemic candidiasis 2. Cryptococcal meningitis 3. Superficial fungal infections resistant to topical antifungals	C

(Contd.)

Table 8.4: Indications of antifungal drugs (Contd.)

Drug	Antifungal spectra	Indication category	Pregnancy
Voriconazole	*Aspergillus, Candida, Fusarium, Scedosporium* spp.	Invasive aspergillosis (superior to amphotericin B), esophageal candidiasis, serious infections caused by Fusarium and *Scedosporium apiospermum*	D
Posacon-azole	*Candida, Aspergillus, Cryptococcus fusarium, Zygomycetes* spp.	Prevention of invasive aspergillosis and Candida infections in immunosuppressed hosts	B
Amphotericin B	*Candida* spp., *Cryptococcus neoformans*, dimorphic fungi (*Histoplasma capsulatum Coccidioides, immitis Blastomyces dermatitidis*), *Aspergillus* spp.	Severe fungal infections including disseminated systemic candidiasis, cryptococcal meningitis, blastomycosis, disseminated histoplasmosis, extracutaneous sporotrichosis and coccidiol-domycosis, paracoccidioidomycosis, mucormy-cosis and aspergillosis	B
Caspofungin acetate	*Aspergillus fumigatus, A. flavus, A. terreus, Candida* spp.	Invasive aspergillosis in patients refractory to or intolerant to other antifungals, candidemia, esophageal candidiasis	

Table 8.5: Important drug interactions of common antifungals

Amphotericin B	Nephrotoxic (aminoglycosides, loop diuretics, cyclosporin, tacrolimus)	Additive nephrotoxicity
	Corticosteroids	**Increased** potassium loss
Itraconazole	Antacids (H$_2$ receptor antagonist, PPI, aluminium hydroxide)	Impair absorption of itraconazole
	CYP3A4 inducers (rifampicin, rifabutin, isoniazid, carbamazepine, phenobarbital, phenytoin, efavirenz, nevirapine)	**Hasten** metabolism of itraconazole	Avoid these drugs 2 weeks before and during treatment
	CYP3A4 inhibitors (macrolides, ciprofloxacin, ritonavir boosted ART, indinavir)	**Retard** metabolism of itraconazole
Fluconazole	CYP3A4 inhibitors (amprenavir, protease inhibitors, paclitaxel)	**Increased** levels of fluconazole
	CYP3A4 inducers	**Decrease** levels of fluconazole
	CCBs	**Increased** risk of hypotension
	Cisapride, pimozide	**Increased** QT prolongation
	Amiodarone, aprepitant, bosentan, budesonide, buspirone, ergotamine, carbamazepine, celecoxib, cyclosporin, digoxin, statins, imatinib, metformin, sulfonylureas, methadone, mifepristone, phenytoin, quinidine, repaglinide, sildenafil, sirolimus, tacrolimus, theophylline, warfarin	**Increased** levels of these drugs
	Pioglitazone	**Increased** hyperglycemia

(Contd.)

Table 8.5: Important drug interactions of common antifungals (*Contd.*)

Ketoconazole (CYP3A4 inhibitor)	Terfenadine, cisapride, quinidine, statins, midazolam, cyclosporin	**Increased** levels of these drugs (metabolised by CYP3A4)
	CYP3A4 inhibitors	**Increased** levels of ketoconazole
Terbinafine	TCAs, theophylline	**Increased** levels of these drugs
	Cyclosporin, codeine	**Decreased** levels of these drugs
	Cimetidine, fluconazole	**Increase** levels of terbinafine
	Rifampicin (enzyme inducer)	**Decreased** levels of terbinafine
Caspofungin	Tacrolimus	Decreased circulating levels of tacrolimus
	Enzyme inducers	Hasten metabolism of caspofungin
Voriconazole (CYP2C19, CYP2C9, CYP3A4 inhibitors)	Enzyme inducers (rifampicin, rifabutin, NNRTIs, efavirenz, phenytoin)	Hasten metabolism of voriconazole
	Cyclosporine, tacrolimus, phenytoin, rifabutin, warfarin, sirolimus, omeprazole	**Increased** levels of these these drugs (by inhibition of metabolism)
	Terfenadine, astemizole, cisapride, pimozide, quinidine	Increased risk of QT prolongation

Table 8.6: Dosing regimens and clinical indications for frequently used systemic antifungal agents

	Clinical Indications	Dosing: Adult			Dosing: Pediatric
		IV	Oral	Notes	
Amphotericin B	Aspergillosis Candidiasis, invasive Candidiasis, mucosal Cryptococcosis Blastomycosis Histoplasmosis Mucormycosis Penicilliosis Phaeohyphomycosis Sporotrichosis	0.7–1 mg/kg/d[a]	NA	—	0.7–1 mg/kg/d[a]
Flucytosine	Cryptococcosis (in combination therapy) Second-line; candidiasis	NA	25 mg/kg 4×/d	GFR <50: Decrease dosing interval to q 12–48 h	25 mg/kg 4 ×/d
Fluconazole	Candidiasis, invasive Candidiasis, mucosal[c] Cryptococcosis Prophylaxis, candidiasis	400–800 mg/d 100–200 mg/d[c]	400–800 mg/d 100–200 mg/d[c]	CrCl <50: Decrease dose by	3–12 mg/kg/d 50%

(Contd.)

Table 8.6: Dosing regimens and clinical indications for frequently used systemic antifungal agents (Contd.)

	Clinical Indications	Dosing: Adult			Dosing: Pediatric
		IV	Oral	Notes	
Itraconazole	Blastomycosis	NA	200 mg 1–3 ×/d	nA	2.5–5 mg/kg 2–3×/d
	Candidiasis, mucosal Coccidioidomycosis Histoplasmosis Onychomycosis Paracoccidioidomycosis Sporotrichosis Second-line: Aspergillosis				
Voriconazole	Aspergillosis Candidiasis, invasive Candidiasis, mucosal Fusariosis Scedosporiosis	6 mg/kg for 2 doses, then 4 mg/kg q 12 h	400 mg bid for 2 doses, then 200 mg q 12 h	CrCl<50: Avoid IV formulation Hepatic impairment Consider 50% reduction	4–7 mg/kg q 12 h
Posaconazole	Candidiasis, mucosal prophylaxis, invasive fungal infection	300 mg/d	Suspension: 800 mg/d divided Tablet: 300 mg bid for 2 doses, then 300 mg/d	GFR < 50: Avoid IV formuation	Age ≥ 13: Suspension 200 mg tid Tablet: 300 mg bid for 2 doses, then 300 mg/d

(Contd.)

Table 8.6: Dosing regimens and clinical indications for frequently used systemic antifungal agents (*Contd.*)

	Clinical Indications	Dosing: Adult			Dosing: Pediatric
		IV	Oral	Notes	
Isavuconazole	Aspergillosis Mucormycosis	372 mg q 8 h for 6 doses, then 372 mg/d	372 mg IV q 8 h for 6 doses, then 372 mg/d	Severe hepatic impairment caution	NA
Caspofungin	Candidiasis, invasive Candidiasis, mucosal Empiric therapy[b] Second-line: Aspergillosis	70 mg for 1 dose, then 50 mg/d	NA	Moderate hepatic impairment: 35 mg/d	50 mg/m²/d
Micafungin	Candidiasis, invasive Candidiasis, mucosal Prophylaxis, invasive[c] fungal infection	100–150 mg/d 50 mg/d[c]	NA	NA	1–3 mg/kg/d
Anidulafungin	Candidiasis, invasive	100–200 mg for 1 dose, then 50–200 mg/d	NA	NA	Age > 16: 100–200 mg for 1 dose, then 50–100 mg/d

Abbreviations: CrCl, creatinine clearance; GFR, glomerular filtration rate; IV, intravenous.

[a]Dosing is listed for the amphotericin B deoxycholate formulation. Dosages for the lipid formulations are higher, L-AmB 3 to 6 mg/kg/d, ABLC 3 to 6 mg/kg/d, and ABCD 3 to 4 mg/kg/d.

[b]For patients with febrile neutropenia.

[c]Lower doses can be administered for the specific indication.

In dermatology as superficial infections are common, a summary of the antifungal spectrum of the commonly used drugs is given in Box 8.1. A summary of the efficacy and some practical tips related to the drugs is given in Box 8.2.

AMPHOTERICIN B

MOA: Binds to ergosterol in the fungal membrane.

Spectrum: Amphotericin B is indicated for treatment of severe, potentially life threatening fungal infections. Unfortunately, it must be given IV and is toxic (due to nonselective action on cholesterol in mammalian cell membranes).

Pharmacokinetics: It is poorly soluble in water and has rapid uptake by RES, then redistributed. More than 90% is bound to serum proteins. Serum t½ is approximately 15 days.

Dose: It is available in four formulations: Amphotericin B colloidal dispersion (ABCD), amphotericin B lipid complex (ABLC), liposomal amphotericin B (L-AMB) and oral amphotericin B (poor absorption).

Adverse Effects

1. Headache, fever, chills, anorexia, vomiting, muscle and joint pain.
2. Pain at site of injection and thrombophlebitis (Drug must never be given intramuscularly).
3. Nephrotoxicity-chronic renal toxicity in up to 80% of patients taking the drug for prolonged periods. It is reversible but can be irreversible in high doses. Test for kidney function regularly. This is the most common limiting toxicity of the drug.
4. Hematologic-hemolytic anemia due to effects on red cell membrane.

Special Groups

- No adjustment required in hepatic/renal impairment/dialysis.
- Pregnancy category B.

For interactions (Table 8.5) and uses (Tables 8.3 and 8.6). A detailed therapy regimen is given in Chapter 7.

GRISEOFULVIN

It is classically the drug of choice for treating dermatophyte infections resistant to topical therapy *in children*. Mycologic cure rates are usually 80 to 95%.

Spectrum: Griseofulvin is active only against dermatophytes; yeast infections, including those caused by Candida organisms and Pityrosporum organisms (tinea versicolor); but deep fungi do not respond.

MOA: Griseofulvin has a fungistatic effect; therefore it works best on actively growing dermatophytes, in which it may inhibit fungal cell wall synthesis.

Box 8.1: Spectrum of activity of common oral antifungal

	Terbinafine	Itraconazole	Fluconazole

Trichophyton species
Microsporum species
Epidermophyton floccosum

Terbinafine—Itraconazole > Fluconazole

Tinea capitis: Endothrix (terbinafine); Ectothrix (azoles, griseofulvin)

C. albicans and
C. parapsilosis

Terbinafine < Itraconazole = Fluconazole

Non-dermatophyte Terbinafine = Itraconazole > Fluconazole

Box 8.2: An overview of the important facts about antifungals

· Safest overall: Griseofulvin and terbinafine
· Safest in **pregnancy:** Griseofulvin and Terbinafine
· Safest in **renal dysfunction:** Fluconazole
· Safest in **liver dysfunction:** Fluconazole
· Maximum **bioavailability:** Fluconazole

Newer Antifungals
· Voriconazole: Invasive aspergillosis, esophageal candidiasis, Fusarium and Scedosporium infections
· Posaconazole: Broadest spectrum amongst azoles (zygomycosis and mucormycosis).
· Caspofungin: Disseminated and mucocutaneous Candida infections, C. glabrata and C. krusei febrile neutropenia patients.

PK: Griseofulvin probably diffuses into the stratum corneum from the extracellular *fluid* and *sweat*. Absorption of griseofulvin is improved when it is administered with fatty *foods*. Drug particle size reduction is done through micronization and ultramicronization.

Dose: In microsize forms, the drug is supplied as 125, 250 and 500 mg tablets; in ultramicrosize forms, it is supplied as 125, 250 and 330 mg tablets. The latter is not available in India. An overview of uses of drugs is given in Box 8.3.

Box 8.3: Dosimetry of griseofulvin	
Indication	*Dose*
Tinea capitis	Microsize: 15–20 mg/kg daily Ultramicrosize: 10–15 mg/kg/d Duration: 6–12 weeks
Tinea corporis, Tinea cruris	Microsize: 0.5 g/d, single or divided doses Ultramicrosize: 330–375 mg/d Duration: 2–4 weeks
Tinea pedis	Duration: 4–8 weeks
Tinea imbricata Onychomycosis	Griseofulvin, 500 mg twice daily for 4–6 weeks Although approved for tinea infection of the nails, its affinity for keratin is low and long-term therapy (at least 9–12 months) is required

Interactions

Decreases levels of warfarin, estrogen, birth control pills. Effect of alcohol is potentiated. Barbiturates depress activity of griseofulvin (*refer* to Table 8.3).

Side Effects

1. *Headaches:* They are the most common side effect. The dosage can be temporarily lowered to see if the side effects dissipate, but sometimes the drug must be discontinued. If a headache occurs, it usually does so during the first few days of treatment and may disappear as treatment is continued.
2. Gastrointestinal symptoms like abdominal pain and nausea.
3. Hepatotoxicity
4. Leukopenia
5. Photosensitivity
6. Avoid concomitant alcohol as effects increase.

Special Groups

- Pregnancy—category C
- Kidney disease—none
- Pediatric—safety has not been determined < 2 years.
- Lactation—no data, best to avoid.
- Liver disease—none

TERBINAFINE

This orally and topically active drug belongs to allylamines class of antifungals.

Discovered in 1983, it is closely related to naftifine. Terbinafine was licensed in Europe in 1991 and in 1996 in the United States. It is an allylamine that inhibits the enzyme squalene epoxidase (Fig. 8.4) and thus depletes the fungal cell wall of ergosterol, a key sterol component in the plasma membrane of the fungal cell. A deficiency of ergosterol results in a fungistatic effect similar to that seen with the azole antifungal compounds. Since the biosynthetic pathway of ergosterol is disrupted, squalene accumulates in the intracellular space, which is believed to exert a further toxic effect on susceptible fungal cells, thereby exerting fungicidal activity.

At standard doses it results in a mycologic cure rate of approximately 70% for onychomycosis of the toenails and 80% for fingernails. In all studies, mycological cure rates were higher at follow-up than at the end of treatment with terbinafine, reflecting the drug's fungicidal mechanism of action and its residual effect in nails. Although not extensively investigated, terbinafine appears to be moderately effective in the treatment of onychomycosis involving non-dermatophytes.

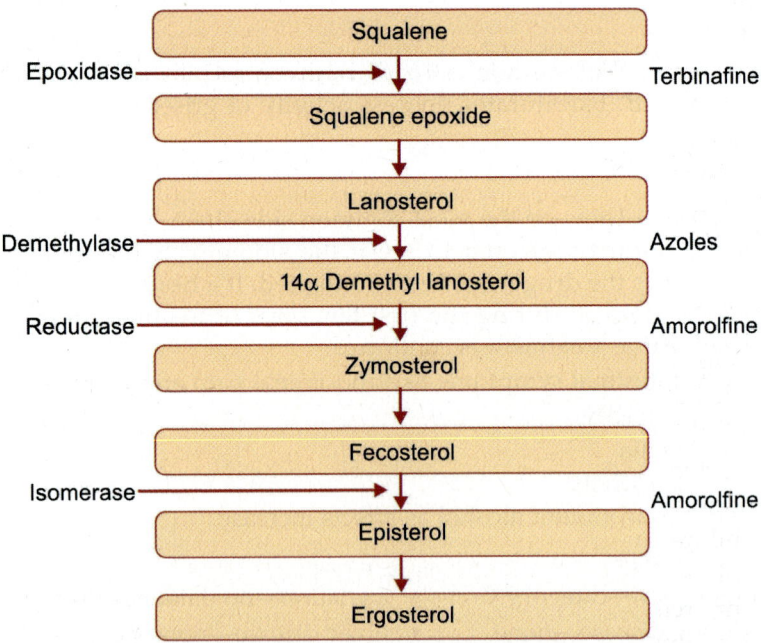

Fig. 8.4: Modes of action of various antifungal drugs

Mycological cure was achieved in 85, 70 and 43% of *C. parapsilosis*, *C. albicans* and *Scopulariopsis brevicaulis* infections, respectively, after 48 weeks' treatment in 1 study. Oral terbinafine is effective in the treatment of superficial dermatophyte infections such as tinea pedis and tinea corporis/cruris, generally achieving mycological cure in > 80% of patients. A typical treatment course of systemic terbinafine is 12 weeks for toenail onychomycosis or 6 weeks for fingernail onychomycosis, and 2–6 weeks for superficial tinea infections resistant to topical antifungal agents. For tinea capitis in children, terbinafine is given continuously 6 to 8 weeks.

MOA: It inhibits squalene epoxidase, a membrane-bound enzyme and is fungicidal to dermatophytes. The initial targets of terbinafine action may be the outer and inner layers of the arthroconidial cell wall, followed by alteration to the cytosol and intracellular organelles. This can produce an inhibitory effect on the morphologic transformation and invasiveness of dermatophytes.

Microbiology: In vitro susceptibility tests have shown terbinafine to have primarily fungicidal activity against dermatophytes, moulds and certain dimorphic fungi, but only fungistatic activity against *Candida albicans*.

PK: Terbinafine is well absorbed and highly *lipophilic* and *keratophilic*, and is distributed throughout adipose tissue, dermis, epidermis, and nails. The drug persists in plasma, dermis-epidermis, hair, and nails for weeks (Table 8.4).

Terbinafine is delivered to the stratum corneum via the sebum and, to a lesser extent, through incorporation into the basal keratino-cytes and diffusion through the dermis-epidermis (Table 8.4). Terbinafine is not found in eccrine sweat. It remains in skin at concentrations above the mean inhibitory concentration (MIC) for most dermatophytes for 2 to 3 weeks after discontinuation of long-term oral therapy. It achieves 70 × times more levels in the stratum corneum as compaired to the plasma. After 6 and 12 weeks of oral therapy, terbinafine has been detected in the nail plate for 30 and 36 weeks, respectively, at a concentration well above the MIC for most dermatophytes.

Dose: Modified in case of liver and kidney failure.
- Adults: 250 mg OD
- Children over 2 years old and under 20 kg: 62.5 mg
- Children over 2 years old and 20–40 kg: 125 mg
- Children over 2 years old and over 40 kg: 250 mg

A summary of the dosimetry in common disorders is given in Box 8.4.

Box 8.4: A summary of the dosimetry of terbinafine in common disorders

Disorder (FDA approved/Unapproved)	Dose/Duration
Aspergillosis,	5–15 mg/kg/d PO for 3–5 months
Black pledra	250 mg for 6 weeks
Chromomycosis	500 mg PO OD for 8–12 months
Dermatophyte Infection	
1. Tinea capitis (oral granule is US FDA approved)	Oral granule < 25 kg, 125 mg daily; 25–35 kg, 187.5 mg daily; >35 kg, 250 mg daily Tablet: 10–20 kg; 62.5 mg; 21–40 kg; 125 mg; 41–50 kg, 250 mg
2. Tinea corporis and tinea cruris	250 mg daily for **4 weeks**
3. Tinea pedis and mannum	250 mg daily for **2–6 weeks**
4. Onychomycosis	250 mg daily for 6 and 12 weeks for fingernail and toenail onychomycosis
5. Seborrheic dermatitis	250 mg—**4 weeks**

Resistance

Resistance has been rarely seen in humans thus far; *in vitro* experiments have shown cross-resistance in C. *tropicalis*, for example, between azoles and terbinafine due to upregulation of efflux transporter genes. In a study, 6 isolates of *Trichophyton rubrum* were found resistant to terbinafine; resistance to terbinafine in these *T. rubrum* isolates appeared to be due to alterations in the squalene epoxidase gene or a factor essential for its activity. Usual MICs are 0.03 mg/ml in susceptible strains of *T. rubrum*; in these resistant strains, MICs were >1.0 mg/ml.

Interactions

In vitro studies have shown that terbinafine inhibits the CYP2D6 liver enzyme and this may be of importance for patients taking tricyclic antidepressants, SSRI antidepressants, MAO inhibitors, and beta-blockers (Table 8.5). Terbinafine can increase serum levels of imipramine and nortriptyline terbinafine blood levels are increased by cimetidine, and decreased by rifampin and rifabutin. See Table 8.5 for more interactions.

SE: Generally considered a safe drug.

In a large uncontrolled post-marketing surveillance study of 25,884 patients, adverse events were reported in 10.4%, mainly from the gastrointestinal system (4.9%) and skin (2.3%).

Skin: The most common reactions in the skin are eczema, pruritus, urticaria, and rash. Others include subacute cutaneous lupus erythematosus, erythema multiforme, exfoliative dermatitis, Stevens-Johnson syndrome and toxic epidermal necrolysis (TEN).

Systemic: **Taste** disturbances were seen in ten patients. Possible risk factors for developing terbinafine associated taste loss include an age greater than 65 years and a body mass index less than 21 kg/m².

Serious adverse drug reactions, most commonly involving the liver and the hematologic system, are only rarely reported with terbinafine use (0.04%). **Hepatotoxicity** ranging from mild transaminitis to fulminant liver failure has been reported as a consequence of oral terbinafine use. It is estimated that 2.2% of patients treated with terbinafine will experience changes in their liver function tests. The onset typically occurs after 3 weeks of therapy and resolution can take as long as 3 months after discontinuation of the drug.

Blood dyscrasias including leucopenia, agranulocytosis, neutropenia and pancytopenia represent the other primary group of severe adverse drug reactions reported with terbinafine use.

While only a few reports exist, **ocular side effects** have been observed with oral terbinafine use. Bilateral anterior optic neuropathy with decreased vision and optic disc edema was reported in a patient 2 weeks after starting terbinafine (500 mg/day). After discontinuing the medication his vision improved.

Special Groups

- Pregnancy category B—this makes it the **safest** oral antifungal in use.
- Lactation—appears in breast milk. Avoid.
- Not recommended in **chronic active** liver disease.
- Avoid if creatinine clearance <50 ml/min.
- Monitor for depressive symptoms.
- Monitor for taste and smell dysfunction.

AZOLES

Fluconazole and itraconazole are the two most commonly used systemic azoles.

MOA: Inhibition of fungal cytochrome P450 dependent enzyme 14α-demethylase, blocking the synthesis of ergosterol, the principal sterol in the fungal cell membrane (Fig. 8.4).

Interactions

Drugs that induce cytochrome P450 enzymes will increase catabolism and reduce plasma concentration of azoles (phenytoin, rifampin, rifabutin, isoniazid, and carbamazepine) (Table 8.5).

Cautions: Atorvastatin, digoxin, quinidine, warfarin, cyclosporine, calcium channel blockers.

Fluconazole

Fluconazole is an orally active bis-triazole antifungal used for the treatment of dermatophyte and Candida infections as well as systemic mycoses. Being an azole it inhibits the same step as other azoles in the ergosterol biosynthesis (Fig. 8.4). This antifungal is dependent on the CYP450 system.

Although the MIC for fluconazole is *high*, it works *well* against most fungi that cause dermatomycoses; *in vitro* drug sensitivities are a poor predictor of antifungal efficacy with this drug. However, drug resistance in Candida species, particularly *C. krusei* and *C. glabrata*, has been described. There is *C. albicans* resistance in patients particularly in those with HIV/AIDS.

PK: Fluconazole is relatively *hydrophilic* compared to other systemic azole antifungal drugs and thus is distributed to the cerebrospinal fluid and can be used to treat fungal meningitis. It is also not dependent on a low gastric pH for absorption. In contrast with many other azoles and terbinafine, fluconazole does not bind strongly to the plasma proteins. It is mostly eliminated unchanged and has a long half-life, which allows once weekly dosing. It is metabolically stable and excreted in urine (91%) and feces (2%).

Fluconazole, as with other azoles, has a *time-dependent kinetics*; the post-antifungal effect is long. The pharmacodynamic target for efficacy is to achieve an AUC (area under the curve)/MIC of ≥ 25.

Dose: Fluconazole is available as 50 mg, 100 mg, 200 mg and 400 mg tablets.

It is given either as a *continuous regimen* of 100–200 mg daily or *intermittently* at 150 mg/week for 2–3 weeks for tinea corporis and tinea cruris and somewhat longer for dry-type tinea pedis.

1. Tinea corporis and tinea cruris—150 mg/week for 2–4 weeks. OR a daily dose 50/100 mg for 2 weeks (ideal for **recalcitrant dermatophytosis** as it achieves the highest intracutaneous levels)
2. Tinea pedis—pulse doses of 150 mg/week for 2–6 weeks
3. Onychomycosis—150 mg/week for 6 months in fingernail and for 12 months in toenail onychomycosis.
4. Tinea capitis and oropharyngeal candidiasis—6 mg/kg on day 1, then 3 mg/kg every 24–72 h for 14 days in adults. In children, 6 mg/kg/day for 2–3 weeks, 200 mg on day 1 then 100 mg for at least 2 weeks.

An overview of the dosimetry is given in Box 8.5.

Box 8.5: An overview of the dosimetry of fluconazole

Disorder	Dose/Duration
Blastomycosis	400–800 mg PO OD for 8 months
candidiasis	
1. Cutaneous candidiasis	150 mg once weekly given for 2–4 weeks.
2. Systemic candidiasis	400 mg IV OD for 7 days, then 400 mg PO OD for 14 days
3. Thrush (oral)	200 mg once or 100 mg PO OD for 5–14 days
4. Oropharyngeal/ Esophagitis	200 mg PO first day, then 100 mg PO OD for 14 days Children: 6 mg/kg on day 1 then 3 mg/kg q24–72 h for 14 days
5. Esophageal	200 mg on day 1 then 100 mg OD for at least 3 weeks Treat for at least 2 weeks after symptoms resolve Children: 6 mg/kg on day 1 then 3 mg/kg q24–72 h for 21 days
6. Vaginal	150 mg PO once stat
Cryptococcosis	400 mg PO/IV OD for 2–6 months **Meningitis** 400 mg on day 1 then 200–400 mg OD continue until 10–12 weeks after spinal fluid is negative **Relapse of cryptococcal meningitis in HIV patients** 20 mg OD
Dermatophyte infection	
Tinea capitis	Continuous regimen: 6 mg/kg daily for 3 weeks can effectively treat tinea capitis Pulse: 8 mg/kg/day 4–8 weeks
Tinea corporis and tinea cruris	150–300 mg once weekly 2–4 weeks 50–100 mg po 2–4 weeks
Tinea pedis and manuum	150 mg once weekly, administered for 2–6 weeks
Tinea pedis and manuum	150 mg once weekly, administered for 2–6 weeks
Tinea versicolor	**Regimen 1:** Fluconazole doses of 300 mg weekly for 1–4 weeks has shown high rates of mycological cure **Regimen 2:** 400 mg PO once
Onychomycosis	**Dermatophytic molds** Fluconazole 150–300 mg once weekly until the abnormal-appearing nail has grown out. The duration is 3–6 months (fingernails) and 9–12 months for toenail **Non-dermatophyte molds and *Candida* species** *Scopulariopsis brevicaulis:* 150 mg daily for 12 weeks *Candida* onychomycosis: 50 mg daily or pulse therapy of 300 mg/week for 6 weeks for fingernails and 3 months for toenails **Children** Dose 5 mg/kg daily for 1 week (2 and 3 pulses for fingernails and toenails)
Sporotrichosis	
Pityriasis versicolor	400 mg PO OD for 6 months

Adverse Reactions

1. *Central nervous system:* Headache, dizziness
2. *Dermatologic:* Skin rash
3. *Gastrointestinal:* Nausea, abdominal pain, vomiting, diarrhea, dysgeusia, dyspepsia.
4. *Hepatic:* Hepatitis, increased serum alkaline phosphatase, increased serum alanine aminotransferase (ALT), increased serum aspartate aminotransferase (AST), jaundice.

Special Groups

- Pregnancy—category C
- Lactation—appears in breast milk. Avoid.
- Hepatic impairment—safer than other antifungals.
- Renal impairment—safer than other antifungals.

Itraconazole

This is an orally absorbed triazole. It has similar activity to the imidazole and ketoconazole, but with less risk of hepatotoxicity. Its mode of action is through the inhibition of the cytochrome P450-dependent demethylation stage in the formation of ergosterol on the fungal cell membrane.

PK: Itraconazole is *lipophilic* and has a high affinity for *keratinizing* tissues. It adheres to the lipophilic cytoplasm of keratinocytes in the nail plate, allowing progressive build-up and persistence in the nail plate. The drug reaches high levels in the nails that persist for at least 6 months after discontinuation of 3 months of therapy and during pulsed cycles. The concentration in the stratum corneum remains detectable for 4 weeks after therapy (Table 8.4). Itraconazole levels in sebum are five times higher than those in plasma and remain high for as long as 1 week after therapy.

Absorption of itraconazole is significantly increased by the presence of food; it should be taken with a full meal acid environment enhances absorption. Absorption is reduced by antacids, histamine-2 blockers (cimetidine, ranitidine) and acid pump inhibitors (omeprazole, lansoprazole).

Itraconazole follows *time-dependent pharmacokinetics* as with other triazoles and has a long post-antifungal effect. The pharmacodynamic target for efficacy is the AUC (area under the curve)/MIC of ≥ 25.

Pharmacokinetics/Pharmacodynamics and Dosimetry

In the pharmacokinetic parameters observed after oral doses of 50, 100, and 200 mg, increases in the AUC and C_{max} are *nonlinear*, suggesting a saturation of the first-pass metabolism process in the liver.

In a human volunteer study, C_{max} for 200 mg was 147% higher on day 1 and 160% higher on day 15 in comparison to 100 mg. This effect was *not* observed between doses of 200 mg per day and 200 mg twice a day, possibly because of the twice daily dosages rather than a single 400 mg dose or the *saturation* of some hepatic metabolic pathway at dosages lower than 200 mg. The mean AUC consistently show three- to fourfold increases for each dosage which is characteristic of nonlinear pharmacokinetic behavior.

Studies have shown that over a wide triazole concentration range (starting below the MIC [sub-MIC] to those more than 200-fold in excess of the MIC), growth of Candida organisms are similarly inhibited. In other words, increasing drug concentrations do not enhance antifungal effect. Furthermore, *in vitro* studies demonstrated organism regrowth soon after drug removal.

The **clinical implications** of this is that there is a little advantage of a dose more than 200 mg a day, but this is dependent on quality MIC studies, which need to be correlated with the dose and AUC levels.

The other clinical implication of this is that even if *in vitro* resistance is there a higher dose may be of a little value.

In vivo studies demonstrated prolonged growth suppression after levels in serum decreased to below the MIC. These prolonged *in vivo* PAFEs have been theorized to be caused by the profound sub-MIC activity of these drugs (i.e. effect of the triazoles after concentrations fall below the MIC *in vivo*). The time kill combination of concentration-independent killing and prolonged PAFEs suggest that the 24 AUC/MIC parameter is most closely tied to treatment effect.

The last ratio is crucial and thus using data from studies from outside India show that a dose of 100 mg a day would be sufficient, but our own work suggest that in recalcitrant cases a justification of a higher dose is there as, the MIC in our work for *T. rubrum* was 0.125 µg/ml as opposed to a level of 0.003 µg/ml from studies outside India.

Bioavailability

Changing the formulation can be useful as an inclusion complex formed with cyclodextrin and the solution form can increase the bioavailability by almost 37% than the oral form.

Dose

1. Pityriasis versicolor: 200 mg for 5–7 days
2. Tinea corporis, tinea cruris 100 mg for 2 weeks or 200 mg for 1 week. A special regimen is reserved for Majocchi granuloma.
3. Tinea pedis 100 mg for 2 weeks or 200 mg for 1 week.

The currently preferred regimen uses 400 mg/day, given as two daily doses of 200 mg. In tinea corporis, 1 week of therapy is sufficient and in tinea pedis, 2 weeks. But this is only in cases of recalcitrant dermatophytosis.

5. Onychomycosis of toenails 200 mg for 12 weeks or 200 mg bd for 1 week, then 3 weeks without treatment, repeated twice more for a total of three pulses of therapy. Onychomycosis of fingernails: 200 mg for 6 weeks or 200 mg bd for 1 week, then 3 weeks without treatment, then 200 mg bd for 1 week.

6. Oropharyngeal candidiasis: Swish and swallow 200 mg for 1–2 weeks. A summary of the dosimetry is given in Box 8.6.

Box 8.6 A summary of the dosimetry of itraconazole

Disorder (FDA approved/ unapproved)	Dose/Duration
Aspergillosis	200 mg PO TDS for 4 days Then 200 mg PO OD 3 months
Blastomycosis	200 mg OD. If there is no improvement or the disease is progressive. The dose may be increased in 100 mg increments. Maximum: 400 mg/d. Children: 100 mg/d
Candidiasis Oral Thrush Stomatitis/Esophagitis/ Vaginitis	200 mg PO OD for 7 days (Swish and swallow) 200 mg PO OD for 14 days (Swish and swallow)
Chromomycosis	100 mg PO OD for 18 months (Adjunctive Rx)
Coccidiodomycosis	200 mg PO BD for 3–12 months
Dermatophyte infection Tinea capitis	5 mg/kg daily for 4–8 weeks, or, in the case of pulse therapy, 5 mg/kg daily for 1 week a month, given for 2–4 months.
Tinea corporis and tinea cruris	100 mg OD 15 days or 200 mg OD 7 days
Tinea pedis and mannum	100 mg/day for 30 days 200 mg daily for **2–4 weeks** (Ideal regimen) 200 mg BID for 7 days
Majocchi's granuloma	200 mg BD for 7 days, then off for 14 days (repeat 3 times total)
Onychomycosis Fingernail	i. 200 mg PO OD for 3 months ii. **Pulse:** 200 mg twice daily (400 mg daily) for 1 week per month. 2 pulses **(FDA approved)**
Toenail	i. 200 mg daily for 12 weeks ii. **Pulse:** 200 mg twice daily (400 mg daily) for 1 week per month. (3–4 pulses)—**not approved by FDA**
Candida onychomycosis	200 mg daily

(Contd.)

Box 8.6 A summary of the dosimetry of itraconazole (*Contd.*)

Disorder (FDA approved/ unapproved)	Dose/Duration
Phaeohyphomycosis	200 mg PO BID until clinical resolution
Tinea versicolor	**Treatment:** 200 mg OD 5–7 days or 100 mg daily for 2 weeks Prophylaxis: A single 400 mg dose of itraconazole— 6 months
Seborrheic dermatitis	Regimen 1: 200 mg OD for 7 days Regimen 2: 200 mg PO OD for first week of month, then first 2 days of every month for 11 months
Sporotrichosis	100–200 mg PO OD for 3–6 months or until 2–4 weeks after all lesions have resolved.

Side Effects

Itraconazole is generally well tolerated. The incidence of side effects is 7% with short-term treatment, but rises to 12.5% with longer duration of therapy. The most common side effects are headache and gastrointestinal symptoms such as nausea, dyspepsia, abdominal pain, diarrhea, and flatulence. Dermatological symptoms such as rash, pruritus, and urticaria and acute generalized exanthematous pustulosis and toxic epidermal necrolysis are less common.

1. Gastrointestinal: Diarrhea, nausea.
2. Cardiovascular: Edema, chest pain, hypertension. Itraconazole may be associated with congestive heart failure. High-dose itraconazole (400 mg/day) causes a significant *decrease* in serum LDL-cholesterol and a significant *increase* in HDL-cholesterol.
3. Central nervous system: Headache, dizziness, anxiety, depression, fatigue, abnormal dreams.
4. Dermatologic: Skin rash, pruritus, diaphoresis.
5. Endocrine and metabolic: Hypertriglyceridemia, hypokalemia.
6. Hepatic: Raised enzyme levels. Elevated liver function tests have been described in 0.3–5% of cases. Very rare cases of serious hepatotoxicity, including some cases of fatal acute liver failure, have been described. Liver function monitoring is recommended in patients receiving treatment with itraconazole of over one month duration.
7. Absorption of itraconazole from capsules is impaired when gastric acidity is reduced in patients with reduced gastric acidity; it is advisable to administer the drug with an acidic beverage and/or a high-fat meal.

Drug interactions: Itraconazole is known to interact with a number of medications. Table 8.5 summarises the important interactions.

Special Groups

Itraconazole is embryotoxic and teratogenic in rats and should not be used during pregnancy. Women of childbearing potential taking itraconazole should use contraceptives. A very small amount of itraconazole is excreted in human milk, and therefore itraconazole should not be given to breastfeeding women.

- Pregnancy —category C
- Lactation—appears in breast milk, avoid.
- Pediatric—safety not been established <3 years.
- Hepatic impairment—use with caution
- Renal impairment—use with caution.

Ketoconazole

Pharmacokinetics/Pharmacodynamics

Peak plasma concentrations are achieved 1–2 h after oral administration. It requires acidity for dissolution and absorption; if patient is receiving antacids, anticholinergics, H2 blockers, they should be given at least 2 h after administration of ketoconazole.

There is a need to acidify the tablet of ketoconazole if given to achlorhydric patients. It is highly protein-bound (99%); although there is distribution to body fluids and tissues, there is only negligible amount in the CSF. About 13% is excreted via urine; majority is excreted via bile.

Ketoconazole demonstrates *time-dependent pharmacokinetics* and has a long post-antifungal effect. The pharmacodynamic target for efficacy is the AUC (area under the curve)/MIC of 25.

Indications

It is used primarily for the topical treatment of tinea corporis, tinea cruris, and tinea pedis; treatment of tinea versicolor; treatment of cutaneous candidiasis and seborrheic dermatitis.

Spectrum of activity: Dermatophyte infections caused by *Trichophyton rubrum, T. mentagrophytes,* and *Epidermophyton floccosum; Candida* spp.; *Malassezia furfur.* Ketoconazole does have in vitro activity against dimorphic fungi and dematiaceous agents of chromoblastomycosis.

Dose

Topically it is used but its systemic use has been restricted and though it is often prescribed by some clinicians in a dose of 200 mg, we cannot jusify its use in view of safer and now cheaper azoles.

Side Effects

a. The major toxicity is that of hepatic toxicity, with an incidence of 1:10,000 and this is usually reversible. Obtaining baseline levels of liver function tests and monitoring these through treatment is important.

b. There have been cases of hypersensitivity in the form of urticaria, lowered serum testosterone levels, and decreased ACTH-induced corticosteroid levels with administration of ketoconazole.

c. There are no known controlled studies in the pregnant patient; teratogenic effects have been seen in animals given large doses of ketoconazole.

d. Cardiac complications have been found with co-administration of terfenadine and astemizole and cisapride.

e. The package contains contraindications for use of ketoconazole along with these agents.

f. Ketoconazole can increase blood levels of cyclosporine, theophylline, and anticoagulants.

Voriconazole

It is a novel azole antifungal.

Indications: Aspergillosis, invasive non-zygomycete filamentous fungal infections, *Pseudallescheria boydii* (*Scedosporium* spp.), *Fusarium* spp., and treatment of positive urine cultures due to resistant *Candida* spp.

Dose:

Loading dose: 6 mg/kg IV/PO q12h × 2 doses

Maintenance dose: 4 mg/kg IV/PO q12h

Oral: 400 mg q12h (wt >40 kg) or 200 mg Q12h (wt)

Drug interactions: Voriconazole is metabolised by and inhibits CYP2C19, CYP2C9, and CYP3A4. Thus it has interactions with all the drugs metabolised by these enzymes. Administration of the following agents with voriconazole is contraindicated: Sirolimus, rifampin, rifabutin, carbamazepine, terfenadine, astemizole, cisapride, pimozide, quinidine, long-acting barbiturates.

Side Effects

1. Visual disturbances (~30%) are usually self-limited. Avoid activities that require keen vision.

2. Rash (6%)

3. Fever

4. Elevation in hepatic enzymes.

Posaconazole

Posaconazole is the azole with the *broadest spectrum*. It has *in vitro* activity against Candida, Aspergillus, Zygomycosis (*Rhizopus* spp.), Mucormycosis (*Mucor* spp.) and *Fusarium* spp. It is an orally administered drug.

Indications

- Salvage treatment of invasive zygomycosis in combination with amphotericin B.
- Monotherapy for zygomycosis after 7 days of combination therapy with amphotericin B.
- Prophylaxis of fungal infections in susceptible patients.

Dose: Each dose should be given with a full high-fat meal or with liquid nutritional supplements if patients cannot tolerate full meals.

Loading dose: 200 mg PO q6h for 7 days

Maintenance dose: 400 mg PO q8–12h drug interactions

Side Effects

1. GI upset
2. Headaches
3. Elevation in hepatic enzymes.
4. Rare but serious effects include QTc prolongation.

ECHINOCANDINS

Echinocandins were discovered as fermentation metabolites with antifungal activity during screening programs for new antibiotics. Three semi-synthetic Echinocandin derivatives have been developed for clinical use: caspofungin, micafungin, and anidulafungin. All three echinocandins are structurally similar: Cyclic hexapeptide antibiotics with modified N-linked acyl lipid side chains, which play a role in anchoring the hexapeptide nucleus to the fungal cell membrane where the drug interacts with the target enzyme complex involved in cell wall synthesis.

Echinocandins target fungal cell glucan synthesis by competitively inhibiting the beta-1,3-D-glucan synthase enzyme complex in susceptible fungi. Beta-glucan depletion causes loss of resistance to osmotic forces and cell lysis among *Candida* spp., thereby having a fungicidal effect. However, in filamentous fungi the bulk of beta-glucan synthesis is concentrated at the apical tips and branching points of hyphae, so echinocandins result in dysmorphic hyphae; and have a fungistatic effect. Echinocandins are primarily effective against *Candida* and *Aspergillus* species, with relatively weak activity *Cryptococcus neoformans*.

Pharmacokinetics

Due to their large molecular weights, echinocandins are minimally absorbed after oral administration and are available only in intravenous formulations. All three echinocandins exhibit a high degree of binding to plasma proteins and distribute minimally to cerebrospinal fluid, urine, and the eye.

Echinocandins are widely used for the treatment of invasive candidiasis, especially in critically ill and neutropenic patients. They are also used for empiric antifungal therapy in patients with neutropenic fever.

Uses

Caspofungin
- Disseminated candidiasis and candidemia
- Empirical antifungal therapy for febrile neutropenia (has replaced AMB)
- Invasive aspergillosis (only as salvage therapy for AMB-resistant patients)

Micafungin
- Mucocutaneous candidiasis
- Candidemia
- Prophylaxis of candida infections in bone marrow transplant patients

Anidulafungin
- Esophageal candidiasis,
- Invasive candidiasis including candidemia

Dose

Caspofungin: 70 mg IV loading dose followed by 50 mg daily dose.

Micafungin: 150 mg/d (Candida esophagitis), 100 mg/d (candidemia), 50 mg/d (prophylaxis of fungal infections).

Anidulafungin: 100 mg/d loading dose followed by 50 mg daily (esophageal candidiasis), 200 mg loading dose followed by 100 mg/d (candidemia).

Adverse Effects

Echinocandins are well tolerated, and all three members of the class have similar types of adverse effects. Serious adverse effects requiring

drug discontinuation occur less frequently with the echinocandins than with other classes of systemic antifungals.
1. Hepatotoxicity
2. Infusion and hypersensitivity reactions.
3. Injection site pain.
4. Gastrointestinal
5. Renal toxicity
6. Hematologic effects
7. Cardiac toxicity

Special Groups

Hepatic impairment: Dose adjustment required only in severe hepatic impairment

Renal impairment: No dose adjustment required

SORDARINS

The sordarins are a new class of antifungal drugs with a novel and unusual mode of action in antifungal therapies. These compounds interfere with protein synthesis through inhibition of protein elongation factor 2. The sordarins have shown *in vitro* activity against *Candida* species, *Pneumocystis carinii*, *Aspergillus* spp., and *Scedosporium apiospermum*.

NIKKOMYCIN

Nikkomycins are nucleoside-peptide antibiotics produced by Streptomyces species with antifungal activity due to the inhibition of chitin synthesis. Since chitin does not exist in mammalian cells, compounds that inhibit chitin biosynthesis are considered potential antifungal drugs of low toxicity for humans. Among the medically important fungi, *Coccidioides immitis* and *B. dermatitidis* are susceptible to nikkomycin Z both *in vitro* and *in vivo*.

CONCLUSIONS

The above overview has to be understood in its relevance to dermatophytosis which is the current concern in India. The almost desperate rush for newer regimens has little science behind its use and reflects a lack of understanding of the PK of these drugs. Instead of focussing on in vitro MIC and blood AUC values, we must focus on the levels of the drug in the skin, which is dependent on the secretion via the sebum, eccrine glands and the blood. The highest levels in the stratum corneum is achieved by fluconazole, while itraconazole and terbinafine are primarily secreted by the sebum. As a corollary in a patient with a little sebum activity the latter two would not be effective. A few principles are laid below:

1. Higher is not better: Thus it is useful to use standard doses initially, but for the proper duration, which in steroid modified cases can extend to 4–6 weeks. This is the commonest cause of the so-called "failure".

2. What drug to use is a matter of choice and comorbidities and most of us use itraconazole which is fair enough, but remember the plethora of interactions. If this is used the dose should not exceed maximum 100 mg twice a day as beyond that dose no added pharmacological effect is achieved. With terbinafine most now use 500 mg, which has evidence, in a BD dose and in HIV positive case, the logic of this dose could be that a steroid modified skin is akin to a localised immunosuppressed!

3. In cases that fail the above, fluconazole is a useful drug. The high MIC, is the property of the drug and does not mean its not clinically useful. In some situations like in xerotic skin, it achieves a higher skin level than the other antifungals.

4. Lastly in some sites, like tinea pedis and non-DTM onycholycosis itraconazole may be ideal.

Lastly quality matters, and there are studies to show that variations in quality affects the results.

Bibliography

1. Andes D, Marchillo K, Conklin R, et al. Pharmacodynamics of a new triazole, posaconazole, in a murine model of disseminated candidiasis. Antimicrob Agents Chemother 2004; 48:137–142.

2. Andes D, Marchillo K, Stamstad T, et al. In vivo pharmacodynamics of a new triazole, ravuconazole, in a murine candidiasis model. Antimicrob Agents Chemother 2003;47:1193.

3. Andes D, Marchillo K, Stamstad T, et al. In vivo pharmacokinetics and pharmacodynamics of a new triazole, voriconazole, in a murine candidiasis model. Antimicrob Agents Chemother 2003;47:3165–3169.

4. Andes D, Van Ogtrop M. Characterization and quantitation of the pharmacodynamics of fluconazole in a neutropenic murine disseminated candidiasis infection model. Antimicrob Agents Chemother 1999;43:2116–2120.

5. Balfour JA, Faulds D. Terbinafine. Drugs. 1992 Feb 1;43(2):259–284.

6. Brodell RT, Elewski BE. Clinical pearl: systemic antifungal drugs and drug interactions. J Am Acad Dermatol. 1995;33:259–260.

7. CLSI document M38A-2 (2008a) Reference method for broth dilution antifungal susceptibility testing of lamentous fungi: approved standard, 2nd edn. Clinical and Laboratory Standards Institute, Wayne, PA).

8. Ernst EJ, Klepser ME, Pfaller MA. Postantifungal effects of echinocandin, azole, and polyene antifungal agents against *Candida albicans* and *Cryptococcus neoformans*. Antimicrob Agents Chemother 2000;44:1008–11.

9. Favre B, Ghannoum MA, Ryder NS (2004) Biochemical characterization of terbinafine-resistant *Trichophyto nrubrum* isolates. Med Mycol 42:525–529.

10. Heykants, J., M. Michiels, W. Meuldermans, J. Monbaliu, K. Lavrijsen, A. Van Peer, J. C. Levron, R. Woestenborghs, and G. Cauwenbergh. 1987. The pharmacokinetics of itraconazole in animals and man: an overview, p. 223–249. In M. A. Fromtling (ed.), Recent trends in the discovery, development and evaluation of antifungal agents. J.R. Prous Science Publishers, Barcelona, Spain.

11. Katz HI, Gupta AK. Oral antifungal drug interactions. Dermatol Clin. 1997;15:535–544.

12. Lamisil SPC. https://www.medicines.org.uk/emc/medicine/1290

13. Lever LR, Dykes PJ, Thomas R, Finlay AY. How orally administered terbinafine reaches the stratum corneum. Journal of Dermatological Treatment. 1990 Jan 1;1(sup2):23–25.

14. Lewis RE, Wiederhold NP, Klepser ME. In vitro pharmacodynamics of amphotericin B, itraconazole, and voriconazole against *Aspergillus, Fusarium,* and *Scedosporium* spp. Antimicrob Agents Chemother 2005;49:945–251.

15. McClellan KJ, Wiseman LR, Markham A. Terbinafine. Drugs. 1999 Jul 1;58(1):179–202.

16. Newland JG, Abdel-Rahman SM. Update on terbinafine with a focus on dermatophytoses. Clinical, cosmetic and investigational dermatology: CCID. 2009;2:49.

17. Stevens DA. Advances in systemic antifungal therapy. Clin Dermatol. 2012;30:657–661.

18. Thomas C. Hardin *et al.* Pharmacokinetics of itraconazole following oral administration to normal volunteers antimicrobial agents and chemotherapy, Sept. 1988, P. 1310–1313.

19. Turnidge JD, Gudmundsson S, Vogelman B, *et al.* The postantibiotic effect of antifungal agents against common pathogenic yeasts. J Antimicrob Chemother 1994;34:83–92.

3. TOPICAL ANTIFUNGAL DRUGS

Surabhi Sinha

Patients with limited fungal infections confined to glabrous skin are usually best treated with topical antifungal drugs. Treatment with topical antifungals has many advantages over systemic treatment including ease of use, fewer side effects, fewer drug interactions and lower cost of therapy. Most topical antifungals belong to one of the three main classes: Imidazoles, allylamines and benzylamines, and polyenes.

Imidazole preparations for topical use, such as clotrimazole, econazole, and ketoconazole, are now well established as effective treatments in ringworm infections with an extremely low incidence of adverse reactions; other drugs in this group, miconazole, isoconazole, tioconazole, and sulconazole, are equally effective. Newer preparations such as sertaconazole, luliconazole, and isoconazole are available in some countries. Generally they are used in cream, solution, or spray formulations at a concentration of 1%. Most are used twice daily for 2–4 weeks although bifonazole is licensed for once-daily use.

The major topical alternative is the topical formulation of **terbinafine**. Terbinafine applied topically has been shown to produce responses in some dermatophyte infections in very short periods of application, e.g. 1–7 days. There is also a topical formulation of terbinafine which is designed for use in infections of the sole of the foot.

Ciclopirox, amorolfine, and bifonazole are available as topical treatments in some but not all countries. The first two agents are available as specially formulated topical nail treatments and the latter as both a cream formulation and as combined treatment in an urea based for nail ablation.

The most recent Cochrane review of topical treatments for foot infections indicates a little difference in efficacy between these different azole compounds and alternatives.

It must be remembered that benzoic acid compound ointment (Whitfield's ointment), full strength, is particularly an irritant and is not used on tender skin sites, such as the scrotum or the groins. Magenta paint (Castellani's paint) is still used in some cases of inflammatory tinea pedis, particularly when bacterial infection coexists, although potassium permanganate followed by a topical antifungal is preferred. Other cream or powder preparations include tolnaftate or zinc undecenoate. An overview of topical antifungal agents is given in Table 8.7.

Table 8.7: Topical antifungal agents commonly used in India*

| Active substance group | Substance | Preparations | Antimicrobial efficacy against | | | |
			Dermatophytes	Yeasts	Molds	Bacteria
Allylamines	Terbinafine*	Cream, gel, solution, spray	✓	✓		✓; Coryne-bacterium minutissimum (erythrasma)
Imidazoles	Bifonazole	Cream, spray, solution, gel, ointment (nail set)	✓	✓		✓; Corynebac-terium minu-tissimum (erythrasma)
	Clotrimazole*	Cream, solution, gel, paste, powder, spray, vaginal tablets, vaginal supposi-tories, vaginal cream, cream	✓	✓	✓	
	Econazole*	Cream, solution, lotion, vaginal suppository and cream	✓	✓	✓	
	Fenticonazole nitrate	Cream, solution, pump, spray, vaginal suppositories				Gram-positive bacteria
	Isoconazole nitrate (only available in combination with diflu-cortolone 21-valerate)	Cream				
	Ketoconazole*	Cream, solution	✓	✓	✓	

(Contd.)

Table 8.7: Topical antifungal agents commonly used in India* (Contd.)

Active substance group	Substance	Preparations	Antimicrobial efficacy against			
			Dermatophytes	Yeasts	Molds	Bacteria
	Miconazole*	Cream, gel, solution, oral gel, paste, buccal tablets, vaginal suppositories, vaginal cream	✓	✓	✓	✓; Gram-positive bacteria (Propioni-bacterium acnes, Staphylo-coccus (S. epidermidis, S. aureus)
	Sertaco-nazole*	Cream, solution	✓	✓	✓ (Asper-gillus, Fusa-rium)	✓; Gram-positive bacteria (staphylococci, streptococci)
	Tioconazole	Cream, lotion, powder, spray	✓	✓	✓	✓; Coryne-bacterium minutissimum
Morpholine derivative	Amoroline* HCl	Nail lacquer, cream	✓	✓	✓	✓; only effec-tive against Actinomyces spp., also mildly effective against Propioni-bacterium acnes

(Contd.)

Table 8.7: Topical antifungal agents commonly used in India* (Contd.)

Active substance group	Substance	Preparations	Antimicrobial efficacy against			
			Dermatophytes	Yeasts	Molds	Bacteria
Polyenes	Nystatin	Suspension, ready-to-use suspension, oral gel, film coated tablets, dragees, paste, ointment, suppositories, vaginal tablets and cream	(X. effective in vitro)	✓	(✓, effective in vitro)	
	Ampho-tericin* B	Lozenge, suspension, tablets, genital cream and vaginal tablets (available only in combination with tetracycline)	✓**	✓	✓ (especially Aspergillus fumigatus)	
	Natamycin	Ophthalmic ointment lozenge	✓	✓	✓	
Pyridone derivative	Ciclopirox* olamine	Cream, gel, solution, nail lacquer, powder, shampoo vaginal cream	✓	✓	✓	
Thiocarba-mate	Tolnaftate	Solution, cream	✓	✓		Also effective against tricho-monads

**Studies have shown that this drug is variably effective with some studies showing superiority over terbinafine

SUMMARY OF INDIVIDUAL DRUGS

Imidazoles

Imidazoles are the largest group of topical antifungals and are the most commonly used agents. They inhibit lanosterol 14α-demethylase, a cytochrome P450 dependent enzyme which converts lanosterol to ergosterol. Depletion of ergosterol results in membrane instability and hyperpermeability which are incompatible with growth and survival of the fungal organisms. Imidazoles are fungistatic. They also possess anti-inflammatory activity via inhibition of neutrophil chemotaxis, calmodulin activity, synthesis of leukotrienes and prostaglandins, and histamine release from mast cells. Ketoconazole is believed to possess anti-inflammatory effects equivalent to 1% hydrocortisone.

Clotrimazole

Classification: Imidazole antifungal

Uses: It is among the first clinically useful azole antifungals. It has excellent activity against *Candida* spp. Because of a lack of systemic effects, it is used only for topical therapy.

Mode of application: To be applied twice daily over the lesions including normal skin for a radius of 2 cm beyond. Treatment should continue for at least 1 week after clinical resolution.

Side effects: Irritant contact dermatitis (worsened by occlusion), allergic contact dermatitis (to active ingredient or more likely to preservatives), and rarely, urticaria.

Special Groups

Pregnancy: Pregnancy class C.

Lactation: Use only if clearly essential.

Children: Safety unknown

Eberconazole

Classification: Imidazole antifungal

Uses: It has a high potency against *Dermatophytes*, *Candida* spp., and *Malassezia furfur*. It is also active against gram-positive bacteria. Another interesting feature of eberconazole is its *anti-inflammatory* activity by the inhibition of the 5-lipo-oxygensae enzyme which is involved in the metabolism of arachidonic acid.It has a documented anti-inflammatory activity, comparable to ketoprofen and acetylsalicylic acid. This activity is seen *"in vivo"* too and is comparable to acetylsalicylic acid.

Mode of application: It is to be applied twice daily for 4 weeks, or for at least one week after there is clinical resolution.

Side effects: The appearance of eczema, desquamation, folliculitis and pustules is rare (1/1000 and< 1/10).

Special Groups

Pregnancy: Safe as clinically insignbificant absorption.

Lactation: Safe as clinically insignbificant absorption.

Children: Unknown safety

Ketoconazole

Classification: Imidazole antifungal

Uses: Ketoconazole is used for treatment of dermatophytoses, pityriasis versicolor, mucocutaneous candidiasis and seborrheic dermatitis.

Mode of application: It is approved for once daily dosing.

Side effects: Irritant and allergic contact dermatitis (unuusal)

Special Groups

Pregnancy: Class C

Lactation: Use only if necessary.

Children: Unknown safety.

Luliconazole

Classification: Imidazole antifungal

Uses: Luliconazole is indicated for the treatment of the following cutaneous mycosis:
1. Tinea: Tinea pedis, tinea corporis, and tinea cruris
2. Candidiasis: Intertrigo and interdigital erosion
3. Pityriasis versicolor

Luliconazole is *superior* to bifonazole, terbinafine and fluconazole.

Mode of application: Luliconazole has to be applied on the affected area once a day.

Side effects:
- Itching, redness, irritation, contact dermatitis, pain, and eczema 0.1 to 5%
- Hot flash, heat sensation and burning sensation <0.1%
- Increase in blood urea nitrogen (BUN) and increase in urinary protein<0.1%

Special Groups

Pregnancy: Safety of luliconazole has not been established during pregnancy and lactation. This product should be used in pregnant women or women who may possibly be pregnant only if the expected benefits outweigh the possible risks associated with treatment.

Lactation: Use only if clearly indicated.

Children: Safety of luliconazole has not been established in pediatric age group.

Miconazole

Classification: Imidazole antifungal

Uses: Dermatophytoses, candidiasis and pityriasis versicolor.

Mode of application: To be applied twice daily for 4 weeks over the affected area with 2 cm radius of surrouinding normal skin too.

Side effects: Rare. Irritant and allergic contact dermatitis, urticaria.

Special Groups

Pregnancy: Class C

Lactation: Safety unknown. Use only if clearly indicated.

Children: Unknown safety.

Oxiconazole

Classification: Imidazole antifungal

Uses: Topical treatment of tinea pedia, tinea cruris and tinea corporis caused by *Trichophyton rubrum, T. mentagrophytesa, Epidermophyton floccosum.* Also pityriasis versicolor caused by *Malassezia furfur.*

Mode of application: Approved for once daily use to affected and immediate surrounding areas for dermatophyte infections and pityriasis versicxolor. Tinea pedis should be treated for 4 weeks to reduce recurrence risk while other infections should be treated for 2 weeks.

Side effects: Pruritus, burning sensation, irritation and rarely allergic contact dermatitis, folliculitis, erythema, fissuring , maceration.

Special Groups

Pregnancy: Class B.

Lactation: Excreted in breats milk, to be apllied with caution.

Children: Unknown safety.

Sertaconazole

Classification: Imidazole antifungal

Uses: Effective against *dermatophytes, Candida* spp., pityriasis versicolor and gram-positive bacteria. Also has an *anti-inflammatory* activity.

Mode of application: To be applied twice daily to affected area and surrounding normal skin for a radius of 2 cm beyond the lesion.

Side effects: Has potential to cause irritant and allergic contact dermatitis.

Special Groups

Pregnancy: Class C.

Lactation: Use only if clearly indicated. Safety unknown.

Children: Unknown safety.

NAFTIFINE

Classification: Allylamine antifungal

Uses: Effective against dermatophytes and pityriasis versicolor. They are known to be fungicidal and possess anti-inflammatory properties.

Mode of application: The cream is applied once daily and the gel is applied twice daily to the affected areas, usually for 2 weeks beyond clinical resolution.

Side effects: Rarely may cause irritant and allergic contact dermatitis.

Special Groups

Pregnancy: Class B.

Lactation: Safety unknown.

Children: Safety unknown.

TERBINAFINE

Classification: Allylamine antifungal

Uses: Very effective against dermatophyte infections caused by Trichopyton (*T. rubrum, T. mentagrophytes, T. verrucosum, T. violaceum*), *Microsporum canis* and *Epidermophyton floccosum*. One week of terbinafine therapy for tinea pedis is as effective as 4 weeks of topical imidazoles.

However, terbinafine demonstrates variable and somewhat poor *in vitro* activity against many yeasts. It generally exhibits fungicidal activity against *C. parapsilosis* but it is fungistatic against *C. albicans* and other *Candida* spp. The in vitro spectrum of activity also includes *Aspergillus* spp., some dimorphic fungi, *S. schenkii*, and others.

Mode of application: Can be applied once or twice daily. Cleanse and dry affected area thoroughly before application.

Side effects: Erythema, itching or stinging sensation may occur transiently at site of application. Allergic contact dermatitis is rare but requires discontinuation. Oral terbinafine has been shown to have myriad side effects.

Special Groups

Pregnancy: Fetal toxicity and fertility studies in animals suggest no adverse effects. Since clinical experience in pregnant women is very limited, it should not be used during pregnancy unless the potential benefits outweigh any potential risks.

Lactation: Terbinafine is excreted in breast milk but with the cream, clinically insignificant amounts are absorbed through skin, unlikely to affect the infant.

Children: Safety unknown.

BUTENAFINE

Classification: Benzylamine antifungal

Uses: Very effective for dermatophytoses; however, efficacy against yeast infections may be variable or reduced in comparison to imidazoles.

Mode of application: Once daily application is enough (except tinea pedis where twice daily dosing may be recommended). For tinea pedis, at least 4 week therapy is required; in other tinea infections, 2 weeks would suffice.

Side effects: Unusual, irritant and allergic contact dermatitis.

Special Groups

Pregnancy: Class B.

Lactation: Safety unknown.

Children: Safety unknown.

NYSTATIN

Classification: Polyene antifungal

Uses: For treatment of mucocutaneous candidiasis caused by susceptible *Candida* species. However, it is less effective than topical imidazoles in treating vulvovaginal candidiasis. It is not effective against dermatophytes or Pityrosporum.

Mode of application: For treating oral candidiasis, nystatin suspension is to be used 4–5 times daily for 2 weeks. For cutaneous infection, the cream, powder or ointment is used twice daily for 2 weeks.

Side effects: Allergic contact dermatitis has been often reported with nystatin. Anaphylaxis has been described with use of nystastin—contining vaginal suppositories but the reaction was due to ingredients other than nystatin.

Special Groups
Pregnancy: Class C.

Lactation: Safety unknown.

Children: Safety unknown.

CICLOPIROX OLAMINE

Classification: Hydroxypyridone antifungal

Uses: Indicated for the treatment of dermatophytoses, onychomysosis, candidiasis, pityriasis versicolor, seborrheic dermatitis and some cutaneous infections with unusual saprophytes.

Mode of application: Tinea pedis requires twice daily dosing for at least 4 weeks; for other tinea infections, candidiasis and pityriasis versicolor, twice daily for 2–4 weeks is enough. Shampoos for seborrheic dermatitis should be used twice weekly for an indefinite duration though improvement is seen in 2 to 4 weeks usually. For onychomycosis, the nail lacquer is applied daily to the nail and hyponychium for 48 weeks and excess medication is removed weekly with alcohol.

Side effects: Rarely, irritant or allergic contact dermatitis.

Special Groups
Pregnancy: Use only if clearly indicated.

Lactation: Unknown safety.

Children: Unknown safety

AMOROLFINE

Classification: Morpholine derivative

Uses:

- Amorolfine has a very broad spectrum of activity against dermatohytes (all 3 species), yeasts (*Candida* spp., *Malassezia* spp.,

Cryptococcus neoformans), Moulds (*Alternaria* spp., *Scopulariopsis brevicaulis, Aspergillus* spp., *Mucor circinelloides, Rhizopus oryzae, Fusarium* spp., *Pseudoallescheria boydii*), Dematiaceous fungi (*Cladosporium carrionii, Fonsecaea pedrosoi, Madurella mycetomatis, Phialophora verrucosa*) and Dimorphic fungi (*Histoplasma capsulatum, Coccidioides dimmitis, Blastomyces dermatitidis, Sporothrix schenckii*).

- It has been shown to be *more* active than azoles and at least as effective as allylamines against dermatophytes.
- Against yeasts, it is *more* active than allylamines and at least as active as the azoles. Thus it is indicated in all infections caused by dermatophytes, and in cutaneous candidiasis and pityriasis versicolor.

Mode of application: Once daily application of the cream and weekly application of the nail lacquer have been shown to have adequate effectiveness. Treatment should generally be continued for 2–3 weeks. For tinea pedis, up to 6 weeks treatment may be required.

Side effects: Most common adverse effects are buring, itching, erythema and scaling.

Special Groups

Pregnancy: There are no adequate data in pregnant women. Studies in animals have shown evidence of reproductive toxicity. The potential risk for humans is unknown. It should thus not be used in pregnancy unless clearly necessary.

Lactation: There are no adequate data in nursing mothers. It should not be used unless clearly necessary.

Children: Unknown safety.

AMPHOTERICIN B

Classification: Macrocyclic, polyene anti-fungal agent.

Mode of action:

- Amphotericin B acts by binding to ergosterol of the cell membrane of the susceptible fungi. It forms transmembrane channels leading to alterations in cell permeability through which monovalent ions (Na^+, K^+, H^+, and Cl^-) leak out of the cell resulting in cell death.
- Amphotericin B has higher affinity for ergosterol than for cholesterol. High affinity of amphotericin B for ergosterol results in its binding predominantly to fungi (and Leishmania spp.)
- The utilization of systemic amphotericin B in clinical practice is restricted due to its severe toxicity to the kidney and RBCs. However, topical application is limited due to its low absorption

through mucosa or skin. Amphotericin B molecule is highly lipophilic and thus cannot be dissolved in aqueous medium. Thus, small size lipid nanoparticles are used as carriers for topical amphotericin B to increase the amount of drug penetrated into the skin.

Spectrum

Candida (Monilia) species for topical preparation, equivalent to most azoles but superior to fluconazole against dermatophyte.

Uses: Regulatory body approved indication—treatment of cutaneous and mucocutaneous fungal infections caused by *Candida* species. Evidence also shows that topical amphotericin is also effective for:

- Non-dermatophyte moulds (NDM) onychomycosis
- Cutaneous leishmaniasis
- Studies have shown it to be effective against dermatophytoses

Mode of application: Once daily, preferably after cleaning/bathing.

Side effects: None or mild, burning sensation, stinging.

Special Groups

Pregnancy: Not many studies but considered safe.

Lactation: Not many studies but considered safe.

Children: Safety unknown.

OTHER AGENTS

1. Benzoic acid and salicylic acid **(Whitfield's)** ointment is a potent keratolytic agent and is used in the treatment of dermatophyte infections. It has, however, a strong potential for causing irritant reactions.

   Dosage: Apply to affected areas bid to tid

2. Carbol-fuchsin solution (**Castellani's** paint) is an aqueous alcohol-acetone solution containing phenol (4.5 g/100 mL), resorcinol (10 g/100 mL), and basic fuschin (300 mg/100 mL). The basic fuschin appears as a dark purple liquid that appears red on the skin and can stain.

   It has local anesthetic, bactericidal, and fungicidal properties. It has also been reported to stimulate granulation and epithelization. It is applied topically in the treatment of subacute and chronic superficial fungal infection. It is particularly effective in intertriginous areas. Carbol-Fuschin is poisonous when ingested and is treated in the same manner as phenol or resorcinol poisoning. Apply to affected areas one to three times a day with swab. Clean skin with soap and water before application.

Bibliography

1. Gupta AK, Sauder DN, Shear NH. Antifungal agents: an overview. Part I. J Am Acad Dermatol. 1994;30:677–98; quiz 698–700.

2. Gupta AK, Sauder DN, Shear NH. Antifungal agents: an overview. PartII. J Am Acad Dermatol. 1994;30:911–933; quiz 934–936.

3. Gupta AK, Shear NH. Terbinafine: an update. Journal of the American Academy of Dermatology. 1997 Dec 31;37(6):979–988.

4. Sardana K. Antifungal Drugs. Systemic Drugs in Dermatology. Jaypee, 2016.

Index